Second Edition

Appleton & Lange's Review for the
USMLE
STEP 3

Appleton & Lange
Stamford, Connecticut

0-8385-0227-X

Copyright © 1997 by Appleton & Lange
A Simon & Schuster Company
Copyright © 1995 by Appleton & Lange
Copyright © 1990 by Appleton & Lange
Copyright © 1985 by Fleschner Publishing Co.

97 98 99 00 01 / 10 9 8 7 6 5 4 3 2

Prentice Hall International (UK) Limited, *London*
Prentice Hall of Australia Pty. Limited, *Sydney*
Prentice Hall Canada, Inc., *Toronto*
Prentice Hall Hispanoamericana, S.A., *Mexico*
Prentice Hall of India Private Limited, *New Delhi*
Prentice Hall of Japan, Inc., *Tokyo*
Simon & Schuster Asia Pte. Ltd., *Singapore*
Editora Prentice Hall do Brasil Ltda., *Rio de Janeiro*
Prentice Hall, *Upper Saddle River, New Jersey*

Library of Congress Cataloging-in-Publication Data

Appleton & Lange's review for the USMLE step 3 / [edited by] Samuel L.
   Jacobs. — 2nd ed.
      p.   cm.
   Includes bibliographical references.
   ISBN 0–8385–0305–5 (pbk. : alk. paper)
   1. Medicine—Examinations, questions, etc.   I. Jacobs, Samuel L.
   [DNLM: 1. Medicine—examination questions.   2. Medicine—outlines.
   W 18.2 A6492 1997]
   R834.5.A662   1997
   610´.76—dc21
   DNLM/DLC
   for Library of Congress   96-36812
                                                                 CIP

Acquisitions Editor: Marinita Timban
Production Editor: Eileen L. Pendagast
Designer: Libby Schmitz

ISBN 0-8385-0305-5

9 780838 503058   90000

PRINTED IN THE UNITED STATES OF AMERICA

Table of Contents

Contributors v

Preface vii

Acknowledgments ix

Introduction xi

Normal Laboratory Values xvii

1. Basic Sciences Review 1

    Anatomy 2
    R. Peter Meyer, PhD

    Biochemistry 13
    Ira Schwartz, PhD

    Microbiology 27
    William W. Yotis, PhD

    Pathology 40
    Thomas K. Barton, MD and Martin Gwent Lewis, MD

    Pharmacology 53
    David A. Johnson, PhD

    Physiology 66
    Andreas Carl, MD, PhD

    Behavioral Sciences 81
    Hoyle Leigh, MD

2. Clinical Sciences Review 93

    Obstetrics and Gynecology 94
    Samuel L. Jacobs, MD

    Pediatrics 114
    Stephan R. Glicken, MD

    Internal Medicine 128
    Catherine E. DuBeau, MD

    Surgery 145
    Morris D. Kerstein, MD and David Coll, MD

Psychiatry 166
Mark Schultz, MD

Preventive Medicine 186
Jocelyn C. White, MD

3. **Clinical Competence Review** 203

4. **Practice Test** 251

Contributors

Thomas K. Barton, MD
Clinical Assistant Professor
Department of Pathology
Palms of Pasadena Hospital
St. Petersburg, Florida

Andreas Carl, MD, PhD
Research Assistant Professor
Department of Physiology & Cell Biology
School of Medicine
University of Nevada
Reno, Nevada

David Coll, MD
Clinical Instructor in Surgery
Allegheny University of the Health Sciences
MCP◆Hahnemann School of Medicine
Philadelphia, Pennsylvania

Catherine E. DuBeau, MD
Instructor in Medicine
Harvard Medical School
Boston, Massachusetts

Stephan R. Glicken, MD
Assistant Pediatrician, Boston Floating Hospital
New England Medical Center
Assistant Professor of Pediatrics
Tufts University School of Medicine
Boston, Massachusetts

Joel S. Goldberg, DO
Clinical Instructor of Family Medicine
Allegheny University of the Health Sciences
MCP◆Hahnemann School of Medicine
Philadelphia, Pennsylvania

Samuel L. Jacobs, MD
Assistant Professor
Department of Obstetrics & Gynecology
Allegheny University of the Health Sciences
MCP◆Hahnemann School of Medicine
Philadelphia, Pennsylvania

David A. Johnson, PhD
Assistant Professor of Pharmacology and
    Toxicology
Duquesne University School of Pharmacy
Pittsburgh, Pennsylvania

Morris D. Kerstein, MD
Professor of Surgery
Department of Surgery
Allegheny University of the Health Sciences
MCP◆Hahnemann School of Medicine
Philadelphia, Pennsylvania

Hoyle Leigh, MD
Professor & Vice Chair
Director, Fresno Division
Department of Psychiatry
University of California, San Francisco
San Francisco, California

Martin Gwent Lewis, MD
Clinical Professor
Department of Pathology
University of South Florida
Tampa, Florida

R. Peter Meyer, PhD
Associate Professor, Biomedical Sciences
Allegheny University of the Health Sciences
MCP♦Hahnemann School of Medicine
Philadelphia, Pennsylvania

Mark Monane, MD
Instructor in Medicine
Harvard Medical School
Associate Physician, Gerontology Division
Brigham & Women's Hospital
Boston, Massachusetts

Stacy Nunberg, MD
Clinical Professor of Emergency Medicine
Albert Einstein College of Medicine
New York, New York
Attending Physician in Emergency Medicine
Long Island Jewish Medical Center
New Hyde Park, New York

Mark Schultz, MD
Clinical Assistant Professor
University of Vermont School of Medicine
Burlington, Vermont

Ira Schwartz, PhD
Professor
Department of Biochemistry and
    Molecular Biology
New York Medical College
Valhalla, New York

Jocelyn C. White, MD
Assistant Professor of Medicine
Oregon Health Sciences University
Faculty Residency Training Program
    in General Internal Medicine
Legacy Portland Hospitals
Portland, Oregon

William W. Yotis, PhD
Professor Emeritus
Department of Microbiology
Loyola University of Chicago
Maywood, Illinois

Preface

Appleton & Lange's Review for the USMLE Step 3 Second Edition is a comprehensive review with cogent explanations and current references, coupled with the self-assessment tool of a practice test. Here the reader can assess strengths and weaknesses as well as review cognitive knowledge, and diagnostic and therapeutic skills. Moreover, all the subjects, question types, techniques, and frameworks encountered on the official examination are presented in this book.

The content has been designed with careful consideration of the appropriate material and is written in a style that is both easy to read and sound in its approach to studying. We enlisted the help of a team of authors and editors of various specialties (involved in both academic and clinical settings) from around the country both to write and review the questions and explanations. Once this process was completed, another team of editors expert in the health-science question-writing field was employed to edit the questions further for style and content to ensure accuracy and readability.

This volume is part of a three-book series designed exclusively for candidates for the United States Medical Licensing Examination Steps 1, 2, and 3. Combined, the three books consist of more than 3200 exam-type questions, including case studies, with detailed explanations.

As a result, we believe you will find the questions, their explanations, the clinical-encounter set-tings, and the general format of the text to be of assistance to you during your review.

Key Features and Use:

- Approximately 330 questions are covered in the basic science review: Anatomy, Physiology, Biochemistry, Microbiology, Pathology, Pharmacology, and Behavioral Sciences.

- Approximately 369 questions are covered in the clinical science review: Obstetrics and Gynecology, Pediatrics, Internal Medicine, Surgery, Psychiatry, and Preventive Medicine.

- Questions are followed by a section with answers and detailed explanations referenced to the most current and popular resources available.

- A subspecialty list at the end of each chapter helps assess your strengths and weaknesses, thus pinpointing areas for concentration during exam preparation.

- A practice test also contains questions organized within clinical-encounter frames as presented on the examination. These are helpful in assessing the physician's abilities in initial work-ups, continuing care, and emergency care within each of the settings.

The Editors and the Publisher

Acknowledgments

I would like to thank the individual contributors for their invaluable effort. I would also like to thank Marinita Timban and Amy Schermerhorn from Appleton & Lange for their editorial assistance, my business partner Gerald V. Burke, MD, and my former administrative assistant Linda McLeer for their help, encouragement, and words of wisdom. Finally, I would like to thank my life partner, Bill Steinberg, for putting up with me while trying to meet manuscript deadlines.

Samuel L. Jacobs
Editor

Introduction

This book is designed for those preparing for the United States Medical Licensing Examination (USMLE) Step 3. It provides a comprehensive review source with 1000 "exam-type" multiple choice questions covering both the basic and clinical sciences. All questions are referenced with detailed explanations for the answers. In addition, the last chapter is an integrated practice test for self-assessment.

THE UNITED STATES MEDICAL LICENSING EXAMINATION, STEP 3

The USMLE Step 3 is a two-day examination. There are 720 test items presented in four booklets. Two booklets are tested each day, each one containing 180 test items.

The test is organized according to the framework of *clinical-encounter frames* and *physician tasks*. It is the third test in the licensure examination and is used to determine the physician's understanding of medical knowledge and its application to the patient in the unsupervised practice of medicine. There is particular emphasis on patient management to include initial work-ups, emergency care, and continued care through the basic physician tasks, comprising physical examinations, diagnostic studies, prognosis, management therapies, and the application of mechanisms of basic science.

As in both the Step 1 and the Step 2 examinations, the categorization and content will vary from test to test. However, the framework will be the underlying structure for those changes, emphasizing the unsupervised practice of medicine.

ORGANIZATION OF THIS BOOK

This book is organized to cover each of the basic and clinical science areas you will encounter on the examination. The individual subject sections present the material in isolation, while the case studies use an integrated clinical approach to the application of that material. Each chapter lists questions first, followed by the answers and explanations, a subspecialty list, and a bibliography for further study. The question formats presented here have been chosen to conform with the style you will encounter on the examination and will help to familiarize you with the styles before you sit for the examination.

Each of the chapters contains multiple-choice questions (or "items"). Most of these are one-best-answer–single-item questions, some are one-best-answer–matching sets, and some are comparison–matching-set questions. In some cases, a group of two or three questions may be related to one situation. In addition, some questions have illustrations (graphs, roentgenograms, tables, or line drawings) that require understanding and interpretation.

One-Best-Answer–Single-Item Question. The majority of the questions are posed in the A-type, or "one-best-answer–single-item" format. This is the most popular question format in most exams. It generally consists of a brief statement, followed by five options of which only ONE is entirely correct. The options on the USMLE are lettered A,B,C,D, and E. Although the format for this question type is straightforward, these questions can be difficult because some of the distractors may be partially right. The instructions you will see for this type of question will generally appear as follows:

DIRECTIONS: Each of the numbered items or incomplete statements in this section is followed by answers or by completions of the statement. Select the ONE lettered answer or completion that is BEST in each case.

The following is an example of this question type:

1. An obese 21-year-old woman complains of increased growth of coarse hair on her lip, chin, chest, and abdomen. She also notes menstrual irregularity with periods of amenorrhea. The most likely cause is

   (A) polycystic ovary disease
   (B) an ovarian tumor
   (C) an adrenal tumor
   (D) Cushing's disease
   (E) familial hirsutism

In the question above, the key word is "most." Although ovarian tumors, adrenal tumors, and Cushing's disease are causes of hirsutism (described in the stem of the question), polycystic ovary disease is a much more common cause. Familial hirsutism is not associated with the menstrual irregularities mentioned. Thus, the most

likely cause of the manifestations described can only be **(A)** polycystic ovary disease.

**STRATEGIES FOR ANSWERING
ONE-BEST-ANSWER–SINGLE-ITEM QUESTIONS**

1. Remember that only one choice can be the correct answer.
2. Read the question carefully to be sure that you understand what is being asked. Pay attention to key words like "most" or "least."
3. Quickly read each choice for familiarity. (This important step is often omitted by test takers.)
4. Go back and consider each choice individually.
5. If a choice is partially correct, tentatively consider it to be incorrect. (This step will help you eliminate your choices and increase your odds of choosing the correct answer.)
6. Consider the remaining choices and select the one you think is the answer. At this point, you may want to quickly scan the item to be sure you understand the question and your answer.
7. Fill in the appropriate circle on the answer sheet.
8. If you do not know the answer, make an educated guess. Your score is based on the number of correct answers, not the number you get incorrect. **Do not leave any blanks.**
9. The actual examination is timed for an average of 50 seconds per question. It is important to be thorough to understand the questions, but it is equally important for you to keep moving.

One-Best-Answer–Matching-Set Questions. This format presents lettered options followed by several items related to a common topic. The directions you will generally see for this type of question are as follows:

DIRECTIONS (Questions 2 through 4): Each group of items in this section consists of a list of lettered headings followed by a set of numbered words or phrases. For each numbered word or phrase, select the ONE best lettered heading that is most closely associated with it. Each lettered heading may be selected once, more than once, or not at all.

Below is an example of this type of question:

For each adverse drug reaction listed below, select the antibiotic with which it is most closely associated.

   (A) tetracycline
   (B) chloramphenicol
   (C) clindamycin

(D) cefotaxime

(E) gentamicin

2. Bone marrow suppression

3. Pseudomembranous enterocolitis

4. Acute fatty necrosis of liver

Note that unlike the single-item questions, the choices in the matching sets *precede* the actual questions. However, as with the single-item questions, only one choice can be correct for a given question.

**STRATEGIES FOR ANSWERING
ONE-BEST-ANSWER–MATCHING-SET QUESTIONS**

1. Remember that the lettered choices are followed by the numbered questions.
2. As with single-item questions, only one answer will be correct for each item.
3. Quickly read each choice for familiarity.
4. Read the question carefully to be sure that you understand what is being asked. Pay attention to key words like "most" or "least."
5. Go back and consider each choice individually.
6. If a choice is partially correct for a particular item, tentatively consider it to be incorrect. (This step will help you eliminate choices and increase your odds of choosing the correct answer.)
7. Consider the remaining choices and select the one you think is the answer.
8. Fill in the appropriate circle on the answer sheet.
9. If you do not know the answer, make an educated guess. Your score is based on the number of correct answers, not the number you get incorrect. **Do not leave any blanks.**
10. Again, the actual examination allows an average of 50 seconds per question.

Extended One-Best-Answer–Matching/Choosing Questions. The USMLE Step 3 uses a new type of matching question that is similar to the one above, but can contain up to 26 lettered options followed by several items. The directions you will see for this type of question will generally read the same as the ones listed for the best answer–matching sets since this is another version of the same question. An example of this type of question is:

(A) sarcoidosis

(B) tuberculosis

(C) histoplasmosis

(D) coccidiomycosis

(E) amyloidosis

(F) bacterial pneumonia

(G) mesothelioma

(H) carcinoma

(I) fibrosing alveolitis

(J) silicosis

627. A right lower lobectomy specimen contains a solitary 1.2-cm diameter solid nodule. The center of the nodule is fibrous. The periphery has granulomatous inflammation. With special stains, multiple 2 to 5 μm budding yeasts are evident within the nodule. Acid-fast stains are negative.

628. A left upper lobectomy specimen is received containing a 4.6-cm nodule with central cystic degeneration. Microscopically, the nodule is composed of anaplastic squamous cells. Similar abnormal cells are seen in a concomitant biopsy of a hilar lymph node.

629. After a long history of multiple myeloma, a 67-year-old male is noted to have abundant acellular eosinophilic deposits around the pulmonary microvasculature at autopsy. A Congo red special stain demonstrates apple green birefringence.

630. A large pleural-based lesion is found on chest roentgenography of an asbestos worker. Electron microscopy of the biopsy shows abundant long microvilli.

Note that, like other matching sets, the lettered options are listed first.

STRATEGIES FOR ANSWERING EXTENDED ONE-BEST-ANSWER–MATCHING/CHOOSING QUESTIONS

1. Read the lettered options through first.
2. Work with one item at a time.
3. Read the item through, then go back to the options and consider each choice individually.
4. As with the other question types, if the choice is partially correct, tentatively consider it to be incorrect.
5. Consider the remaining choices and select the answer.
6. Fill in the appropriate circle on the answer sheet.
7. Remember to make a selection for each item.
8. Again, the test allows for 50 seconds per item.

Answers, Explanations, and References

In each of the sections of this book, the question sections are followed by a section containing the answers, explanations, and references to the questions. This section (1) tells you the answer to each question; (2) gives you an explanation and review of why the answer is correct, background information on the subject matter, and why the other answers are incorrect; and (3) tells you where you can find more in-depth information on the subject matter in other books or journals. We encourage you to use this section as a basis for further study and understanding.

If you choose the correct answer to a question, you can then read the explanation (1) for reinforcement and (2) to add to your knowledge about the subject matter (remember that the explanations usually tell not only why the answer is correct, but also why the other choices are incorrect). **If you choose the wrong answer** to a question, you can read the explanation for a learning and reviewing discussion of the material in the question. Furthermore, you can note the reference cited (eg, Last, pp 478–484), look up the full source in the bibliography at the end of the section (eg, Last JM, Wallace RB, Barrett-Connor E. *Maxcy-Rosenau-Last Public Health and Preventive Medicine*. 13th ed. Norwalk, Conn: Appleton & Lange; 1992.), and refer to the pages cited for a more in-depth discussion.

Subspecialty Lists

At the end of each section of this book is a subspecialty list for each subject area. These subspecialty lists will help point out your areas of relative weakness, and thus help you focus your review.

For example, by checking off your incorrect answers on, say, the preventive medicine list, you may find that a pattern develops in that you are incorrect on most or all of the biostatistics questions. In this case, you could note the references (in the explanation section) for your incorrect answers and read those sources. You might also want to purchase a biostatistics text or review book to do a much more in-depth review. We think that you will find these subspecialty lists very helpful, and we urge you to use them.

Practice Test

The last chapter is a 180-question Practice Test consisting of 120 single items and 60 case study questions arranged in the clinical encounter setting categories. It presents the material from each of the subject areas in an integrated fashion, with like question types grouped together. This format attempts to present the material in a format similar to what you will encounter on examination day. In using the test, we suggest you simulate examination conditions to the best of your ability to help you prepare for the actual exam. Once you have taken the Practice Test, you can check your results for strengths and weaknesses using the subspecialty list provided at the end.

HOW TO USE THIS BOOK

There are two logical ways to get the most value from this book. We will call them Plan A and Plan B.

In **Plan A,** you go straight to the practice test and complete it according to the instructions on page 251. After taking the practice test, you check your answers and then tick off the ones you got wrong on the subspecialty list on pages 312 through 314. The *number* of questions you got wrong will be a good indicator of your initial knowledge state, and the *types* of questions you got wrong will help point you in the right direction for further preparation and review. At this point, you can use the first and second chapters of the book, with the lists and discussions, to help you improve your areas of relative weakness.

In **Plan B,** you go through the basic and clinical science sections, checking off your answers, and then compare your choices with the answers and discussions in the book. Once you've completed this process, you can take the practice test, check your answers as described above, and see how well prepared you are at this point. If you still have a major weakness, it should be apparent in time for you to take remedial action.

In Plan A, by taking the practice test first, you get quick feedback regarding your initial areas of strength and weakness. You may find that you know all of the material very well, indicating that perhaps only a cursory review is necessary. This, of course, would be good to know early on in your exam preparation. On the other hand, you may find that you have many areas of weakness (say, for example, in all of pediatrics and psychiatry and in some of the subspecialties of preventive medicine). In this case, you could then focus on these areas in your review—not just with this book, but also with textbooks of pediatrics and psychiatry.

It is, however, unlikely that you will not do some studying prior to taking the USMLE Step 3 (especially since you have this book). Therefore, it may be more realistic to take the practice test *after* you have reviewed the basic and clinical science sections (as in Plan B). This, of course, will probably give you a more realistic test-type situation since very few of us just sit down to a test without studying. In this case, you will have done some reviewing (from superficial to in-depth), and your practice test will reflect this studying time. If, after reviewing the basic and clinical science sections and taking the practice test, your scores still indicate some weaknesses, you can then go back into the subject review sections and supplement your review with your texts.

SPECIFIC INFORMATION ON THE STEP 3 EXAMINATION

The official source of all information with respect to the United States Medical Licensing Examination is the National Board of Medical Examiners (NBME), 3930 Chestnut Street, Philadelphia, PA 19104. Established in 1915, The NBME is a voluntary, nonprofit, independent organization whose sole function is the design, implementation, distribution, and processing of a vast bank of question items, certifying examinations, and evaluative services in the professional medical field.

To sit for the Step 3 examination, you must have obtained the MD degree (or its equivalent) and meet the requirements imposed by the licensing authority that is administering the exam.

In applying for Step 3, you must use forms supplied by NBME. Remember that registration closes *10 weeks* before the scheduled examination date. Some United States and Canadian medical schools require their students to take Step 3 even if they are noncandidates. Such students can register as noncandidates at the request of their school. A person who takes Step 3 as a noncandidate can later change to candidate status and after payment of a fee, receive certification credit.

Physical Conditions

The NBME is very concerned that all their examinations be administered under uniform conditions in the numerous centers that are used. Except for several No. 2 pencils and an eraser, you are not permitted to bring anything (books, notes, calculators, etc) into the test room. All examinees receive the same questions at the same session. However, the questions are printed in different sequences in several different booklets, and the booklets are randomly distributed. In addition, examinees are moved to different seats at least once during the test. And, of course, each test is policed by at least one proctor. The object of these maneuvers is to frustrate cheating or even the temptation to cheat.

Normal Laboratory Values

BLOOD, PLASMA, SERUM	NORMAL VALUE
Ammonia, blood	80–110 μ/dL
Amylase, serum	60–180 Somogyi units/dL
Bicarbonate, serum	21–30 mEq/L
Bilirubin, serum (total)	0.1–1.0 mg/dL
Calcium, serum	9–11 mg/dL
Chloride, serum	98–106 mEq/L
CO_2 content, blood	24–30 mEq/L
Cortisol, fasting	5–20 μ/dL
Creatinine, serum	<1.5 mg/dL
Dehydrogenase, lactate, serum	200–450 units/mL
Electrolytes, serum	
Sodium	136–145 mEq/L
Chloride	98–106 mEq/L
Potassium	3.5–5.0 mEq/L
Bicarbonate	21–30 mEq/L
Folate, serum	6–15 ng/mL
Gases, arterial blood (room air)	
Po_2	75–100 mm Hg
Pco_2	35–45 mm Hg
pH	7.38–7.44
Glucose, plasma	Fasting: 70–105 mg/dL; 2-h postprandial: >140mg/dL is abnormal
Osmolality, serum	280–295 mosmol/kg H_2O
Phosphatase (alkaline), serum	21–91 IU/L
Phosphorus (inorganic), serum	3.0–4.5 mg/dL
Potassium, serum	3.5–5.0 mEq/L
Proteins, serum	
Total	5.5–8.0 g/dL
Albumin	3.5–5.5 g/dL
Globulin	2.0–3.5 g/dL
Sodium, serum	136–145 mEq/L

BLOOD, PLASMA, SERUM   NORMAL VALUE

Thyroxine (T_4), serum	4–12 µg/dL
Transaminase, serum glutamic oxaloacetic (SGOT)	10–40 Karmen units/mL
Transaminase, serum glutamic pyruvic (SGPT)	10–40 Karmen units/mL
Triiodothyronine (T_3) resin uptake	25%–35%
Urea nitrogen, blood (BUN)	10–20 mg/dL
Uric acid, serum	3.0–7.0 mg/dL
Vitamin B_{12}, serum	200–600 pg/mL

CEREBROSPINAL FLUID

Cell count	1–4 mononuclear cells/mm^3
Glucose	44–100 mg/dL
Pressure (initial)	10–20 cm H_2O
Total proteins	15–45 mg/dL

HEMATOLOGIC

Hematocrit	Male: 42%–52%
	Female: 38%–47%
Hemoglobin	Male: 14–18 g/dL
	Female: 12–16 g/dL
Leukocytes	4300–10 000/mm^3
Neutrophils, band	1%–21%
Neutrophils, segmented	25%–62%
Lymphocytes	20%–53%
Monocytes	2.4%–11.8%
Eosinophils	0.3%–5.0%
Basophils	0.6%–1.8%
Mean corpuscular hemoglobin concentration	32–36 g/dL
Platelet count, blood	150 000–400 000/mm^3
Prothrombin time, plasma	<2 s from control
Reticulocyte count	0.5%–2.0%
Sedimentation rate, erythrocyte (Westergren)	Male: 0–15 mm/h
	Female: 0–20 mm/h

URINE

Creatinine clearance	90–140 mL/min
Osmolality	38–1400 mosmol/kg H_2O
Protein	<100 mg/24 h
Specific gravity	1.002–1.028

CHAPTER 1

Basic Sciences Review

Anatomy

R. Peter Meyer, PhD

DIRECTIONS (Questions 1 through 23): Each of the numbered items or incomplete statements in this section is followed by answers or completions of the statement. Select the ONE lettered answer or completion that is BEST in each case.

1. Which of the following arteries arise from the mandibular portion of the maxillary artery?

   (A) masseteric
   (B) buccal
   (C) sphenopalatine
   (D) descending palatine
   (E) deep auricular

2. The pterygoid plexus communicates with the cavernous sinus of the cranial dura mater by an emissary vein that passes through which of the following foramina?

   (A) foramen rotundum
   (B) foramen ovale
   (C) foramen lacerum
   (D) jugular foramen
   (E) foramen spinosum

3. Which of the following statements correctly applies to the tongue?

   (A) it is composed of an anterior one third and a posterior two thirds separated by the sulcus terminalis
   (B) the muscles of the tongue are innervated by the vagus nerve
   (C) the vallate papillae lie posterior to the sulcus terminalis
   (D) the apex of the sulcus terminalis is directed anteriorly

   (E) the mobility of the tongue is enhanced by its suspension from three bilateral attachments

4. The muscles of the palate include all of the following EXCEPT

   (A) the palatoglossus
   (B) the tensor veli palatini
   (C) the styloglossus
   (D) the palatopharyngeus
   (E) the levator veli palatini

5. All of the muscles of the palate are innervated by the vagus nerve EXCEPT

   (A) the palatopharyngeus
   (B) the palatoglossus
   (C) the musculus uvulae
   (D) the tensor veli palatini
   (E) the levator veli palatini

6. The nasolacrimal duct drains into which of the following structures?

   (A) the sphenoethmoidal recess
   (B) the inferior meatus
   (C) the hiatus semilunaris
   (D) the bulla ethmoidalis
   (E) the orifice of the auditory tube

7. All of the statements concerning the maxillary sinus are correct EXCEPT

   (A) it is the largest of the paranasal sinuses
   (B) its floor is formed by the alveolar process of the maxilla

(C) it communicates with the nasal cavity via the hiatus semilunaris

(D) the maxillary division of the trigeminal nerve supplies the lining of the maxillary sinus

(E) the drainage of the maxillary sinus is most efficient in the erect posture

8. All of the following foramina are associated with the maxillary division of the trigeminal nerve and its branches EXCEPT

(A) the incisive
(B) the greater palatine
(C) the infraorbital
(D) the mental
(E) the lesser palatine

9. All of the following are diagnostic signs of cervical sympathetic trunk injury EXCEPT

(A) ptosis
(B) dilated pupil
(C) miosis
(D) anhidrosis
(E) enophthalmos

10. All of the following structures refract light entering the eye EXCEPT

(A) the pupil
(B) the cornea
(C) the aqueous humor
(D) the lens
(E) the vitreous humor

11. All of the following statements concerning the stapedius muscle are correct EXCEPT

(A) it inserts on the neck of the stapes
(B) it is innervated by the facial nerve
(C) the contraction of this muscle tends to dampen the vibrations of the stapes
(D) it has a protective function
(E) it takes origin from the anterior process of the malleus

12. The smooth, depressed area between the two superciliary arches is which of the following?

(A) the pterion
(B) the supraorbital margin
(C) the glabella
(D) the zygoma
(E) the crista galli

13. All of the following bones were formed from the cartilaginous neurocranium EXCEPT

(A) the occipital
(B) the maxilla
(C) the sphenoid
(D) the ethmoid
(E) the petrous portion of the temporal

14. All of the following muscles develop from the mesodermal germ layer EXCEPT

(A) the muscles of the iris
(B) the muscles of facial expression
(C) the muscles of mastication
(D) the muscles of the lower limb
(E) the muscles of the pharynx

15. The free margin of the falciform ligament contains a remnant of which of the following structures?

(A) the bile duct
(B) the portal vein
(C) the hepatic artery
(D) the hepatic vein
(E) the umbilical vein

16. All of the following are associated with the tetralogy of Fallot EXCEPT

(A) pulmonary stenosis
(B) right ventricular hypertrophy
(C) interventricular septal defect
(D) overriding aorta
(E) patent ductus arteriosus

17. The fourth aortic arch forms which of the following arteries?

    (A) the maxillary
    (B) the right common carotid
    (C) the proximal segment of the right subclavian
    (D) the proximal segment of the right pulmonary
    (E) the ductus arteriosus

18. Which of the following is one of the most frequently seen abnormalities of the great vessels?

    (A) a patent ductus arteriosus
    (B) a double aortic arch
    (C) abnormal position of the pulmonary trunk
    (D) a right aortic arch
    (E) a double superior vena cava

19. The closure of the distal parts of the umbilical arteries after birth forms which of the following structures?

    (A) the ligamentum venosum
    (B) the medial umbilical ligaments
    (C) the ligamentum teres hepatis
    (D) the ligamentum arteriosum
    (E) the urachus

20. The main pancreatic duct is formed by which of the following?

    (A) the distal part of the dorsal pancreatic duct and the entire ventral pancreatic duct
    (B) the prominal part of the dorsal pancreatic duct and the distal portion of the ventral pancreatic duct

    (C) the entire dorsal pancreatic duct
    (D) the entire dorsal and ventral pancreatic ducts
    (E) the proximal parts of both the dorsal and ventral pancreatic ducts

21. Whenever the intestinal midgut loop fails to return from the umbilical cord into the abdominal cavity, the defect is known as which of the following?

    (A) gastroschisis
    (B) an omphalocele
    (C) Meckel's diverticulum
    (D) a vitelline fistula
    (E) a left-sided colon

22. The mesonephric duct persists to form which of the following structures?

    (A) the prostate
    (B) the testes
    (C) the seminal vesicle
    (D) the ovary
    (E) the uterine tube

23. An undescended testis that remains in the pelvic cavity or somewhere in the inguinal canal is known as which of the following?

    (A) a hydrocele
    (B) hypospadias
    (C) epispadias
    (D) cryptorchidism
    (E) hermaphroditism

DIRECTIONS (Questions 24 through 33): Each set of matching questions in this section consists of lettered headings followed by a set of words or phrases. For each numbered word or phrase, select the ONE lettered heading that is most closely associated with it. Each lettered heading may be selected once, more than once, or not at all.

Questions 24 through 33

(A) first pharyngeal arch
(B) head somites
(C) third pharyngeal arch
(D) second pharyngeal arch
(E) first pharyngeal pouch
(F) second pharyngeal pouch
(G) fourth and sixth pharyngeal arches
(H) third pharyngeal pouch
(I) fourth pharyngeal pouch

24. Which of the above structures gives rise to the stapes?

25. Which of the above structures gives rise to the stylopharyngeal muscle?

26. The superior parathyroid gland is formed from which of the above structures?

27. The malleus and incus are formed from which of the above structures?

28. The thyroid, arytenoid, corniculate, and cuneiform cartilages of the larynx are formed from which of the above structures?

29. The auditory tube is formed from which of the above structures?

30. The muscles of facial expression are formed from which of the above structures?

31. The muscles of mastication are formed from which of the above structures?

32. The thymus gland is formed from which of the above structures?

33. The anterior two thirds of the tongue is formed from which of the above structures?

DIRECTIONS (Questions 34 through 43): Each of the numbered items or incomplete statements in this section is followed by answers or completions of the statement. Select the ONE lettered answer or completion that is BEST in each case.

34. All of the following statements apply to a synovial joint EXCEPT

(A) the cartilage is usually the hyaline type
(B) the cartilage has nerves and blood vessels
(C) the synovial membrane produces synovial fluid
(D) the articular capsule envelops the articulation or joint
(E) the cartilage is nourished by the synovial fluid

35. All of the following types of joints are classified as synovial EXCEPT

(A) hinge
(B) condyloid
(C) saddle
(D) symphysis
(E) ball and socket

36. All of the following statements concerning ribs are correct EXCEPT

(A) the first seven pairs of ribs are called true ribs
(B) the 8th to 12th pairs of ribs are vertebrochondral ribs
(C) the third to ninth ribs are typical
(D) the second rib has a prominent scalene tubercle
(E) the first rib is the broadest and most curved of all ribs

37. Which of the following nerves are parasympathetic?

(A) the greater splanchnic
(B) the lesser splanchnic
(C) the pelvic splanchnic
(D) the hypogastric plexuses
(E) the trigeminal nerve

38. All of the following statements concerning the coracobrachialis are correct EXCEPT

(A) it arises from the coracoid process
(B) it inserts into the humerus
(C) it is innervated by the median nerve
(D) it arises with the short head of the biceps
(E) it both adducts and flexes the arm

39. All of the following statements concerning the cruciate ligaments are correct EXCEPT

(A) the anterior cruciate attaches to the lateral side of the medial condyle of the femur
(B) the posterior cruciate arises from the posterior intercondylar area of the tibia
(C) both cruciate ligaments are tense during full extension
(D) both cruciate ligaments are tense during full flexion
(E) the anterior cruciate ligament is longer than the posterior cruciate

40. The bare area of the liver is in contact with all of the following structures EXCEPT

(A) the aorta
(B) the diaphragm
(C) the inferior vena cava
(D) the right suprarenal gland
(E) the right kidney

41. The external surface of the tympanic membrane is supplied by which of the following nerves?

(A) the zygomatic branch of the facial
(B) the auriculotemporal
(C) the temporal branch of the facial
(D) the great auricular
(E) the tympanic

42. All of the following statements concerning the otic ganglion are correct EXCEPT

(A) it contains postganglionic parasympathetic cells
(B) it is located in the pterygopalatine fossa
(C) it is located medial to the mandibular nerve

(D) it is posterior to the medial pterygoid muscle
(E) it contains cells that are secretory to the parotid gland

43. All of the following statements concerning the thoracic duct are correct EXCEPT

(A) it is the main lymphatic duct
(B) it begins in the cisterna chyli
(C) it ascends through the aortic hiatus
(D) it ascends in the posterior mediastinum
(E) it drains into the azygos system of veins

DIRECTIONS (Questions 44 through 50): Each group of items in this section consists of lettered headings followed by a set of numbered words or phrases. For each numbered word or phrase, select the ONE lettered heading that is most closely associated with it. Each lettered heading may be selected once, more than once, or not at all.

Questions 44 through 50

(A) the azygos vein
(B) the pulmonary veins
(C) the coronary sinus
(D) the superior vena cava
(E) the anterior cardiac veins
(F) the anterior intercostal veins
(G) the hemiazygos veins
(H) the great cardiac vein
(I) the internal thoracic veins
(J) the posterior intercostal veins

44. The posterior intercostal veins anastomose with which of the above veins?

45. Which of the above veins empty into the left atrium?

46. Which of the above veins is the main vein of the heart?

47. Which of the above veins drain the apex of the heart?

48. Which of the above veins connects the superior and inferior venae cavae?

49. Which of the above veins are located in the superior mediastinum?

50. The coronary sinus drains all of the venous blood from the heart except that carried by which of the above veins?

ANSWERS AND EXPLANATIONS

1. **(E)** The branches of the mandibular portion of the maxillary artery include the deep auricular, the anterior tympanic, the middle meningeal, the accessory meningeal, and the inferior alveolar. The pterygoid portion of the maxillary artery includes the masseteric and the buccal arteries. The pterygopalatine portion of the maxillary artery includes the descending palatine and the sphenopalatine arteries. *(Woodburne and Burckel, pp 268–269)*

2. **(B)** The pterygoid plexus communicates with the cavernous sinus of the cranial dura mater by an emissary vein that passes through the foramen ovale. The foramen rotundum contains the maxillary division of the trigeminal nerve. The foramen lacerum contains cartilage and minor vessels. The jugular foramen contains cranial nerves IX, X, and XI. The foramen spinosum contains the middle meningeal artery. *(Woodburne and Burckel, pp 270,322)*

3. **(E)** The mobility of the tongue is enhanced by its suspension from three well-separated bilateral attachments: the mandible, the styloid process, and the hyoid bone. The muscles of the tongue are innervated by the seventh, ninth, tenth, and twelfth cranial nerves. The tongue is composed of an anterior two thirds and a posterior one third. The anterior part is separated from the posterior part by a V-shaped sulcus terminalis. The apex of the V is directed posteriorly and ends in a median pit, the foramen cecum of the tongue. The vallate papillae lie anterior to the sulcus terminalis. *(Woodburne and Burckel, pp 274–275)*

4. **(C)** The styloglossus is a muscle of the tongue. The muscles of the palate include the levator veli palatini, tensor veli palatini, muscular uvulae, palatoglossus, and palatopharyngeus. *(Woodburne and Burckel, pp 275–276)*

5. **(D)** The tensor veli palatini muscle is supplied by the mandibular division of the trigeminal nerve. All other palatal muscles are supplied by the contributions of the vagus nerve to the pharyngeal plexus. *(Woodburne and Burckel, p 278)*

6. **(B)** The inferior meatus receives the slitlike termination of the nasolacrimal duct. The sphenoid sinus empties into the sphenoethmoidal recess. The bulging mass in the middle meatus is known as the bulla ethmoidalis. The hiatus semilunaris is the deep groove anterior to and inferior to the bulla. The orifice of the auditory tube is posterior to the opening of the nasolacrimal duct. *(Woodburne and Burckel, pp 282–283)*

7. **(E)** The drainage of the maxillary sinus is very poor in the erect position, and the dependent drainage of the sinuses requires the laying of the head on one side. The communication of the maxillary sinus with the nasal cavity is via the hiatus semilunaris. It is the largest of the paranasal sinuses, and its floor is formed by the alveolar process of the maxilla. *(Woodburne and Burckel, pp 284–285)*

8. **(D)** The mental nerve, a branch of the inferior alveolar nerve, emerges onto the face through the mental foramen. The nasopalatine nerves, branches of the maxillary division of the trigeminal nerve, pass through the incisive canal, where they communicate with terminals of the greater palatine nerves. The greater palatine nerve emerges onto the oral surface of the palate at the greater palatine foramen. The lesser palatine emerges at the lesser palatine foramen. *(Woodburne and Burckel, pp 265–268,285–288)*

9. **(B)** The superior tarsal muscle is innervated by fibers traveling through the cervical sympathetic trunk and the internal carotid plexus. If the trunk is interrupted, the muscle is paralyzed, causing drooping of the eyelid

(ptosis). This is one of the signs of cervical sympathetic trunk injury. The affected pupil is smaller than the pupil of the opposite eye. It does not dilate when the pupil is shaded (miosis). The face is dry (anhidrosis), red, and warm. *(Woodburne and Burckel, p 294)*

10. **(A)** The iris is a thin, contractile membrane having a central aperture, the pupil. Light rays are bent at the interfaces of materials of different densities. The refractive media in the course of light entering the eye are at the cornea, the aqueous humor, the lens, and the vitreous humor. *(Woodburne and Burckel, pp 300–301)*

11. **(E)** The pyramidal eminence is hollow, and its walls give rise to the fibers of the stapedius muscle, whose central tendon emerges at an aperture on the summit of the eminence and inserts in the posterior surface of the neck of the stapes. The facial nerve sends a small branch into the muscle at the base of the pyramidal eminence. The contraction of the stapedius muscle tilts the footplate of the stapes, tending to dampen its vibrations, and thereby serves a protective function. *(Woodburne and Burckel, pp 306–307)*

12. **(C)** The smooth, depressed area between the two superciliary arches is the glabella. The pterion is located at the junction of the sphenoid, frontal, parietal, and temporal bones. The frontal bone of the forehead turns into the orbits below, forming the supraorbital margins. The zygoma forms the prominence of the cheek. The crista galli is part of the ethmoid bone and gives attachment to the falx cerebri. *(Woodburne and Burckel, pp 310,313–316,320)*

13. **(B)** The cartilaginous neurocranium is a number of separate cartilages that fuse and ossify to form the base of the skull. The occipital bone is formed by the parachordal cartilage. Rostrally, the hypophyseal cartilages and the trabeculae cranii fuse to form the sphenoid and ethmoid bones. The periotic capsule gives rise to the petrous and mastoid parts of the temporal bone. The viscerocranium consists of the bones of the face and is

formed mainly by the cartilages of the first two arches. The first arch gives rise to a dorsal part, the maxillary process, which gives rise to the maxilla. *(Sadler, pp 150–151)*

14. **(A)** The muscular system develops from the mesodermal germ layer (with the exception of the muscles of the iris, which form from the optic cup ectoderm) and consists of skeletal, smooth, and cardiac muscle. *(Sadler, p 166)*

15. **(E)** The free margin of the falciform ligament contains a remnant of the umbilical vein. The free margin of the lesser omentum contains the bile duct, the portal vein, and the hepatic artery. The hepatic veins empty into the inferior vena cava. *(Sadler, pp 250–251)*

16. **(E)** An unequal division of the conus results in a narrow right ventricular outflow region known as a pulmonary stenosis. A large defect of the interventricular septum places the aorta directly above the septal defect from both ventricular cavities, and the resulting higher pressure on the right side causes hypertrophy of the right ventricular wall. The ductus arteriosus is the distal part of the left sixth arch during intrauterine life. *(Sadler, pp 201–208)*

17. **(C)** The fourth aortic arch, on the right, forms the proximal segment of the right subclavian artery. The first arch largely disappears; however, a small portion persists as the maxillary artery. The third arch forms the common carotid. The sixth arch forms the proximal segment of the right pulmonary artery and the ductus arteriosus. *(Sadler, pp 212–215)*

18. **(A)** A patent ductus arteriosus is one of the most frequently seen abnormalities of the great vessels (8/10 000 births), especially in premature infants, and may occur either as an isolated abnormality or in combination with other heart defects. *(Sadler, p 216)*

19. **(B)** The closure of the distal parts of the umbilical arteries form the medial umbilical ligaments. After obliteration of the umbilical

vein and ductus venosus, the umbilical vein forms the ligamentum teres hepatis in the lower margin of the falciform ligament. The ductus venosus is also obliterated to form the ligamentum venosum. The obliterated ductus arteriosus forms the ligamentum arteriosum. The lumen of the allantois is obliterated to form the urachus, to become the median umbilical ligament. *(Sadler, pp 224–228,283–284)*

20. **(A)** The main pancreatic duct (of Wirsung) is formed by the distal part of the dorsal pancreatic duct and the entire ventral pancreatic duct. The proximal part of the dorsal pancreatic duct either is obliterated or persists as a small channel, the accessory pancreatic duct. *(Sadler, pp 256–257)*

21. **(B)** When the midgut loop fails to return from the umbilical cord into the abdominal cavity and is covered only by amnion, the defect is known as an omphalocele. In the most severe cases, there is a defect in the anterior abdominal wall and all the viscera, including the liver, may be found outside the abdominal cavity. This is known as Meckel's diverticulum. The vitelline duct may remain patent over its entire length to form a vitelline fistula. A left-sided colon is related to malrotation. *(Sadler, pp 258–266)*

22. **(E)** The mesonephric duct elongates to form the ductus epididymis, ductus deferens, ejaculatory ducts, and the epididymis. The testes and ovary develop from the genital or gonadal ridges. The uterine tubes develop from the paramesonephric duct. *(Sadler, pp 286,291–297)*

23. **(D)** One or both testes may remain in the pelvic cavity or somewhere in the inguinal canal and this condition is known as cryptorchidism. Connections between the coelomic cavity and the vaginal process may remain open with irregular obliteration of this passageway, leaving small cysts known as hydroceles. Hermaphroditism is a condition in which the gonads and external genitalia of both sexes are present. Abnormal openings of the urethra may be found along the inferior aspect or dor-

sum of the penis, and this is known as either hypospadias or epispadias, according to the aspect on which the opening occurs. *(Sadler, pp 299–301,303–304,309)*

24. **(D)** The cartilage of the second, or hyoid, arch (Reichert's cartilage) gives rise to the stapes, styloid process of the temporal bone, the stylohyoid ligament, lesser horn, and the upper part of the body of the hyoid bone. *(Sadler, pp 315–316)*

25. **(C)** The cartilage of this arch produces the lower part of the body and greater horn of the hyoid bone. The musculature is limited to the stylopharyngeal muscle. *(Sadler, pp 315–316)*

26. **(I)** The epithelium of the dorsal wing of the fourth pharyngeal pouch forms the superior parathyroid gland. *(Sadler, p 322)*

27. **(A)** The first pharyngeal arch forms the maxillary and mandibular processes. Part of the mandibular process persists to form the incus and malleus. *(Sadler, pp 313–315)*

28. **(G)** The cartilaginous components of the fourth and sixth pharyngeal arches fuse to form the thyroid, cricoid, arytenoid, corniculate, and cuneiform cartilages of the larynx. *(Sadler, p 317)*

29. **(E)** The first pharyngeal pouch forms a stalklike diverticulum, the tubotympanic recess, which comes in contact with the epithelial lining of the first pharyngeal cleft, the future external auditory meatus. The distal portion of the outpocketing widens to form the middle ear cavity, whereas the proximal part forms the auditory tube. *(Sadler, p 319)*

30. **(D)** The muscles of the second (hyoid) pharyngeal arch are the stapedius, the stylohyoid, the posterior belly of the digastric, the auricular, and the muscles of facial expression. *(Sadler, pp 315–316)*

31. **(A)** The musculature of the first pharyngeal arch is formed by the muscles of mastication (temporalis, masseter, pterygoids), the ante-

rior belly of the digastric, the mylohyoid, the tensor tympani, and tensor veli palatini. *(Sadler, pp 313–315)*

32. **(H)** The ventral part of the third pharyngeal pouch forms the thymus. *(Sadler, pp 321–322)*

33. **(A)** The tongue appears in the form of two lateral lingual swellings, and one medial swelling, the tuberculum impar. These three swellings originate from the first pharyngeal arch. The swellings merge to form the anterior two thirds. *(Sadler, pp 326–329)*

34. **(B)** The articular cartilage is usually of the hyaline type. This cartilage has no nerves or blood vessels. It is nourished by the synovial fluid. The articular capsule envelops the articulation or joint. The synovial fluid lubricates the joint. *(Moore, pp 17–18)*

35. **(D)** Both the pubic symphysis and the mandibular symphysis are examples of secondary cartilaginous joints where bone is united by either hyaline cartilage or fibrocartilage. There are six types of synovial joint, all classified according to the shape of the articulating surfaces or the type of movement they permit. They include plane, hinge, condyloid, saddle, ball and socket, and pivot joints. *(Moore, pp 17,19)*

36. **(D)** The first rib is the broadest and most curved of all the ribs. It is flat and has a prominent scalene tubercle on its superior surface. The first seven pairs of ribs are called true or vertebrosternal ribs. The 8th to 12th pairs of ribs are false or vertebrochondral ribs. The 3rd to 9th ribs are typical, and the 1st, 2nd, and 10th to 12th pairs of ribs are atypical. *(Moore, p 35)*

37. **(C)** The pelvic splanchnic nerves represent the sacral portion of the craniosacral (parasympathetic) portion of the autonomic nervous system. The greater and lesser splanchnic nerves are sympathetic. The hypogastric plexuses are formed by the superior mesenteric plexus. *(Woodburne and Burckel, pp 562, 502–507)*

38. **(C)** The coracobrachialis muscle arises with the short head of the biceps from the coracoid process and passes downward to insert into the medial border of the body of the humerus. It is innervated by the musculocutaneous nerve. The coracobrachialis both adducts and flexes the arm. *(Hollinshead, pp 209,211)*

39. **(A)** The longer anterior cruciate ligament arises from the anterior intercondylar area of the tibia, adjacent to the medial condyle, and extends obliquely upward, backward, and laterally to attach to the medial side of the lateral condyle of the femur. The posterior cruciate ligament arises from the posterior intercondylar area of the tibia and attaches the lateral surface of the medial condyle. Both ligaments are most tense during full extension and full flexion. *(Hollinshead, pp 437–438)*

40. **(A)** Most of the bare area of the liver is in direct contact with the diaphragm and, in addition, with the inferior vena cava and, just to its right, with the right suprarenal gland and a small area of the right kidney. *(Hollinshead, p 648)*

41. **(B)** The external surface of the tympanic membrane is supplied by the auriculotemporal nerve, a branch of the mandibular division of the trigeminal nerve. Some innervation is supplied by a small auricular branch of the vagus nerve. This may contain some glossopharyngeal and facial fibers. The zygomatic and temporal branches of the facial serve only those areas designated by the name. The great auricular is from the cervical plexus. The tympanic nerve is a branch of the glossopharyngeal and is located on the interior of the tympanic membrane. *(Moore, pp 766,769)*

42. **(B)** The otic ganglion is a parasympathetic ganglion located in the infratemporal fossa, just inferior to the foramen ovale, medial to the mandibular nerve, and posterior to the medial pterygoid muscle. Preganglionic parasympathetic fibers travel with the glossopharyngeal nerve and synapse in the otic gan-

glion. The postganglionic parasympathetic fibers are secretory to the parotid gland. *(Moore, p 731)*

43. **(E)** The thoracic duct opens near or at the angle of union of the internal jugular and subclavian veins. The thoracic duct is the main lymphatic duct. It begins in the cisterna chyli and ascends through the aortic hiatus in the diaphragm to the thorax. *(Moore, p 237)*

44. **(F)** The posterior intercostal veins anastomose with the anterior intercostal veins, which are tributaries of the internal thoracic veins. *(Moore, p 59)*

45. **(B)** Four pulmonary veins (two superior and two inferior) enter the posterior wall of the left atrium. *(Moore, p 94)*

46. **(C)** The coronary sinus is the main vein of the heart. *(Moore, p 102)*

47. **(H)** The great cardiac vein is the main tributary of the coronary sinus. It begins near the apex of the heart and ascends in the anterior interventricular groove with the anterior interventricular artery. *(Moore, p 102)*

48. **(A)** The azygos vein connects the superior and inferior venae cavae, either directly by joining the inferior vena cava or indirectly by the hemiazygos and accessory hemiazygos veins. *(Moore, p 115)*

49. **(D)** The superior vena cava, the great vein draining blood from the head and neck, is located in the superior mediastinum. *(Moore, p 109)*

50. **(E)** The coronary sinus drains all of the venous blood from the heart, except that carried by the anterior cardiac vein and the venae cordis minimae. *(Moore, p 102)*

REFERENCES

Hollinshead WH, Rosse C. *Textbook of Anatomy.* 4th ed. Philadelphia: Harper & Row Publishers Inc; 1985.

Moore KL. *Clinically Oriented Anatomy.* 3rd ed. Baltimore: Williams & Wilkins; 1992.

Noback CR, Strominger NL, Demarest RJ. *The Human Nervous System.* 5th ed. Philadelphia: Lea & Febiger; 1996.

Sadler TW. *Langman's Medical Embryology.* 7th ed. Baltimore: Williams & Wilkins; 1995.

Woodburne RT, Burckel WE. *Essentials of Human Anatomy.* 9th ed. New York: Oxford University Press; 1994.

SUBSPECIALTY LIST: ANATOMY

Question Number and Subspecialty
1. Cardiovascular system
2. Skeletal system
3. Digestive system
4. Muscular system
5. Peripheral nervous system
6. Respiratory system
7. Respiratory system
8. Peripheral nervous system
9. Autonomic nervous system
10. Special sensory—eye
11. Special sensory—ear
12. Skeletal system
13. Embryology
14. Embryology
15. Embryology
16. Cardiovascular system
17. Cardiovascular system
18. Cardiovascular system
19. Embryology
20. Digestive system
21. Embryology
22. Embryology—urogenital system

23. Embryology—urogenital system
24. Special senses
25. Muscular system
26. Embryology—endocrine system
27. Embryology—special senses
28. Embryology—respiratory system
29. Embryology—special sensory
30. Embryology—muscular system
31. Embryology—muscular system
32. Embryology—lymphatic system
33. Embryology—digestive system
34. Cardiovascular system
35. Cardiovascular system
36. Cardiovascular system
37. Autonomic nervous system
38. Muscular system
39. Skeletal system
40. Digestive system
41. Special senses
42. Autonomic nervous system
43. Lymphatic system
44. Cardiovascular system
45. Cardiovascular system
46. Cardiovascular system
47. Cardiovascular system
48. Cardiovascular system
49. Cardiovascular system
50. Cardiovascular system

Biochemistry

Ira Schwartz, PhD

DIRECTIONS (Questions 51 through 76): Each of the numbered items or incomplete statements in this section is followed by answers or by completions of the statement. Select the ONE lettered answer or completion that is BEST in each case.

51. Which of the following interactions are involved in the maintenance of protein secondary structure?

    (A) hydrophobic interactions
    (B) peptide bonds
    (C) hydrogen bonds
    (D) polar interactions
    (E) disulfide bonds

52. All the following bonding reactions are important in the stabilization of the tertiary structure of proteins EXCEPT

    (A) peptide bonds
    (B) hydrophobic interactions
    (C) ionic bonds
    (D) hydrogen bonds between peptide groups
    (E) hydrogen bonds between side chains of amino acids

53. Which of the following clotting factors is present only in the intrinsic pathway of coagulation?

    (A) fibrinogen (factor I)
    (B) accelerin (factor V)
    (C) prothrombin (factor II)
    (D) antihemophilic factor (factor VIII)
    (E) Stuart factor (factor X)

54. The active sulfhydryl group of coenzyme A (CoA) is derived from

    (A) lipoic acid
    (B) pantothenate
    (C) cysteine
    (D) hyaluronic acid
    (E) folic acid

55. The free-energy change ($\Delta G^{\circ\prime}$) for the hydrolysis of phosphoenolpyruvate is $- 14.8$ kcal/mol and that of ATP hydrolysis to ADP and orthophosphate (P_i) is -7.3 kcal/mol. Which of the following values represents the standard free-energy change for the production of phosphoenolpyruvate by the reaction shown below?

    $$ATP + pyruvate \rightleftharpoons$$
    $$phosphoenolpyruvate + ADP + P_i$$

    (A) $+ 7.5$ kcal/mol
    (B) $- 7.5$ kcal/mol
    (C) $+22.1$ kcal/mol
    (D) -22.1 kcal/mol
    (E) -14.8 kcal/mol

56. The ATPase activity required for muscle contraction is located in

    (A) myosin
    (B) troponin
    (C) myokinase
    (D) sarcoplasmic reticulum
    (E) actin

57. Which of the following saccharides enters glycolysis at the level of three-carbon intermediates?

   (A) lactose
   (B) mannose
   (C) galactose
   (D) maltose
   (E) fructose

58. All the following statements regarding protein synthesis in eukaryotes are true EXCEPT that

   (A) most eukaryotic mRNAs may contain a modified "cap" structure at the 5' end
   (B) a "Shine-Dalgarno" sequence is required upstream of the translation initiation site
   (C) AUG is the initiation codon
   (D) the mRNA is monocistronic
   (E) most eukaryotic mRNAs contain a poly A sequence at their 3' end

59. All the following statements about enzymes are true EXCEPT that enzymes

   (A) alter reaction equilibria
   (B) are highly specific in choice of substrates
   (C) decrease activation energies of reactions
   (D) bind substrate in the first step of catalysis
   (E) may assist in transforming one kind of energy to another

60. Quaternary structure is important in the function of all of the following proteins EXCEPT

   (A) hemoglobin
   (B) bovine ribonuclease
   (C) immunoglobulin G
   (D) collagen
   (E) insulin

61. The effect of aspirin is to inhibit

   (A) endorphin synthesis
   (B) conversion of essential fatty acids into arachidonic acid
   (C) essential fatty acid synthesis

   (D) arachidonic acid release
   (E) prostaglandin cyclooxygenase

62. Which of the following base pair sequences is palindromic?

   (A) TCC
       AGG
   (B) CCTAGG
       GGATCC
   (C) CTCT
       GAGA
   (D) CCAGGG
       GGTCCC
   (E) ACTGT
       TGACA

63. During intense muscular activity the glycolytic end product that increases significantly is:

   (A) pyruvate
   (B) phosphoenolpyruvate
   (C) lactate
   (D) 3-phosphoglycerate
   (E) 2-phosphoglycerate

64. The ingestion of candy immediately before or during marathon running is thought to be deleterious to the efforts of a long-distance runner because it may lead to

   (A) stimulation of glucagon secretion
   (B) inhibition of glycogen synthesis
   (C) stimulation of insulin secretion
   (D) inhibition of glycolysis
   (E) hypoglycemia

65. Concerning the structure of the plasma membranes of mammalian cells, all of the following statements are correct EXCEPT

   (A) cholesterol influences the fluidity of membranes
   (B) membrane proteins do not undergo transverse diffusion (flip-flop) across bilayers
   (C) proteins may span the entire width of a membrane

(D) membrane lipids undergo lateral diffusion within the plane of the membrane

(E) sugar residues of glycoproteins and glycolipids are usually located on the cytoplasmic surface

66. The central processing system for intracellular and plasma membranes is the

(A) Golgi apparatus
(B) lysosome
(C) nuclear membrane
(D) rough endoplasmic reticulum
(E) smooth endoplasmic reticulum

67. The action of morphine is mediated through receptors for

(A) histamine
(B) endorphins
(C) alloxan
(D) thyroxine
(E) acetylcholine

68. All of the following cell events are stimulated by epinephrine EXCEPT

(A) glycogenolysis
(B) lipolysis
(C) ketogenesis
(D) glucose oxidation
(E) gluconeogenesis

69. In the formation of methionine, a methyl group derived from serine is transferred to homocysteine. The coenzyme involved in this reaction is derived from the vitamin

(A) folate
(B) biocytin
(C) pyridoxine
(D) lipoate
(E) cyanocobalamin

70. Up to one third of the amino acid residues of collagen are

(A) serine
(B) hydroxyproline
(C) valine

(D) proline
(E) glycine

71. Which of the following compounds is an essential fatty acid?

(A) oleic acid
(B) stearic acid
(C) linoleic acid
(D) palmitoleic acid
(E) arachidonic acid

72. In the posttranslational modification of collagen, ascorbate (vitamin C) acts as

(A) a carrier of amino acids
(B) a reducing agent
(C) a carrier of hydroxyl groups
(D) an oxidizing agent
(E) an enzyme

73. Medium-chain fatty acids are transported from the cytoplasm of cells into the inner matrix of mitochondria in the form of

(A) esters of glycerol
(B) lipoprotein complexes
(C) acyl CoA thioesters
(D) free fatty acids
(E) acyl carnitine esters

74. Which of the following fatty acids has the highest melting point?

(A) 14:0 (14 carbons, 0 double bonds)
(B) 16:0
(C) 18:0
(D) 18:1
(E) 18:2

75. Sickle cell anemia can be characterized by all of the following features EXCEPT

    (A) sickling occurs when there is a high concentration of the deoxygenated form of hemoglobin S (HbS)

    (B) a single amino acid residue in the β chain is altered

    (C) sickling is promoted by high oxygen levels

    (D) the solubility of deoxygenated HbS is abnormally low

    (E) HbS has an abnormal electrophoretic mobility

76. All of the following reactions may increase in rate during strenuous physical exercise EXCEPT

    (A) fatty acid + CoA + ATP → acyl CoA + AMP + P_i

    (B) ATP + H_2O → ADP + P_i

    (C) fructose 6-phosphate + ATP → fructose 1,6-bisphosphate + ADP

    (D) pyruvate + NADH + H^+ → lactate + NAD^+

    (E) 2 ADP → ATP + AMP

DIRECTIONS (Questions 77 through 88): Each group of items in this section consists of lettered headings followed by a set of numbered words or phrases. For each numbered word or phrase, select the ONE lettered heading that is most closely associated with it. Each lettered heading may be selected once, more than once, or not at all.

Questions 77 through 79

For each principle below, select the phenomenon that provides the best proof.

    (A) a substitution mutation changes only one specific amino acid of the protein coded

    (B) a codon codes for one specific amino acid

    (C) deletions or insertions cause frame shifts starting at the codon for the amino acid affected

    (D) the sum of purines in double-stranded DNA is equal to the sum of pyrimidines

    (E) most of the 64 possible base triplets have been shown to code for 1 of about 20 amino acids

E 77. The genetic code is degenerate

A 78. The genetic code is nonoverlapping

C 79. The sequence of bases in DNA is read sequentially from a fixed starting point

Questions 80 and 81

For each disease condition, choose the affected enzyme.

    (A) thymidylate synthase

    (B) xanthine oxidase

    (C) hypoxanthine-guanine phosphoribosyl transferase

    (D) adenine phosphoribosyl transferase

    (E) adenosine deaminase

C 80. Lesch-Nyhan syndrome

E 81. Severe combined immunodeficiency

Questions 82 through 84

For each reaction described below, choose the enzyme that catalyzes it.

    (A) glucokinase

    (B) glucose 6-phosphate dehydrogenase

    (C) glycogen phosphorylase

    (D) glucose 6-phosphatase

    (E) glycogen synthase

C 82. Inorganic phosphate is a substrate

E 83. UDP-glucose is a substrate

A 84. ATP is a substrate

Questions 85 through 88

For each statement below, choose the reaction from the pathway which best applies.

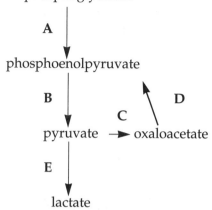

2-phosphoglycerate

A

phosphoenolpyruvate

B   D
C
pyruvate → oxaloacetate

E

lactate

C 85. ATP is required

B 86. ATP is formed

E 87. NADH is required

D 88. CO_2 is released

DIRECTIONS (Questions 89 through 97): Each of the numbered items or incomplete statements in this section is followed by answers or completions of the statement. Select the ONE lettered answer or completion that is BEST in each case.

89. Vitamin D is correctly described by all of the following statements EXCEPT

(A) it promotes absorption of calcium from the gut

(B) it is modified into an active form by the kidney

(C) it participates in carboxylation of glutamate residues

(D) it stimulates the synthesis of specific proteins

(E) it is derived from 7-dehydrocholesterol

90. The terminal step of protein glycosylation occurs in which of the following structures?

(A) Golgi apparatus

(B) plasma membrane

(C) endoplasmic reticulum

(D) lysosomes

(E) endosomes

91. Allopurinol is a drug that is employed in the treatment of gout. This drug

(A) causes a decrease in hypoxanthine and xanthine excretion

(B) inhibits hypoxanthine phosphoribosyl transferase

(C) inhibits xanthine oxidase

(D) causes an increase in uric acid excretion

(E) inhibits de novo purine biosynthesis

92. The effects of diisopropylphosphofluoridate (DFP) on chymotrypsin can be characterized as

(A) competitive inhibition

(B) feedback inhibition

(C) reaction with a histidine at the active site

(D) reaction with a serine at the active site

(E) reaction with a lysine at the active site

93. The catabolism of amino acids may involve

(A) amidation

(B) transamination

(C) nitrogenation

(D) phosphorylation

(E) carboxylation

94. Integral membrane proteins are correctly described by all of the following statements EXCEPT

(A) they can be exposed by freeze-fracture

(B) they extend into the lipid bilayer

(C) they bind noncovalently to the hydrophobic chains of lipids

(D) they bind primarily by electrostatic and hydrogen bond interactions

(E) they contain extensive regions of nonpolar amino acid residues

95. Which of the following will not be a cause of diabetes mellitus?

(A) stimulation of glycolysis
(B) secretion of proinsulin instead of insulin
(C) secretion of structurally abnormal insulin
(D) defective insulin receptors
(E) lack of pancreatic beta cells

96. The number of moles of ATP (and/or GTP) produced by complete oxidation of one mole of pyruvate in mitochondria is

(A) 3
(B) 4
(C) 12
(D) 15
(E) 24

97. The synthesis of messenger RNA in eukaryotic cells is catalyzed by

(A) RNA polymerase I
(B) RNA polymerase II
(C) RNA polymerase III
(D) reverse transcriptase
(E) poly A polymerase

ANSWERS AND EXPLANATIONS

51. **(C)** The secondary structure of a protein is maintained by virtue of hydrogen bonding between the α-amino and α-carboxyl groups of the substituent amino acids. The secondary structure of a protein can assume either an α-helical or a β-pleated sheet conformation. Hydrophobic interactions, polar interactions, and disulfide bonds are involved in the stabilization of the tertiary folding of a protein. The primary structure of a protein is defined by the sequential attachment of amino acids via peptide bonds. *(Stryer, pp 27–37)*

52. **(A)** Although peptide bonds define the primary structure (the sequence of amino acids) and, hence, supply the information necessary to specify the three-dimensional structure of a protein, they play no active role in stabilizing the tertiary structure of proteins. Four major types of weak bonds are important in tertiary structure—hydrogen bonds between R groups of the amino acids composing the protein, hydrogen bonds between the peptide groupings of α-helical and β-pleated sheet regions, ionic bonds between positively and negatively charged R groups, and hydrophobic interactions between nonpolar R groups. Study has revealed that hydrophobic interactions are the most important forces involved in maintaining the tertiary structure of proteins. *(Stryer, pp 33–39)*

53. **(D)** The activation of factor X is the final reaction of both the extrinsic and intrinsic pathways of clotting. Activated factor X proteolytically cleaves prothrombin to thrombin, which in turn cleaves fibrinogen to fibrin. Accelerin stimulates the activation of factor X, and fibrin-stabilizing factor (factor XIII) stabilizes the clot by cross-linking fibrin. All of these factors are part of the common pathway. The defect in hemophilia is a deficiency in factor VIII, or antihemophilic factor. This factor acts at the last step of the intrinsic pathway. Factor VIII acts in concert with factor IX, a proteolytic enzyme, to activate factor X. *(Stryer, pp 252–255)*

54. **(C)** Coenzyme A (CoA) is synthesized from cysteine, AMP, and the vitamin pantothenate. Its major function is the transfer of acyl groups. To attach acyl groups, CoA forms a thioester linkage between the carboxyl of the acyl group and the sulfhydryl of the β-mercaptoethylamine moiety derived from the amino acid cysteine. *(Stryer, pp 451–452,754–755)*

55. **(A)** During glycolysis, pyruvate is synthesized from phosphoenolpyruvate with the concomitant production of ATP from ADP. The equilibrium of this reaction lies far to the left for the reaction as written:

$$ATP + pyruvate \rightleftharpoons$$
$$phosphoenolpyruvate + ADP + P_i$$

The standard free-energy change ($\Delta G^{\circ\prime}$) for the hydrolysis of ATP is –7.3 kcal/mol, whereas the $\Delta G^{\circ\prime}$ for the phosphorylation of pyruvate to phosphoenolpyruvate is +14.8 kcal/mol (the opposite of the $\Delta G^{\circ\prime}$ for the hydrolysis of phosphoenolpyruvate). Thus, the calculated $\Delta G^{\circ\prime}$ for the thermodynamically unfavorable production of phosphoenolpyruvate is +7.5 kcal/mol. *(Stryer, pp 444–446,491)*

56. **(A)** Myosin contains the ATPase activity that hydrolyzes ATP and allows contraction to proceed. The binding of actin to myosin enhances the ATPase activity of myosin. In fact, actin alternately binds to myosin and is released from myosin as ATP is hydrolyzed. This reaction, which requires magnesium ion, is the driving force of contraction. Although troponin is not directly involved in the ATPase reaction, it binds calcium released by the sarcoplasmic reticulum; this action allows conformational changes in tropomyosin and actin to occur, permitting contraction. Myokinase catalyzes the formation of ATP and AMP from two molecules of ADP. *(Stryer, pp 392–404)*

57. **(E)** Of the monosaccharides and disaccharides listed in the question, only fructose enters the glycolytic pathway at the level of three-carbon intermediates. Fructokinase catalyzes the phosphorylation of fructose by ATP to fructose 1-phosphate, which is then cleaved to glyceraldehyde and dihydroxyacetone phosphate by aldolase. The glyceraldehyde is phosphorylated to glyceraldehyde 3-phosphate. Thus, two intermediates of glycolysis are formed from one molecule of fructose. In contrast, galactose and mannose enter glycolysis at the level of glucose 1-phosphate and fructose 6-phosphate, respectively. The breakdown products of maltose (ie, glucose) and lactose (ie, glucose and galactose) enter glycolysis at the level of six-carbon sugars. *(Stryer, pp 491–493)*

58. **(B)** Most eukaryotic mRNAs are modified at both the 5′ and 3′ ends. The modification at the 5′ end involves attachment of a 7-methylguanylate residue by an unusual 5′-5′ phosphodiester bond. This is referred to as the 5′ cap structure. At the 3′ end the mRNA is modified by the sequential addition of up to 250 adenylate residues by the enzyme poly A polymerase. This modification is referred to as the poly A tail. Essentially all eukaryotic mRNAs have a single initiation site for protein synthesis and thus direct the synthesis of a single polypeptide chain; they are monocistronic. The initiation codon is almost always AUG. Protein synthesis is initiated by binding of the 40S ribosomal subunit to mRNA at the 5′ cap. The ribosome then migrates along the mRNA to the first AUG codon and protein synthesis begins. In contrast, mRNA binding to ribosomes during initiation of protein synthesis in prokaryotes is mediated by an rRNA–mRNA interaction. This involves the association of a specific sequence, the so-called Shine–Dalgarno sequence, on the 5′ side of the AUG initiation codon in mRNA and a complementary sequence at the 3′ end of the 16S rRNA. The Shine–Dalgarno interaction occurs only in prokaryotes. *(Stryer, pp 858–859,895–896,903–905)*

59. **(A)** As a catalyst, an enzyme cannot alter the equilibria of chemical reactions. In catalyzing a reaction, however, enzymes do increase the rate at which equilibrium is attained, by decreasing the energy of activation. During the first step of a reaction, enzymes specifically bind to substrate to form a complex. In many reactions, enzymes transform the energy of reactants into a different form of energy. For example, in photosynthesis, light energy is changed to the energy of chemical bonds; in respiration, the free energy of small molecules is stored as ATP; and in contraction, the energy in ATP is converted into mechanical energy. *(Stryer, pp 181–190)*

60. **(B)** Quaternary structure of a protein refers to the way that the chains in oligomeric proteins interact. Obviously, if a protein is composed of one uninterrupted chain, it has no quaternary structure. Except for ribonuclease, all the proteins listed in the question are composed of two or more subunits. Hemo-

globin and immunoglobulin G are tetramers with two pairs of unlike chains. Collagen has three chains, which may be identical or unlike, depending on the type of collagen. Insulin has two unlike chains. *(Stryer, pp 25, 31–32,37–39,154–157,367–369)*

61. **(E)** Arachidonic acid (eicosatetraenoic acid) derived from the diet or obtained by modification of the essential fatty acid linoleate is stored as a part of cell membrane phospholipids. It serves as the precursor for most of the prostaglandins synthesized in humans. When prostaglandin synthesis is stimulated, arachidonic acid is released for use as a precursor by the action of phospholipase A_2. A cyclopentane ring is formed, and three oxygen atoms are introduced by the action of prostaglandin cyclooxygenase (also called prostaglandin synthetase). Aspirin (acetylsalicylate) inhibits the oxygenase activity of this enzyme by acetylating the terminal group of one of its subunits. The inhibition of prostaglandin biosynthesis is thought to be the main pharmacologic activity of aspirin. *(Stryer, p 624–625)*

62. **(B)** Restriction endonucleases recognize specific base pair sequences usually of four to six base pairs when they possess twofold rotational symmetry. Such a symmetrical placement of base pairs leading to an identical reading from 5′ to 3′ on one strand and from 3′ to 5′ on the other strand is called a palindrome. Of the sequences shown in the question, only CCTAGG GGATCC contains a palindrome. The exact center of symmetry lies between the complementary TA–AT base pairs. *(Stryer, pp 120–121)*

63. **(C)** Under anaerobic conditions, such as intense muscular activity, the rate of formation of pyruvate during glycolysis exceeds its oxidation by the citric acid cycle. As a result, pyruvate is converted to lactate by the action of lactate dehydrogenase. This enzyme employs NADH as a cofactor. Phosphoenolpyruvate, 3-phosphoglycerate, and 2-phosphoglycerate do not accumulate under these conditions. *(Stryer, pp 490–491,497–498,577)*

64. **(C)** The ingestion of candy leads to increased blood glucose levels, which in turn stimulate the α cells of the pancreas to release insulin. Insulin antagonizes the actions of glucagon and epinephrine, which stimulate glycogenolysis and lipolysis. The major energy source in long-distance running is fatty acid metabolism, which spares glucose utilization. Carbohydrate loading—ie, the ingestion of carbohydrates long before a race—is thought to be the best method for building up glycogen stores. These stores will then be released gradually during the race without a dramatic build-up of insulin, which would interfere with fatty acid release through lipolysis. *(Stryer, pp 773–774)*

65. **(E)** The plasma membranes of all cells are functionally and structurally asymmetrical. Sugars and complex carbohydrates of glycoproteins and glycolipids are usually exposed to the external environment on the outer cell surface. This results in a glycocalyx or carbohydrate coating of most cells. Sphingomyelin and phosphatidyl choline are preferentially localized to the outer leaflet of the lipid bilayer, and phosphatidyl serine and phosphatidyl ethanolamine are primarily in the inner leaflet. Proteins are asymmetrically oriented so that polarized functions may occur. Some proteins, such as those that form channels, span the entire bilayer of the membrane, with different parts of their polypeptide chain exposed to the cytoplasm and the external surface. The lipid milieu of the bilayers is fluid. This fluidity is dependent on the length and number of double bonds present in the fatty acyl chains of the phospholipids. The amount of cholesterol present in plasma membranes regulates their fluidity. Increasing amounts of cholesterol decrease membrane fluidity. Both lipids and proteins diffuse laterally in the plane of the membrane, but proteins do not diffuse transversely (flip-flop) across the bilayer. *(Stryer, pp 263–281)*

66. **(A)** The Golgi apparatus sorts membranes and proteins that are transported from the endoplasmic reticulum to the cell surface.

During this process, glycoproteins are modified. Lysosomal membranes and proteins route through the Golgi apparatus. Endocytotic vesicles and their contents that derive from the cell surface also interact with the Golgi apparatus. The Golgi apparatus is a stack of flattened membrane sacs that receive membrane from the endoplasmic reticulum as vesicles fusing with the concave face. Plasma membrane vesicles interact with the convex face of the Golgi apparatus. *(Stryer, pp 922–924)*

67. **(B)** Opiate receptors in brain tissue are, in fact, receptors for endorphins. Endorphins are peptide hormones that are released by the anterior pituitary and are natural analgesics. They are thought to regulate perception of pain. Morphine, which is an opiate alkaloid derived from the juice of poppy seeds, interacts with the same receptors, thus mimicking endorphin action. The actions of both endorphins and morphine are blocked in the presence of the antagonist naloxone. *(Stryer, 3rd ed., pp 992–993)*

68. **(D)** Epinephrine promotes the formation of blood glucose from glycogenolysis in the liver and the release of fatty acids by stimulation of lipolysis in adipose tissue. Epinephrine, which is released when blood glucose levels are low, promotes glucose sparing by encouraging lipolysis and gluconeogenesis. Increased fatty acid levels also lead to increased ketogenesis in the liver. The ketone bodies released into the bloodstream further spare glucose utilization. In contrast, insulin is secreted when blood glucose levels are high. Insulin stimulates the entry of glucose into cells and encourages the utilization and storage of glucose. Thus, increased glucose oxidation and glycogen synthesis would be expected in the presence of insulin but not in the presence of its antagonist, epinephrine. *(Stryer, pp 773–774)*

69. **(A)** Tetrahydrofolate, which is derived from the vitamin folate, is a major intermediate carrier of hydroxymethyl, formyl, and methyl groups. Folate is widely distributed in plants. Dietary deficiency results in an inhibition of growth and a variety of anemias. The one-carbon transfers with which it is involved include the synthesis of purines and pyrimidines and the intermediary metabolism of amino acids. *(Stryer, pp 719–723)*

70. **(E)** Collagens are a unique class of proteins in several respects. The amount of glycine in collagen is unusually high, composing as much as 35% of the amino acid residues. In addition, collagen contains two other amino acids that are present in few other proteins found in nature, hydroxyproline and hydroxylysine. These residues are important in the cross-linking of collagen fibers. *(Stryer, pp 31–32)*

71. **(C)** Mammals lack the ability to synthesize linoleic or linolenic acid. Because these compounds serve as the precursors for the synthesis of other fatty acids they must be provided in the diet. *(Stryer, p 623)*

72. **(B)** Ascorbate (vitamin C) is a cofactor necessary for the action of the enzymes prolyl hydroxylase and lysyl hydroxylase, which catalyze the posttranslational modification of proline and lysine in collagen to hydroxyproline and hydroxylysine. At their active sites these enzymes contain a ferrous atom, which must be kept in a reduced state. Because ascorbate is used as a reducing agent, it activates the enzymes. A deficiency of vitamin C leads to scurvy, a disease characterized by skin lesions and blood vessel fragility. Citrus fruits, which are rich in vitamin C, supply a sufficient amount of the vitamin when eaten regularly. *(Stryer, p 454–455)*

73. **(D)** Approximately 10% of the fatty acids obtained from the diet are short (2 to 4 carbon atoms) or medium (5 to 10 carbon atoms) in chain length. Unlike long-chain fatty acids (> 10 carbon atoms), short-chain and medium-chain fatty acids are freely diffusible across the mitochondrial membranes. Once inside the mitochondrial matrix, these free fatty acids are activated to fatty acyl CoA complexes by mitochondrial matrix fatty acyl

CoA synthetases (thiokinases). In contrast, long-chain fatty acids are activated into acyl CoA thioesters by thiokinases located on the outer mitochondrial membranes. These activated long-chain fatty acids are transferred from the sulfur atom of CoA to the hydroxyl group of carnitine to form acyl carnitine, which diffuses across the inner mitochondrial membrane. On the matrix side, the acyl group is transferred from carnitine back to CoA. This carnitine-mediated transfer of activated long-chain fatty acids is catalyzed by the enzyme fatty acyl CoA:carnitine fatty acyl transferase. Activated fatty acyl CoA derivatives present in the mitochondrial matrix are the substrates of β oxidation. Triacylglycerols (fatty acyl esters of glycerol) are storage forms of fatty acids. They are transported in the blood packaged as lipoprotein complexes. *(Stryer, pp 606–608)*

74. **(C)** The degree of unsaturation and the chain length of fatty acids contribute to their physical properties. The melting point of fatty acids decreases with the degree of unsaturation; each double bond kinks the otherwise saturated hydrocarbon chain of a fatty acid, producing a fixed angle of about 30°. The melting point of fatty acids increases with increasing chain length. Long, saturated fatty acids are hard waxes, whereas shorter, polyunsaturated fatty acids are oils. Of the fatty acids listed in the question, 18:0 is the longest saturated fatty acid. *(Stryer, pp 604–605)*

75. **(C)** In the genetic disease known as sickle cell anemia, homozygous persons suffer from hemolytic anemia caused by the presence of sickled erythrocytes in the venous circulation. The sickle effect is a result of the change of one amino acid (glutamate to valine) at position 6 of the β chain of hemoglobin. This amino acid substitution results in aggregation of deoxygenated Hb S. The solubility of the deoxygenated Hb S is lower than normal, and precipitation of the aggregates causes the observed sickle shape. This occurs when oxygen levels are low. The substitution of the highly polar glutamate with nonpolar valine leads to a change in the electrophoretic mo-

bility of Hb S when compared with normal Hb. *(Stryer, pp 168–172)*

76. **(A)** The hydrolysis of ATP to ADP and inorganic phosphate by interacting filaments of actin and myosin is the driving force of muscle contraction. As the level of ATP drops in active muscle, a variety of mechanisms come into play to increase cell ATP. Phosphocreatine, the reservoir of high-energy phosphate bonds in muscle, donates its phosphoryl group to ADP to form ATP. Adenylate kinase (myokinase) produces ATP and AMP from ADP. In addition, the lowered energy charge of exercising muscle stimulates the rates of glycolysis, the citric acid cycle, and oxidative phosphorylation. Hence, production of fructose 1,6-bisphosphate and ADP is increased. Lactate production also is increased, because the rate of production of pyruvate by glycolysis exceeds the rate of oxidation of pyruvate by the citric acid cycle. Likewise, the rate of NADH production in glycolysis is greater than the rate of its oxidation by the respiratory chain. Subsequently, lactate is produced by lactate dehydrogenase and NAD^+ is regenerated. Lactate diffuses from muscle into the blood and is carried to the liver, where it is converted to glucose. The glucose may then be transported back to muscle. This manner of interaction between the liver and actively contracting muscle is referred to as the Cori cycle. By contast, in resting muscle the major energy source is derived from the oxidation of fatty acids. *(Stryer, pp 393–394,447–448,497–498,577–578,771–772)*

77–79. **(77–E, 78–A, 79–C)** The genetic code defines the relationship between the sequence of bases in DNA and the corresponding sequence of amino acids in proteins. Three bases form a codon that codes for an amino acid. Since it has been demonstrated that most of the 64 possible arrangements of bases into codons do code for specific amino acids, and since there are only 20 amino acids, the code is degenerate (ie, the same amino acid may be coded for by more than one codon). If a single base pair is substituted, only one amino acid is changed (provided, of course, that the new codon does not also code for the original amino acid). This phenomenon demonstrates that the code is not overlapping but that codons are read sequentially, one after the other. Finally, deletions or additions of a single base pair cause a shift of the reading frame subsequent to the point of change. Consequently, all amino acids in the coded protein subsequent to that point will be altered. This change demonstrates a sequential reading of bases from a fixed starting point. *(Stryer, pp 103–104)*

80–81. (80–C, 81–E) Lesch-Nyhan syndrome is caused by a decrease or lack of hypoxanthine-guanine phosphoribosyl transferase (HGPRT) activity. HGPRT is a salvage pathway enzyme that catalyzes the synthesis of inosinate (IMP) or guanylate (GMP) from hypoxanthine or guanine. Lesch-Nyhan syndrome is characterized by compulsive, self-destructive behavior. Adenosine deaminase catalyzes the conversion of adenosine to inosine and normally functions in the breakdown of adenine-containing nucleotides to uric acid. Adenosine deaminase deficiency results in severe combined immunodeficiency. This is due to the buildup of dATP, which inhibits cellular DNA synthesis because it blocks the biosynthesis of deoxyribonucleotides. Thymidylate synthase catalyzes the synthesis of thymidine monophosphate, xanthine oxidase catalyzes the conversion of hypoxanthine to xanthine and uric acid, and adenine phosphoribosyl transferase is a salvage pathway enzyme that catalyzes the synthesis of AMP from adenine. *(Stryer, pp 744, 749–750,755–758)*

82–84. (82–C, 83–E, 84–A) Glycogen phosphorylase catalyzes the sequential removal of glucose residues from glycogen yielding glucose 1-phosphate. The reaction is

$$\text{Glycogen}_{(n)} + P_i \rightarrow \text{glucose 1-phosphate} + \text{glycogen}_{(n-1)}$$

The synthesis of glycogen is mediated by glycogen synthase, which catalyzes the addition of glucose residues to a growing glyco-

gen chain. The glucose must be in the activated form of UDP-glucose.

$$\text{Glycogen}_{(n)} + \text{UDP-glucose} \rightarrow \text{glycogen}_{(n+1)} + \text{UDP}$$

Glucokinase catalyzes the formation of glucose 6-phosphate from glucose and ATP. Glucose 6-phosphate dehydrogenase catalyzes the first step of the pentose phosphate pathway. The reaction is

$$\text{Glucose 6-phosphate} + NADP^+ \rightarrow \text{6-phosphoglucono-}\delta\text{-lactone} + NADPH + H^+$$

Glucose 6-phosphatase catalyzes the hydrolysis of glucose 6-phosphate to glucose and inorganic phosphate. This enzyme occurs in liver and allows for the release of free glucose from the liver. *(Stryer, pp 495,560,585–587)*

85–88. (85–C, 86–B, 87–E, 88–D) Reactions A, B, and E are part of the glycolytic pathway, whereas C and D are steps in gluconeogenesis. Pyruvate kinase catalyzes the conversion of phosphoenolpyruvate to pyruvate (reaction B) with the release of ATP. Under anaerobic conditions (eg, muscle during strenuous exercise), pyruvate is reduced to lactate in a reaction requiring NADH as a cofactor. The first phase of gluconeogenesis is the conversion of pyruvate to phosphoenolpyruvate via oxaloacetate. The reactions are

$$\text{Pyruvate} + CO_2 + ATP + H_2O \rightarrow \text{oxaloacetate} + ADP + P_i + 2\,H^+$$

$$\text{Oxaloacetate} + GTP \rightarrow \text{phosphoenolpyruvate} + GDP + CO_2$$

The sum of these two reactions permits the conversion of pyruvate to phosphoenolpyruvate in gluconeogenesis. In glycolysis, formation of pyruvate from phosphoenolpyruvate is essentially irreversible. *(Stryer, pp 490,497–498,569–572)*

89. (C) Vitamin D can be obtained by ingestion or formed by the action of ultraviolet light on 7-dehydrocholesterol, an intermediate in the pathway of cholesterol synthesis. It is stored in the kidneys as 25-hydroxycholecalciferol. When calcium levels are low, parathyroid hormone stimulates the kidneys to modify 25-hydroxycholecalciferol to 1,25-dihydroxy-cholecalciferol, the active form of vitamin D. This compound induces the synthesis of specific proteins that participate in the transport of calcium from the gut. Poor exposure to sunlight and absence of fish products in the diet can lead to a deficiency of vitamin D. In growing children vitamin D deficiency causes rickets, a disease of improper calcification of bones. Adults may develop osteomalacia, a condition characterized by bone fragility. The carboxylation of glutamate residues is mediated by vitamin K. *(Stryer, pp 707)*

90. **(A)** Core glycosylation of proteins occurs on the luminal side of the endoplasmic reticulum membrane. Dolichol phosphate, a lipid carrier of oligosaccharides, transfers oligosaccharides to either asparagine, serine, or threonine residues of proteins. Terminal glycosylation (trimming and remodeling of the attached oligosaccharide units) occurs after transfer of the nascent glycoprotein to the Golgi apparatus. Lysosomes, which contain hydrolytic enzymes, and the plasma membrane are not sites of biosynthesis of glycoproteins. Endosomes are vesicles formed during the process of endocytosis. *(Stryer, pp 920–924)*

91. **(C)** Gout is characterized by an elevation in the serum levels of uric acid (hyperuricemia). This condition may be caused by a variety of metabolic factors that lead to increased intracellular levels of nucleotides, eg, increased synthesis of ribonucleoside monophosphates or impairment in salvage pathway function. Because uric acid is the end product of purine degradation, elevation of purine nucleotide levels results in overproduction of uric acid. The enzyme xanthine oxidase catalyzes the last two reactions of purine degradation, ie, the conversion of hypoxanthine to xanthine to uric acid. Allopurinol is a substrate analogue of hypoxanthine and is a competitive inhibitor of xanthine oxidase.

The result of allopurinol administration is an inhibition of xanthine oxidase activity, a decrease in uric acid production, and a concomitant increase in hypoxanthine and xanthine formation, since these latter compounds cannot be metabolized further. Allopurinol has no direct effect on de novo purine biosynthesis. *(Stryer, pp 755–757)*

92. **(D)** DFP is a reagent that reacts covalently with active site serines. Because the reagent forms a covalent bond with the enzyme, chymotrypsin is irreversibly inhibited. Chymotrypsin is among a group of proteolytic enzymes referred to as serine proteases because they possess an active site serine that is required for enzymatic activity. Other members of this group include trypsin, thrombin, and elastase. Competitive inhibition involves reversible binding of a structural analogue of the substrate to the active site. Feedback inhibition is characterized by inhibition of the first reaction of a metabolic pathway by the end product of that pathway. *(Stryer, pp 196–197,222–225)*

93. **(B)** Catabolism of amino acids involves removal of the α-amino group followed by conversion of the resulting carbon skeleton into a major metabolic intermediate. Deamination of most amino acids is accomplished by transfer of the α-amino group to α-ketoglutarate to form glutamate (transamination), followed by oxidative deamination of glutamate to yield ammonium ion and α-ketoglutarate. *(Stryer, pp 629–631)*

94. **(D)** Membrane proteins are classified as either integral or peripheral. Integral membrane proteins extend into the bilayer of membranes, and some may extend across the entire width of the membrane. They are fixed in the membrane by hydrophobic interactions between regions of nonpolar amino acid residues and the fatty acyl residues of phospholipids. In contrast, peripheral or extrinsic membrane proteins do not extend into the bilayer. They are attached to the surface of membranes by electrostatic or hydrogen bond interactions. It is thought that most peripheral proteins are bound to the exposed

surfaces of integral membrane proteins. When frozen cells are fractured by the impact of a microtome knife, cleavage preferentially occurs in the middle of the membrane bilayer, thereby exposing those membrane proteins extending well into the membrane proper. By definition, only integral membrane proteins can be so exposed. *(Stryer, pp 275–276)*

95. **(A)** The complex disease known as diabetes mellitus may be caused by a variety of underlying molecular defects. Any defect that prevents the action of insulin will yield the clinical symptoms of diabetes. These defects include (1) a lack of insulin resulting from destruction of the beta cells of the pancreas, (2) a defective conversion of proinsulin to insulin prior to secretion, (3) structurally abnormal and functionless insulin molecules as a result of mutation, and (4) abnormal insulin receptors. Inhibition of glycolysis, rather than its stimulation, is a hallmark of diabetes. *(Stryer, pp 779–780)*

96. **(D)** Pyruvate is converted to acetyl-CoA in an oxidative decarboxylation reaction catalyzed by pyruvate dehydrogenase.

$$\text{Pyruvate} + \text{CoA} + \text{NAD}^+ \rightarrow \text{acetyl CoA} + \text{CO}_2 + \text{NADH}$$

The acetyl CoA then enters the citric acid cycle. The overall stoichiometry of the cycle can be represented as follows:

$$\text{Acetyl CoA} + 3\,\text{NAD}^+ + \text{FAD} + \text{GDP} + \text{P}_i + 2\,\text{H}_2\text{O} \rightarrow 2\,\text{CO}_2 + 3\,\text{NADH} + \text{FADH}_2 + \text{GTP} + 2\,\text{H}^+ + \text{CoA}$$

Thus, from one mole of pyruvate a total of 4 moles of NADH and 1 mole each of FADH_2 and GTP are produced. Each NADH yields 3 moles of ATP via mitochondrial electron transport and oxidative phosphorylation. The same processes result in the production of 2 moles of ATP per mole of FADH_2. In sum, the complete mitochondrial oxidation of 1 mole of pyruvate yields 15 moles of ATP (+GTP). *(Stryer, pp 513–514,551–552)*

97. **(B)** Eukaryotic cells contain three different DNA-dependent RNA polymerases that are responsible for the synthesis of different types of RNA. RNA polymerase I catalyzes the synthesis of ribosomal RNA, RNA polymerase II is responsible for synthesis of messenger RNA, and RNA polymerase III mediates the production of transfer and 5S RNA. Most eukaryotic mRNAs contain poly A tails of varying lengths at their 3′ ends. This is synthesized by poly A polymerase. Reverse transcriptase is found in most retroviruses and is responsible for synthesis of DNA from the genomic RNA of these viruses. *(Stryer, pp 91–93,853–854,859)*

REFERENCE

Stryer L. *Biochemistry*. 4th ed. New York: WH Freeman Co Publishers; 1995.

SUBSPECIALTY LIST: BIOCHEMISTRY

Question Number and Subspecialty

51. Protein
52. Protein
53. Blood
54. Vitamins
55. Thermodynamics
56. Muscle contraction
57. Carbohydrates
58. Molecular biology
59. Enzymes
60. Protein
61. Lipids
62. Molecular biology
63. Carbohydrate metabolism
64. Integration of metabolism
65. Membranes
66. Membranes
67. Hormones
68. Hormones
69. Vitamins
70. Proteins
71. Lipids
72. Vitamins

73. Energy metabolism
74. Lipids
75. Blood
76. Muscle contraction
77. Molecular biology
78. Molecular biology
79. Molecular biology
80. Nucleotide metabolism
81. Nucleotide metabolism
82. Carbohydrate metabolism
83. Carbohydrate metabolism
84. Carbohydrate metabolism
85. Carbohydrate metabolism

86. Carbohydrate metabolism
87. Carbohydrate metabolism
88. Carbohydrate metabolism
89. Vitamins
90. Proteins
91. Nucleotide metabolism
92. Enzymes
93. Small molecule metabolism
94. Membranes
95. Hormones
96. Energy metabolism
97. Molecular biology

Microbiology

William W. Yotis, PhD

DIRECTIONS (Questions 98 through 130): Each of the numbered items or incomplete statements in this section is followed by answers or by completions of the statement. Select the ONE lettered answer or completion that is BEST in each case.

98. Methods that would blunt T-cell-mediated reactions include all of the following EXCEPT

    (A) lymphocyte elimination
    (B) x-ray irradiation
    (C) antithymocyte serum
    (D) postneonatal tolerization
    (E) induction of anti-idiotypic antibodies to T cells that recognize the graft

99. The virulence of *Haemophilus influenzae* is directly related to its

    (A) possession of an antiphagocytic protein capsule
    (B) possession of an antiphagocytic polysaccharide capsule
    (C) ability to produce an exotoxin
    (D) production of hyaluronidase, which helps it to spread through the host tissues
    (E) ability to hemolyze erythrocytes

100. The predominant cause of bacterial meningitis in children between the ages of 6 months and 6 years is

    (A) *Escherichia coli*
    (B) *Haemophilus influenzae*
    (C) *Listeria monocytogenes*
    (D) *Neisseria meningitidis*
    (E) *Streptococcus faecalis*

101. All the following antiviral agents would be effective against DNA viruses EXCEPT

    (A) interferon
    (B) amantadine
    (C) iododeoxyuridine
    (D) ribavirin
    (E) adenosine arabinoside

102. The virus that has been associated with progressive multifocal leukoencephalopathy is

    (A) SV 40
    (B) polyomavirus
    (C) human papilloma virus
    (D) BK virus
    (E) JC virus

103. Attenuated live-virus vaccines are useful in the prevention of all the following diseases EXCEPT

    (A) mumps
    (B) measles
    (C) poliomyelitis
    (D) hepatitis B
    (E) rubella

104. The inclusion body seen in cells infected with rabies virus is called

    (A) a Negri body
    (B) a Quarnieri body
    (C) a reticulate body
    (D) an elementary body
    (E) an Ammon's body

105. A virus that does not encode a DNA-dependent DNA polymerase is

    (A) adenovirus
    (B) herpes simplex virus type 1
    (C) herpes simplex virus type 2
    (D) papovavirus
    (E) vaccina virus

106. Individuals with hereditary angioneurotic edema have a deficiency in

    (A) C1 esterase inhibitor
    (B) C3b inactivator
    (C) C3 activator
    (D) β-1H-globulin
    (E) carboxypeptidase

107. Immunoglobulin E (IgE), the antibody involved in atopic allergies, can be described by which of the following statements?

    (A) it can cross the placenta
    (B) it has an affinity for cells of the host
    (C) it can activate complement by the classical pathway
    (D) it contains J chains
    (E) it contains α heavy chains

108. Activated macrophages

    (A) cannot kill facultative intracellular pathogens such as listeria and mycobacteria
    (B) do not participate in granuloma formation and tissue damage during delayed-type hypersensitivity reaction
    (C) stain negative for many esterases
    (D) have increased C3b receptors
    (E) are incapable of killing any type of tumor cell

109. Monoclonal antibody

    (A) has antigen-combining sites that are not identical
    (B) may belong only to the IgM, IgA, or IgG classes
    (C) may be present in the serum of patients with multiple myeloma

    (D) cannot be obtained by the hybridoma technique
    (E) shows a lower level of specificity than the polyclonal antibody

110. Class I major histocompatibility complex determinants are

    (A) nucleoproteins
    (B) found only on T cells
    (C) not involved in the recognition of virally infected cells by CD4 + cytotoxic T cells
    (D) the heterodimers of a heavy chain that is covalently bound to beta-2 microglobulin
    (E) not involved in transplant rejection

111. Which of the following disorders is an autoimmune disease with a characteristic antibody response to autologous immunoglobulin G (IgG)?

    (A) pernicious anemia
    (B) rheumatoid arthritis
    (C) Goodpasture's syndrome
    (D) myasthenia gravis
    (E) Wiskott-Aldrich syndrome

112. Antibiotics that may be used in the treatment of gonorrhea caused by penicillinase-producing strains include

    (A) methicillin
    (B) cephalothin
    (C) oxacillin
    (D) spectinomycin
    (E) all of the above

113. Lysogenic conversion is responsible for which of the following phenomena?

    (A) production of erythrogenic toxin
    (B) production of botulinus toxin type C
    (C) production of diphtheria toxin
    (D) antigenic conversions in certain strains of *Salmonella*
    (E) all of the above

114. The pilus, a bacterial organelle found on the cell surface, can be described by which of the following statements?

(A) it is involved in attachment to host membranes

(B) it is found on all gram-positive and gram-negative organisms

(C) it does not play a role in conjugation

(D) it can be an organelle of locomotion

(E) none of the above

115. A single-stranded nucleic acid core is found in which of the following viruses?

(A) adenovirus

(B) reovirus

(C) herpesvirus

(D) paramyxovirus

(E) none of the above

116. A 16-year-old otherwise healthy woman is complaining of frequent and painful urination. A urine specimen is obtained and sent to the laboratory for culture and sensitivity. The laboratory reports back 10^5 *Escherichia coli* and 10^3 *Staphylococcus epidermidis* per mL. A suitable course of action will be to

(A) reculture for staphylococci

(B) admit and catheterize the patient

(C) treat for *S. epidermidis*

(D) treat for *E. coli*

(E) treat with penicillin

117. The following toxin is produced by *Staphylococcus aureus:*

(A) enterotoxin

(B) erythrogenic toxin

(C) excruciating toxin

(D) verotoxin

(E) none of the above

118. Gene transfer between bacteria of the same species can occur by all of the following EXCEPT

(A) transformation

(B) conjugation

(C) transduction

(D) complementation

(E) plasmids

119. Aseptic meningitis may be caused by which of the following viruses?

(A) herpesvirus

(B) coxsackievirus

(C) poliovirus

(D) arenavirus

(E) all of the above

120. The human immunodeficiency virus (HIV)

(A) is a single-stranded RNA virus

(B) is a member of the retrovirus group

(C) contains reverse transcriptase

(D) destroys T_4 lymphocytes

(E) all of the above

121. A 25-year-old male patient is experiencing inability to swallow and has speech difficulty. The patient was in perfect health prior to the consumption of home-canned green beans. He also stated that the jar lid was swollen prior to being opened. Which of the following is the most likely method of treatment?

(A) administration of staphylococcal enterotoxin antiserum

(B) penicillin administration

(C) immunization with *Staphylococcus aureus* enterotoxin toxoid

(D) administration of trivalent botulinum antitoxin

(E) placement of the patient in a hyperbaric oxygen chamber

122. All of the following statements about class I and class II MHC proteins are true EXCEPT

(A) they are integral membrane proteins

(B) they restrict immune responses to T lymphocytes

(C) they are codominantly expressed

(D) they are expressed on all nucleated cells

(E) they are glycoproteins

123. The figure given represents the death curve of microorganisms. According to this graph, the percentage of cells dying every 10 minutes is

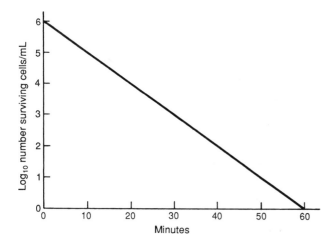

(A) 100%

(B) 0.1%

(C) 9%

(D) 10%

(E) 90%

124. The AIDS virus (HIV) differs from the RNA tumor viruses in that it

(A) does not require T4 receptor protein for adsorption to host cells

(B) contains two copies of single-stranded RNA in its virion

(C) contains the *gag* gene

(D) contains the *pol* gene

(E) lyses the host cells

125. A rapid method using molecular biology techniques that may be useful for the specific diagnosis of cytomegalovirus infections in the clinical laboratory is the use of

(A) gram stain

(B) labeled DNA probe and DNA hybridization

(C) agglutination using latex particles tagged with virus

(D) acid-fast stain

(E) silver stain to detect capsid antigens

126. A 10-month-old baby was vaccinated against smallpox virus. He developed a progressive necrotic lesion of the skin, muscles, and subcutaneous tissue. The growth of the attenuated virus and subsequent reaction resulted from

(A) B-lymphocyte deficiency

(B) reaction to the adjuvant

(C) complement deficiency

(D) immediate hypersensitivity produced by IgE reactivity to the virus

(E) T-lymphocyte deficiency

127. You are examining a 38-month-old white male showing lethargy, fever, painful cervical dorsiflexion and an inflamed throat. The LEAST likely approach you will take is

(A) perform a spinal tap and send the specimen to the clinical laboratories for culture and sensitivity, CIE (or agglutination with monoclonal antibody), and chemistry.

(B) perform a Gram stain on sediment from CSF.

(C) after drawing the CSF, begin treatment with penicillin G.

(D) obtain several throat swabs and send them to the laboratory for culture and sensitivity.

(E) consult with public health officials to see if there is an outbreak of similar cases in the area.

128. The most likely component responsible for the production of overwhelming septic shock complicating bacteremia with *Neisseria meningitidis* is the

(A) capsular polysaccharide

(B) pili

(C) lipopolysaccharide in the outer membrane

(D) low-molecular-weight outer membrane proteins

(E) peptidoglycan

129. The etiologic agent of infectious mononucleosis is

(A) Epstein–Barr virus
(B) varicella-zoster virus
(C) variola virus
(D) herpes simplex virus
(E) rubeola

130. Q fever is an acute infectious disease of worldwide occurrence that

(A) is caused by *Rickettsia akari*
(B) stimulates the production of proteus agglutinins
(C) involves a rash that spreads from the trunk to the extremities
(D) is acquired by inhaling dust containing infected animal excreta
(E) is usually acquired by tick bites

DIRECTIONS (Questions 131 through 139): Each group of items in this section consists of lettered headings followed by a set of numbered words or phrases. For each numbered word or phrase select the ONE lettered heading that is most closely associated with it. Each lettered heading may be selected once, more than once, or not at all.

Question 131

For the description below, select the type of immunoglobulin with which it is most likely to be associated.

(A) immunoglobulin A
(B) immunoglobulin D
(C) immunoglobulin E
(D) immunoglobulin G
(E) immunoglobulin M

131. The immunoglobulin cytotropic for mast cells

Question 132

For the description below, choose one of the following:

(A) *Clostridium perfringens*
(B) *Bacteroides melaninogenicus*

(C) *Bacillus stearothermophilus*
(D) *Streptococcus pyogenes*
(E) *Neisseria meningitidis*

132. Spore-forming anaerobe

Questions 133–134

(A) interferon-γ
(B) interleukin-2
(C) tumor necrosis factor
(D) transfer factor
(E) blastogenic factor

133. Substance responsible for hypotension induced in a 24-year-old patient with septicemia caused by *Salmonella typhi*

134. May be employed to briefly restore specific cellular immunity to an immunocompromised patient

Questions 135 and 136

(A) *Leishmania donovani*
(B) *Aspergillus fumigatus*
(C) *Entamoeba histolytica*
(D) *Trypanosoma cruzi*
(E) *Histoplasma capsulatum*
(F) *Toxoplasma gondii*
(G) *Cryptococcus neoformans*
(H) *Trichophyton rubrum*
(I) *Trichomonas vaginalis*
(J) *Coccidioides immitis*
(K) *Plasmodium falciparum*
(L) *Sporothrix schenckii*

135. An 11-year-old boy is hospitalized with anemia, pigmentation, hypertrophy of spleen, and a prolonged fever of 41°C that fails to remit. Giemsa stain blood smears show kidney-bean–shaped gametocytes with round, pointed ends. Treatment with chloroquine resulted in marked improvement of the patient.

136. A middle-aged, male, immunocompromised patient, living in an area infested with pigeons, is admitted to the hospital. He has fever, headache, stiff neck, and disorientation. His spinal fluid is clear, but it has mononuclear cells. An india ink staining of the spinal fluid and culture on Sabouraud's agar at 37° C following staining show encapsulated yeast cells.

Questions 137 through 139

(A) variable regions of light and heavy chains

(B) constant regions of light and heavy chains

(C) constant region of heavy chain

(D) J chain

(E) hinge region

(F) HLA-A

(G) HLA-B

(H) HLA-C

(I) C5a

(J) Fc

137. Macrophage and neutrophil attractant

138. Determines isotypes

139. Determines idiotypes

ANSWERS AND EXPLANATIONS

98. (D) Neonatal tolerization (administration of antigens to neonates and in utero) leads to immunologic tolerance. Postneonatal tolerization cannot blunt T-cell-mediated reactions. Similarly, lymphocyte removal and x-rays will eliminate T lymphocytes that are needed for T-cell-mediated reactions. Anti-thymocyte serum, in the presence of complement, damages and lyses thymocytes, precursors of T cells. Finally, another immunosuppressive technique is the induction of anti-idiotypic antibodies to T cells that recognize the graft. These antibodies block the recognition of the major histocompatibility complex antigens on the graft. (*Joklik et al, pp 256–262, 274–283*)

99. (B) The capsule of *Haemophilus influenzae* type B is considered the key virulence factor of this microorganism. The capsule is a polymer of ribose-ribitol phosphate (PRP), and it inhibits phagocytosis. Immunization with PRP is now proposed for mothers at high risk of infection who lack antibodies against PRP, as well as children over 2 years old and those between 18 and 23 months old who attend day care centers or those with asplenia. *H. influenzae* has not been shown to produce hemolysins, exotoxins, or hyaluronidase. (*Jawetz et al, pp 237–239*)

100. (B) *Haemophilus influenzae* is the most common cause of bacterial meningitis in the age group 2 to 60 months. Two common fecal organisms, *Escherichia coli* and *Streptococcus faecalis,* are associated with meningitis in the very young (less than 2 months of age). *Neisseria meningitidis* can cause meningitis in adults; it is also associated with epidemics of the disease in army recruits and others sharing close quarters. *Listeria monocytogenes* causes meningitis in individuals of all age groups. (*Joklik et al, p 466*)

101. (B) Interferon is a very broad-spectrum antiviral agent that interferes with the translation of messenger RNA by inducing the cell to produce an adenine trinucleotide that activates a cellular endonuclease. It also causes inactivation of elongation factor 2 (EF-2) by induction of a protein kinase that phosphorylates the factor. Iododeoxyuridine, ribavirin, and adenosine arabinoside all interfere with viral DNA synthesis. Amantadine is effective in inhibiting the multiplication of myxoviruses, rubella, and some other RNA viruses; it is not effective against DNA viruses. (*Joklik et al, pp 863–865*)

102. (E) Progressive multifocal leukoencephalopathy is an uncommon, generally fatal, demyelinating disease that occurs in compromised hosts. It is caused by infection of oligodendrocytes by JC virus. There is no known treatment for this viral disease. (*Joklik et al, p 978; Ryan, pp 559–560*)

103. **(D)** Vaccines against mumps, measles, polio, smallpox, yellow fever, rubella, and adenovirus are available as live, attenuated viral preparations. The rabies vaccine used in humans is a killed virus preparation; however, veterinary vaccines against the virus are live, attenuated strains of the agent. Hepatitis B virus has not been grown successfully in cell cultures in quantities sufficient for vaccine production. The vaccine now used for the prevention of this disease is purified viral antigen obtained from the blood of individuals with a persistent viremia. This preparation is then inactivated before it is administered as a vaccine. *(Jawetz et al, pp 403–406)*

104. **(A)** The Negri bodies associated with rabies are large cytoplasmic granules containing rabies virus. They are the most abundant in the area known as Ammon's horn of the hippocampus. They are best detected by special stains (eg, Seller's stain), which reveal the granules as cherry red in color with dark blue spots; immunofluorescence is another reliable method of identifying these inclusions. Quarnieri bodies are seen in poxvirus-infected cells. Reticulate and elementary bodies are seen in chlamydial infections. *(Joklik et al, pp 719,950,1029)*

105. **(D)** Papovaviruses are the smallest double-stranded DNA viruses. In these viruses, viral DNA replicates using the host's DNA-dependent DNA polymerase. *(Joklik et al, pp 796–798; Levinson and Jawetz, pp 163–164)*

106. **(A)** Individuals with an inherited deficiency of C1 esterase inhibitor have the disease known as hereditary angioneurotic edema. These individuals experience acute episodes of local accumulation of edema fluid. The disease is inherited as an autosomal dominant trait. Administration of ε-aminocaproate, an inhibitor of plasmin activation of C1, reduces the frequency of the episodes. *(Joklik et al, p 294)*

107. **(B)** IgE antibodies have an affinity for host cells, particularly basophils and tissue mast cells. The antibodies react with the cell membrane through the Fc portion of the molecule. When a specific allergen reacts with the cell-bound molecule, it triggers the release from the cell of various pharmacologic mediators, such as histamine, serotonin, slow-reacting substance of anaphylaxis, heparin, and an eosinophil chemotactic factor. *(Joklik et al, pp 224,352)*

108. **(D)** The histologic picture of delayed hypersensitivity reactions shows an intense mononuclear cell (granulomatous) inflammatory infiltrate comprised of lymphocytes and macrophages. Certain cell-surface receptors (C3b) or markers (esterase) are more pronouncedly demonstrated in activated macrophages. Only activated macrophages can effectively kill the facultative intracellular pathogens, such as mycobacteria and listeria. Activated macrophages also kill some tumor cells. *(Joklik et al, pp 254–255,292,322–323)*

109. **(C)** Monoclonal antibodies may be present in the serum of patients with multiple myeloma; have antigen-combining sites that are identical; may belong to the IgM, IgA, IgE, IgD, or IgG classes; are ordinarily obtained by the hybridoma technique; and show a higher level of specificity than the polyclonal antibodies. *(Joklik et al, p 206; Levinson and Jawetz, pp 327–328)*

110. **(D)** Class I major histocompatibility complex (MHC) determinants, intimately involved in transplant rejection, are found on activated T cells as well as on virtually all cells of the body. The structure of the class I MHC determinants consists of an alpha-glycosylated polypeptide heavy chain of molecular weight about 45,000, which is noncovalently associated with a nonglycosylated beta-microglobulin having an approximate molecular weight of 12,000. *(Joklik et al, pp 271–277; Levinson and Jawetz, p 340; Ryan, p 112)*

111. **(B)** One of the autoantibodies commonly found in persons with rheumatoid arthritis is rheumatoid factor. This antibody, usually of the immunoglobulin M (IgM) class, is specific for IgG immunoglobulins. Affected persons also may have anti-DNA antibodies, and levels of complement may be depressed, particularly during a disease exacerbation. Antiinflammatory therapy is recommended: lymphotoxic drugs (eg, cortisone) are used only when other, nonsteroidal modalities have failed. *(Joklik et al, p 211)*

112. **(E [all])** Methicillin and oxacillin are semisynthetic penicillin antibiotics that are resistant to beta lactamase. They can therefore be used to treat infections caused by organisms having a plasmid that carries the lactamase gene. Cephalothin is another semisynthetic antibiotic with a mode of action similar to that of penicillin (ie, it blocks the cross-linking reaction in cell wall synthesis). Like penicillin, cephalothin contains a lactam ring; however, this ring is resistant to hydrolysis by beta lactamase. Spectinomycin is commonly used to treat gonorrhea caused by penicillinase-producing gonococci. It does not contain a lactam ring and is actually an aminocyclitol antibiotic that acts on the bacterial ribosome to effect its antimicrobial action. *(Joklik et al, pp 160–163)*

113. **(E [all])** The genetic information needed for the manufacture of any product, be it an exotoxin or a new cell-surface antigen, resides in the genome of the bacteriophage. If the phage is able to establish a lysogenic (temperate) relationship, these genes will be expressed in the host bacterium. This phenomenon is called lysogenic conversion. *(Joklik et al, pp 145,422,650)*

114. **(A)** Pili are found on some gram-negative bacteria. They have two known functions: adherence to host cell surfaces and transfer of genetic material. Somatic pili are involved in surface adherence, and conjugal pili are involved in gene transfer. *(Joklik et al, pp 21–23)*

115. **(D)** Most DNA viruses, including the adenoviruses and the herpesviruses, are composed of double-stranded DNA. Most RNA viruses are composed of single-stranded nucleic acid; however, the reovirus group contains segmented, double-stranded RNA. Para-

myxoviruses contain single-stranded RNA. *(Joklik et al, pp 769–781)*

116. **(D)** *Escherichia coli* is the most common cause of urinary tract infections, both hospital and community acquired. Women are more likely to have urinary tract infections at a young age because of differences in anatomic structure, sexual maturation, or other reasons. Urinary tract infections are associated with frequent, painful urination and *E. coli* counts of 10^5 or more organisms per milliliter of urine. The bacterial concentration is a key diagnostic feature for urinary tract infections, and thus it must be well documented. For this reason a repeat sample of urine must be taken and the number of *E. coli* be redetermined by viable plate counts. The diagnosis of urinary tract infections is based on the examination of the normally sterile urine for evidence of bacteria or accompanying inflammation. Critical to this examination is the use of appropriate techniques for specimen collection. Voided urine is invariably contaminated with *Staphylococcus epidermidis* or other urethral flora and, in women, vaginal secretions that can confound the laboratory tests results. Although contaminants can never be completely eliminated, their quantity may be diminished by carefully cleansing the periurethral area before voiding and allowing the initial part of the urine to flush the urethra before collection of a specimen for culture. This clean-voided midstream urine collection procedure is preferred to catheterization for routine purposes because it avoids the risk of introducing bacteria into the bladder. Treatment should be directed against the causative agent of the urinary tract infection, that is, *E. coli* and not the contaminant *S. epidermidis*. *(Joklik et al, p 547)*

117. **(A)** The majority of *Staphylococcus aureus* strains isolated from clinical specimens produce various types of enterotoxins, known as A, B, C_1, C_2, D, E, that are responsible for food poisoning. Staphylococcal food poisoning is the most common form of microbial food intoxication. It is caused by the ingestion of food that contains preformed entero-

toxin. The symptoms include abdominal pain, nausea, vomiting, diarrhea and appear 2 to 6 hours after the ingestion of food containing enterotoxin. Erythrogenic toxin is produced by *Streptococcus pyogenes* and is responsible for the development of scarlet fever. Verotoxins are produced by some strains of *Escherichia coli*. (*Joklik et al, pp 408–409, 422,546*)

118. **(D)** Gene transfer can occur in bacteria by transformation, conjugation, or transduction. Transformation occurs when foreign DNA gains entry into a competent cell and is expressed. During the process of conjugation, genetic material is exchanged between the donor strain and the recipient. In transduction, the vector carrying the genetic material is a bacteriophage; foreign bacterial genes are injected into the recipient along with the viral chromosome. Complementation is a condition in which two mutant genes present in the same cell have mutations at different sites in the gene; therefore, affected cells function normally in regard to that particular gene's product, because the two mutant genes have "complemented" each other. (*Joklik et al, pp 136–141*)

119. **(E [all])** All the viruses listed can cause aseptic meningitis in humans. Although herpesviruses are not particularly neurotropic, both herpes simplex and the varicella virus can cause meningoencephalitis. Group B coxsackieviruses are isolated commonly from the cerebrospinal fluid of patients with aseptic meningitis. Poliovirus usually is limited in its pathogenesis to the alimentary tract; and an even smaller number (probably less than 1%) develop paralytic poliomyelitis. Lymphocytic choriomeningitis virus, the Tacaribe viruses, and the agent of Lassa fever are classified as arenaviruses. (*Joklik et al, pp 779,957,960, 983,984*)

120. **(E)** The human immune virus (HIV) is the causative agent of acquired immune deficiency syndrome (AIDS). The virus is a member of the retrovirus group, which contains single-stranded RNA viruses, and an enzyme that synthesizes DNA from RNA (reverse transcriptase). The virus multiplies in CD4+ lymphocytes and this multiplication leads to severe lymphopenia as a result of the lysis of CD4+ lymphocytes. (*Joklik et al, pp 1050–1051*)

121. **(D)** The patient described in this question is showing the typical symptoms of botulism, which is commonly caused by types A, B, or E *Clostridium botulinum* toxin. Therefore, early administration of potent botulinum antitoxin containing antibodies to toxins A, B, and E constitutes the most appropriate type of treatment. (*Joklik et al, pp 652–653*)

122. **(D)** Class I and II MHC proteins are integral membrane glycoproteins, restrict T lymphocyte immune responses, and are codominantly expressed. Class II molecules are *not* expressed on all nucleated cells. (*Joklik et al, p 268*)

123. **(E)** An examination of the death curve of the microorganisms indicates that for every 10 minutes that elapse there is a drop of one log in the number of surviving cells per milliliter. That is, at zero time there are 1 000 000 surviving cells per milliliter ($\log_{10} = 6$); 10 minutes later there are 100 000 ($\log_{10} = 5$) cells per milliliter; at 20 minutes there are 10 000 ($\log_{10} = 4$) surviving cells per milliliter. In each case the percentage of cells dying every 10 minutes is 90%, eg 90% of 1 000 000 is 900 000 deaths with 10%, or 100 000 surviving. (*Jawetz et al, p 43*)

124. **(E)** An important difference between the AIDS (HIV) virus and the RNA tumor viruses is that HIV lyses the host cells, whereas RNA tumor viruses transform the cells that they invade but do not possess cytolytic activity. The tropism of the AIDS virus for the T4 lymphocytes depends upon the presence of the T4 protein on the surface of the T4 lymphocyte. This protein serves as the receptor for the adsorption of the AIDS virus to T4 lymphocytes. The AIDS virus is a member of the retroviruses. Retroviruses contain two copies of the genome's RNA molecule. The genomic RNA molecule contains the *gag*, *pol*, and *env* genes. Therefore, the AIDS virus

cannot be expected to differ from the RNA tumor retroviruses. *(Joklik et al, p 1052)*

125. **(B)** DNA homology (in case of DNA viruses such as cytomegalovirus) is most accurately determined by the DNA-DNA hybridization technique using labeled DNA probes. DNA from a suspected viral strain is denatured by heating or treatment with alkali, so as to separate the two strands. These are then adsorbed on some supporting matrix. To them we add some small, broken, denatured DNA oligonucleotide strands derived from a known strain of cytomegalovirus, which is radioactively labeled. The mixture is then heated and allowed to anneal by cooling slowly. If the two DNA samples are entirely homologous, radioactively labeled DNA is hybridized and is then converted to the DNAase-resistant form. If they are completely dissimilar, all radioactive DNA remains DNAase sensitive. Retention of radioactivity with the supporting matrix after DNAase treatment and washing becomes a measure of hybridization and DNA homology. The acid-fast stain is used in the diagnosis of mycobacteria, whereas the silver stain is used in the diagnosis of spirochetes. *(Joklik et al, pp 945–946)*

126. **(E)** In general, establishment of delayed hypersensitivity and destruction of intracellular parasites such as viruses, fungi, some protozoa, and certain bacteria depends upon the presence of a complete array of T cells. T cells are involved in the production of interferon-γ and lymphotoxins that stimulate the macrophages and natural killer cells that are active participants in the destruction of virus-infected cells. Furthermore, T cells play a regulatory role in T-cell-dependent antibody production by B cells against viruses and other intracellular parasites. Thus, T-lymphocyte deficiency is revealed by enhanced susceptibility to infection by viruses, or other intracellular parasites, and absence of delayed type hypersensitivity reactions. The development of progressive necrotic lesions in skin, muscles, and subcutaneous tissues following vaccination with vaccinia virus is a good example of T-lymphocyte deficiency. *(Jawetz et al, pp 116–117)*

127. **(C)** Given the circumstances of age (38 months) the case history most probably represents meningitis due to *Haemophilus influenzae*. Chloramphenicol should be used initially, not penicillin G, which is susceptible to destruction by *H. influenzae* strains producing beta lactamase. Diagnosis of meningitis due to *H. influenzae* requires spinal tap specimen sent to clinical laboratory for the following: Gram stain, culture, antibiotic sensitivity, detection of capsular polysaccharide of *H. influenzae* in the spinal fluid by counter-immune electrophoresis (CIE), or agglutination by monoclonal antibody, tests for sugar and protein levels in the spinal fluid. Meningitis caused by *H. influenzae* leads to a decreased concentration of glucose and an elevated protein level due to the presence of bacteria in the spinal fluid. Throat swabs and cultivation are intended for the detection of carriers and/or initial stages of infection. Consultation with public health officials are advised to determine if an epidemic of meningitis is starting and the infection is not due to *H. influenzae*. *(Ryan, pp 364–365; Levinson and Jawetz, pp 112–113; Joklik et al, pp 466–468)*

128. **(C)** The lipopolysaccharide, or endotoxin, in the outer membrane is the most likely *Neisseria meningitidis* component responsible for the production of overwhelming septicemic shock during meningococcemia. It causes intravascular activation of the complement system, the kallikreinkinin system (hypotension) and the clotting cascade (hemorrhage). *(Joklik et al, pp 446–449; Ryan, pp 310–313)*

129. **(A)** The majority of normal individuals living in the United States possess antibodies against Epstein–Barr virus. Conversion from the seronegative to the seropositive state occurs during the acute phase of infectious mononucleosis. *(Levinson and Jawetz, pp 191–193).*

130. **(D)** Q (query) fever is a zoonosis caused by *Coxiella burnetii*. It is a respiratory disease that may be severe enough to develop into

interstitial pneumonia. The microorganism is a natural parasite of cattle and sheep, and humans are incidental hosts, being infected by inhalation of infected excreta or contact with animal tissues. *C. burnetii* is spread from animal to animal by ticks and remains as an inapparent infection in the mammalian host until parturition. The organisms multiply readily in the placenta and other birth tissues and are found in the urine and stool. These wastes contaminate the soil and serve as the source of infection for humans. *(Joklik et al, pp 713–714; Ryan, pp 436–437)*

131. **(C)** Immunoglobulin E (IgE) antibodies are cytotropic for mast cells and basophilic leukocytes of the peripheral blood. When these cell-bound antibodies react with their specific allergen, the cells degranulate and secrete vasoactive amines. Among the pharmacologically active substances released by these cells are histamine, serotonin, eosinophil chemotactic factor of anaphylaxis, heparin, and several enzymes (eg, chymase and arylsulfatase). After the interaction of allergen and antibody occurs at the cell membrane, the synthesis of other pharmacologically active compounds, called secondary mediators, occurs. The most important of these products is SRS-A (slow-reacting substance of anaphylaxis). In addition various kinins and platelet-activating substances are also synthesized by the mast cells and basophils after allergen contact.

IgA antibodies are the secretory immunoglobulins and are found in highest concentrations in the secretions that bathe certain body surfaces. They are a primary line of defense in tears, saliva, bronchial fluids, and intestine contents. In addition, milk contains high concentrations of IgA. IgM is the immunoglobulin first produced in any immune response. It is the only antibody that is present in the serum of neonates and is of endogenous origin. In contrast, IgG present in fetal blood is of maternal origin. *(Joklik et al, pp 173–174,312; Jawetz et al, pp 110–112)*

132. **(A)** *Clostridium perfringens* is a gram-positive, spore-forming rod unable to grow in the presence of oxygen (ie, it is a strict anaerobe). It ranks second only to staphylococci as the leading cause of food poisoning in the United States. The organism produces an enterotoxin in certain foods, particularly meat products allowed to sit out at room temperature for a considerable period of time after cooking.

Neisseria meningitidis is a gram-negative coccus that can cause meningitis. During fulminant meningococcemia, adrenal insufficiency associated with bilateral adrenal hemorrhage may occur (Waterhouse-Friderichsen syndrome). Vasomotor collapse and shock often lead to death.

Bacteroides melaninogenicus is part of the normal flora throughout the upper portion of the alimentary canal. This gram-negative rod may be found in mixed infections in the mouth (Vincent's angina) or other areas of the body (eg, pulmonary and brain abscesses).

Streptococcus pyogenes is a gram-positive coccus that grows either aerobically or anaerobically (ie, it is a facultative anaerobe). This organism causes many different infections in humans. It is the etiologic agent of scarlet fever and is also associated with erysipelas, puerperal sepsis, and diseases of brain, lungs, and other organs of the body. Two nonsuppurative sequelae of streptococcal infection are rheumatic fever and glomerulonephritis.

Bacillus stereothermophilus is a gram-positive heat-tolerant aerobic rod found in the hot springs of Yellowstone National Park and other similar environments. *(Joklik et al, pp 418–426,445–450,619,637,642,690–691)*

133–134. **(133-C, 134-E)** Tumor necrosis factor is a cytokine produced mostly by macrophages following stimulation by the endotoxins of gram-negative bacteria such as *Salmonella typhi*. Tumor necrosis factor is associated with endotoxin-induced hypotension that can lead to shock and death. Interferon-γ is another cytokine produced by T lymphocytes, and it can influence natural killer cells, macrophages, or other cells. Interleukin-2 stimulates the growth of T cells. Transfer factor is a lymphocyte-derived cytokine, which is used to transfer specific delayed-type hypersensitivity to a nonreactive individual. Blastogenic factor causes the transformation of some lymphocytes into actively dividing blast cells. Furthermore, blastogenic factor may be employed to briefly restore specific cellular immunity to an immunocompromised patient. *(Jawetz et al, p 117)*

135. **(K)** *Plasmodium falciparum* is the etiologic agent of malaria, the most outstanding features of which is anemia (resulting from the destruction of red blood cells by the parasite), pigmentation (resulting from the deposition of the hemozoin, a red blood cell pigment), hypertrophy of spleen and liver, and a prolonged fever of 41° C to 42° C. Definitive diagnosis of malaria caused by *P. falciparum* is made with Giemsa stain. Blood smears will show kidney-bean–shaped gametocytes with round or pointed ends. None of the other microorganisms listed in this question produce diseases that can be definitely diagnosed by the presence of kidney-bean gametocytes in blood smears. *(Joklik et al, pp 1180–1182)*

136. **(G)** Cryptococcosis is a fungal disease caused by *Cryptococcus neoformans*, which is found in the soil and in pigeon droppings. The incidence of this disease is higher in immunocompromised individuals than in persons whose immunologic system is intact. Thus, such patients as those with AIDS, lymphoma, or leukemia are particularly susceptible to cryptococcus, as well as many other fungal parasitic, viral, or bacterial diseases. Disseminated cryptococcosis is a meningitis in which patients have fever, headache, stiff neck, and disorientation. Examination of india ink stains of spinal fluid from such patients and culture on Sabouraud agar at 37° C show yeast cells with large capsules. The other microorganisms listed may produce meningitis in immunosuppressed patients, but india ink stains or culture of their spinal fluids will not reveal yeast cells with large capsules. *(Joklik et al, pp 1146–1147)*

137. **(I)** C5a is a component of complement. Chemically it is a protein found in the nor-

mal human and animal serum. Activation of complement by immune complexes or endotoxins produces C5a, which is a macrophage and neutrophil attractant. Intradermal administration of C5a induces vasodilation and local accumulation of neutrophils and macrophages. The variable regions, the constant regions of light and heavy chains, the J chains, and the hinge region represent moieties of the immunoglobulin molecule and do not possess chemotactic properties for macrophages. HLA-A, HLA-B, and HLA-C are the three genes for the human leukocyte antigens (HLA) and they control the synthesis of class I antigens. The success of tissue and organ transplants depends on the donor's and recipient's HLA complex encoded by the HLA-A, HLA-B, and HLA-C genes. The Fc is the crystallizable fragment of the immunoglobulin molecule which lacks the ability to bind antigen. It is involved in complement fixation, in placental transfer and attachment for various cells. *(Joklik et al, pp 223–235,264–282,292–293)*

138. **(C)** Based on the structure of their heavy-chain constant regions, immunoglobulins are divided into major classes such as immunoglobulin G (IgG), IgA, IgM, IgD, and IgE. These classes can be distinguished not only by their amino acid sequences of the constant regions of their heavy chains but also by the antigenic structures that these sequences produce. For example, by injecting human IgG myeloma protein into a rabbit, it is possible to produce an antiserum that can be absorbed by mixtures of myelomas of other classes to remove cross-reacting antibodies and that will then be able to react with IgG, but not IgM, IgA, IgD, or IgE. Since all the heavy-chain constant region structures produce the immunoglobulin, classes are called isotypes or isotypic variants. Viability in the variable regions of the light and heavy chains determines immunoglobulin idiotypes; constant regions of light and heavy chains determine immunoglobulin allotypes. *(Joklik et al, pp 223–235,264–282,292–293)*

139. **(A)** It has been stated in the previous answer that it is feasible to produce antibodies that recognize isotypic variants. It is also possible to produce antisera that are specific for individual antibody molecules and distinguish between one monoclonal antibody and another, independently of isotypic structures. Such antisera delineate the individual determinants unique to each antibody, collectively called the idiotype. The idiotypic determinants are located in the variable regions of the light and heavy chains of the immunoglobulins. Anti-idiotypic sera constitute useful reagents for demonstrating the same variable region on different heavy chains and on different cells. For reasons why the other choices listed are inappropriate, see answer to previous question. *(Joklik et al, pp 223–235, 264–282,292–293)*

REFERENCES

Jawetz E, Melnick JL, Adelberg EA, et al. *Review of Medical Microbiology.* 19th ed. Norwalk, Conn: Appleton & Lange; 1991.

Joklik WK, Willett HP, Amos DB, et al. *Zinsser Microbiology.* 20th ed. Norwalk, Conn: Appleton & Lange; 1992.

Levinson WE, Jawetz E. *Medical Microbiology and Immunology.* 4th ed. Stamford, Conn: Appleton & Lange; 1996.

Ryan KJ. *Sherris Medical Microbiology*, 3rd ed. Norwalk, Conn: Appleton & Lange, 1994.

SUBSPECIALTY LIST: MICROBIOLOGY

Question Number and Subspecialty

98. Immunology
99. Pathogenic bacteriology
100. Pathogenic bacteriology
101. Virology
102. Virology
103. Virology
104. Virology
105. Virology
106. Immunology
107. Immunology
108. Immunology
109. Immunology
110. Immunology
111. Immunology
112. Physiology
113. Microbial genetics
114. Physiology
115. Virology
116. Pathogenic bacteriology
117. Pathogenic bacteriology
118. Microbial genetics
119. Virology
120. Virology
121. Pathogenic bacteriology
122. Immunology
123. Physiology
124. Virology
125. Molecular microbiology
126. Immunology
127. Pathogenic bacteriology
128. Pathogenic bacteriology
129. Virology
130. Pathogenic bacteriology
131. Immunology
132. Pathogenic bacteriology
133. Immunology
134. Immunology
135. Parasitology
136. Mycology
137. Immunology
138. Immunology
139. Immunology

Pathology

Thomas K. Barton, MD and Martin Gwent Lewis, MD

DIRECTIONS (Questions 140 through 165): Each of the numbered items or incomplete statements in this section is followed by answers or by completions of the statement. Select the ONE lettered answer or completion that is BEST in each case.

140. The major pathologic change found in the hearts of persons with hypertensive heart disease is

    (A) right ventricular dilation
    (B) right ventricular hyperplasia
    (C) right ventricular hypertrophy
    (D) left ventricular dilation
    (E) left ventricular hypertrophy

141. Which of the following is the most common cause of spontaneous subarachnoid hemorrhage?

    (A) primary brain tumors
    (B) blood dyscrasias
    (C) arteriovenous malformations
    (D) intracranial congenital aneurysms
    (E) tumors metastatic to the brain

142. An elderly male expires with a clinical diagnosis of adult respiratory distress syndrome. At autopsy a pathologic diagnosis of diffuse alveolar damage is rendered. All of the following would support these diagnoses EXCEPT

    (A) heavy, wet, meaty lungs on gross examination
    (B) clinical history of relative unresponsiveness to oxygen therapy
    (C) intra-alveolar hyaline membrane formation

    (D) sloughing and loss of type I pneumocytes
    (E) numerous large areas of gross abscess formation

143. Niacin deficiency is associated with

    (A) night blindness
    (B) bleeding diathesis
    (C) altered formation of connective tissues
    (D) neuromuscular and cardiac problems
    (E) dementia

144. Diverticulosis occurs most frequently in the

    (A) cecum
    (B) ascending colon
    (C) transverse colon
    (D) descending colon
    (E) sigmoid colon

145. The histologic changes seen in the connective tissue from the joint space of the great toe shown in the photomicrograph below are pathognomonic for

    (A) rheumatoid arthritis
    (B) suppurative arthritis

(C) gout

(D) osteoarthritis

(E) ankylosing spondylitis

146. The occurrence of malignant mesothelioma has been correlated with industrial exposure to

(A) beryllium

(B) silica

(C) coal dust

(D) asbestos

(E) nitrogen dioxide

147. The changes seen in the kidney shown in the photograph below most likely were produced by

(A) postrenal obstruction

(B) renal infarct

(C) hypertension

(D) renal cell carcinoma

(E) abuse of analgesics

148. Down syndrome is produced by the genotype

(A) trisomy 13

(B) trisomy 18

(C) trisomy 21

(D) XO

(E) XXY

149. A red (hemorrhagic) infarct rather than a pale infarct is most likely to occur in which of the following sites:

(A) kidney

(B) brain

(C) lung

(D) heart

(E) spleen

150. Cells that exhibit neoplastic transformations may show all of the following changes EXCEPT

(A) increased sensitivity to contact inhibition of growth

(B) decreased sensitivity to density-dependent inhibition

(C) loss of anchoring ability for growth

(D) infinite potential for replication and survival

(E) the ability to produce malignant transformations in synergistic hosts

151. In which of the following populations is pulmonary tuberculosis *most* frequently encountered?

(A) US whites

(B) US blacks

(C) Scandinavians

(D) Black Africans

(E) Japanese

152. Which of the following statements describing toxemia of pregnancy is true?

(A) it occurs in 50% of pregnant women

(B) deficient placental production of prostaglandins may play a causative role

(C) symptoms become manifest in the first trimester

(D) hypotension is a prominent feature

(E) the presence of disseminated intravascular coagulation (DIC) is diagnostic of preeclampsia

Figure for use with question 154.

153. Polyarteritis nodosa typically involves

   (A) large elastic arteries
   (B) medium-size muscular arteries
   (C) arterioles
   (D) capillaries
   (E) venules

154. The most likely cause of the pathologic findings in the spleen pictured above is

   (A) amyloidosis
   (B) metastatic carcinoma
   (C) septic infarct
   (D) Hodgkin's disease
   (E) traumatic rupture

155. Which of the following diseases is *not* caused by a fungus?

   (A) aspergillosis
   (B) toxoplasmosis
   (C) candidiasis
   (D) histoplasmosis
   (E) cryptococcosis

156. Mutations of the p53 gene are associated with

   (A) carcinogenesis
   (B) micrognathia
   (C) cystic fibrosis
   (D) pulmonary fibrosis
   (E) essential hypertension

157. What is the term used to describe an abnormal toxic yellow pigmentation found in the brains of neonates exposed to excessive unconjugated hyperbilirubinemia?

   (A) kernicterus
   (B) mucoviscidosis
   (C) zellballen
   (D) cholestasis
   (E) sequestrum

158. Which statement is FALSE concerning breast cancer:

   (A) incidence is lower in Japan than in United States
   (B) increased incidence with early menarche or late menopause

Figure for use with question 161.

(C) increased incidence with high fat diet

(D) decreased incidence with atypical ductal or lobular hyperplasia

(E) increased incidence with family history of breast cancer

159. Tumors arising from the germinal epithelium of the seminiferous tubules include all of the following EXCEPT

(A) seminoma

(B) choriocarcinoma

(C) embryonal carcinoma

(D) Leydig's cell tumor

(E) teratoma

160. Which of the following is *most* likely to be associated with systemic effects produced by products of the tumor?

(A) osteogenic sarcoma

(B) follicular adenoma of thyroid

(C) papillary carcinoma of thyroid

(D) pheochromocytoma

(E) anaplastic carcinoma of thyroid

161. The photomicrograph pictured above is of a bone biopsy. The most likely diagnosis is

(A) benign neoplasm

(B) cellular hyperplasia

(C) osteogenic sarcoma

(D) metastatic lesion

(E) chronic leukemia

162. All of the following are true statements concerning Burkitt's lymphoma EXCEPT

(A) it is a neoplasm of B lymphocytes

(B) it is considered a high-grade lymphoma of the small, noncleaved cell type

(C) nonendemic cases are more frequently associated with Epstein-Barr virus than are endemic African cases

(D) in some cases of Burkitt's lymphoma a chromosomal 8-14q translocation has been identified

(E) examination of the tumor at low-power light microscopy reveals a "starry-sky" appearance

163. Irreversible morphologic changes associated with cell death include all of the following EXCEPT

    (A) karyorrhexis
    (B) hydropic swelling
    (C) pyknosis
    (D) apoptosis
    (E) rupture of the nuclear membrane

164. All of the following are known adverse factors that increase the risk of coronary artery disease EXCEPT

    (A) obesity and physiologic inactivity
    (B) high levels of HDL cholesterol
    (C) diabetes mellitus
    (D) hypertension
    (E) cigarette smoking

165. Fibrocystic disease of the breast is characterized by all of the following EXCEPT

    (A) congo red birefringence
    (B) apocrine metaplasia
    (C) epitheliosis
    (D) stromal fibrosis
    (E) cyst formation

DIRECTIONS (Questions 166 through 187): Each group of items in this section consists of lettered headings followed by a set of numbered words or phrases. For each numbered word or phrase, select the ONE lettered heading that is most closely associated with it. Each lettered heading may be selected once, more than once, or not at all.

Questions 166 through 169

    (A) metaplasia
    (B) hypertrophy
    (C) hyperplasia
    (D) dysplasia
    (E) atrophy

166. A nonmitotic increase in cell size

167. An atypical potentially precancerous cellular alteration

168. Shrinkage of cell substance from inactivity, lack of trophic stimuli, or senescence

169. The replacement of one adult cell type by another adult cell type

Questions 170 through 172

    (A) coarctation of the aorta
    (B) ventricular septal defect
    (C) Ebstein's anomaly
    (D) patent ductus arteriosus
    (E) tetralogy of Fallot

170. Most common congenital cardiac defect

171. Congenital abnormality of tricuspid valve

172. Abnormal persistent communication between pulmonary artery and aorta

Questions 173 through 176

    (A) *Yersinia pestis*
    (B) *Treponema pallidum*
    (C) *Rickettsia typhi*
    (D) *Bordetella pertussis*
    (E) *Rickettsia rickettsii*

173. Etiologic agent of Rocky Mountain spotted fever

174. Etiologic agent of syphilis

175. Etiologic agent of plague

176. Etiologic agent of whooping cough

Questions 177 through 180

    (A) systemic lupus erythematosis
    (B) primary biliary cirrhosis
    (C) amyloidosis
    (D) pemphigus
    (E) pernicious anemia

177. Autoantibodies against parietal cells or intrinsic factor

178. Autoantibodies against surface antigens in keratinocytes

179. Autoantibodies against mitochondria

180. Autoantibodies against nuclear antigens

Questions 181 through 184

(A) hemophilia A
(B) thalassemia
(C) myeloma
(D) methemoglobinemia
(E) megaloblastic anemia

181. Usually seen with folate deficiency

182. X-linked hereditary disorder with inadequate factor VIII activity

183. Malignant proliferation of plasma cells

184. Hereditary disorder with discordant globin chain synthesis

Questions 185 through 187

(A) benign hyperplasia
(B) sinus histiocytosis
(C) metastatic carcinoma
(D) non-Hodgkin's disease
(E) metastatic melanoma
(F) Hodgkin's disease
(G) sarcoidosis
(H) angiosarcoma
(I) lipid granuloma
(J) tuberculosis

185. A 4-cm lymph node is removed from an otherwise healthy 32-year-old dentist. Microscopically the nodal architecture is effaced by a polymorphous infiltrate of neutrophils, plasma cells, eosinophils, and Reed–Sternberg cells.

186. Numerous enlarged inguinal lymph nodes are removed from a 45-year-old female. Microscopically the nodal architecture is effaced by anaplastic noncohesive cells with prominent nucleoli and cytoplasmic melanin. Two

years earlier the woman had a "black" lesion removed from the ipsilateral foot.

187. An enlarged axillary lymph node is removed from a 61-year-old female. Microscopically the nodal architecture is effaced by anaplastic gland-forming cells. Special studies on the tissue confirm the presence of estrogen and progesterone receptor proteins.

ANSWERS AND EXPLANATIONS

140. **(E)** Hypertensive heart disease is a common form of heart disease in the elderly population, affecting men more often than women and blacks more often than whites. The majority of cases are of idiopathic origin, but some cases are secondary to renal, cerebral, endocrine, or cardiovascular disease. Because of the increased resistance to blood flow, the most significant pathologic change is left ventricular hypertrophy with increasing size of the myocardial cells. There is no actual increase in cell number (hyperplasia). There is thickening of the left ventricular muscle wall concentrically, with narrowing of the chamber. Endocardial fibrous thickening may also occur. Left ventricular wall thickness is increased as much as 2 cm, and the heart weight may be doubled. With long-standing hypertrophic heart disease, there is gradual dilatation and hypertrophy of the right ventricle and dilatation of the right and left atria. Enlargement of the myocardial cells, an increased number of nuclei per cell (boxcar nuclei), degenerative changes, and fibrosis may be seen microscopically. *(Cotran, pp 541–542)*

141. **(D)** The most common cause of spontaneous subarachnoid hemorrhage, and the cerebrovascular lesion most often responsible for death in young adults, is a ruptured intracranial aneurysm. Intracranial congenital aneurysms (berry aneurysms) account for 85% of spontaneous subarachnoid hemorrhages. Such aneurysms are seen in 4% of adults at autopsy; in 20% of these cases they are multiple. Aneurysm formation is thought

to be related to a combination of congenital and acquired factors. A defect in the media of the artery wall is believed to be the major congenital defect and is particularly significant at arterial bifurcation sites. Atherosclerosis and hypertension appear to be the most significant acquired factors causing fragmentation of the elastic lamina. Other causes of spontaneous subarachnoid hemorrhage include arteriovenous malformations (10% of cases) and tumors, blood dyscrasias, and mycotic aneurysms (5% of cases combined). *(Rubin and Farber, pp 1390–1397)*

142. (E) Diffuse alveolar damage is a nonspecific reaction pattern of the peripheral lung to an acute insult. Grossly, the lungs are heavy, meaty, and wet. They cut with increased consistency and weep only a small amount of bloody fluid. With microscopic examination fibrin membranes are found adherent to the alveolar walls, the type I pneumocytes are sloughed, and there may be ongoing organization if the insult is old enough. Clinically, there is respiratory insufficiency which is relatively unresponsive to oxygen therapy. *(Rubin and Farber, pp 576–579)*

143. (E) A wide variety of afflictions may be caused by vitamin deficiencies. Niacin deficiency, also known as pellagra, is associated with dermatitis, diarrhea, and dementia. Papular dermatitis and night blindness (nyctalopia), with or without keratomalacia, suggest vitamin A deficiency. Vitamin K deficiency may manifest itself as a bleeding diathesis because of the role of vitamin K in the formation of prothrombin and clotting factors VII, IX, and X. Scurvy, or vitamin C deficiency, results in the altered formation of connective tissues such as collagen, osteoid, dentin, and intercellular cement substance. Thiamine deficiency, or beriberi, presents in three ways that generally overlap to some extent in any given patient. Neuromuscular signs and symptoms alone are known as "dry beriberi" but in association with edema are known as "wet beriberi." Heart failure, generally high-output failure, accounts for so-called cardiac beriberi. *(Chandrasoma and Taylor, pp 144–157)*

144. (E) Clinically detectable diverticulosis is seen in about 1 in 8 patients older than 45 years of age; in autopsy series, the incidence estimate is higher. Diverticulosis occurs in the sigmoid colon in 95% of affected individuals. Other segments of the large bowel become involved by diverticulosis as follows: descending colon, 30%; transverse colon, 4%; and entire colon, 16%. The sigmoid is the only region of the colon involved with disease in about 41% of cases. In underdeveloped and tropical countries, as well as in Japan, diverticulosis is rare, apparently partially because of the high-residue diets in these regions of the world. The most consistent abnormality seen in diverticulosis is an abnormality of the muscle wall, which leads to herniation of the colonic mucosa and submucosa through the muscularis and eventually into the pericolic adipose tissue. Fecal material may become trapped in the diverticulum, leading to ulceration, inflammation, and rarely perforation. *(Cotran, pp 806–808)*

145. (C) The pathognomonic lesion of gout is the tophus—a collection of crystalline or amorphous urates surrounded by an inflammatory response consisting of macrophages, lymphocytes, fibroblasts, and foreign body giant cells. In the photomicrograph that accompanies the question, the darker stellate deposits denote the center of the tophus. These urate deposits would appear golden brown, in contrast to the pink-staining tissue about them on hematoxylin-eosin staining. Gout is a systemic disorder of uric acid metabolism resulting in hyperuricemia. Urates precipitate out of the supersaturated blood and deposit in the joints and soft tissues. Rheumatoid arthritis, which includes ankylosing spondylitis, is characterized by a diffuse proliferative synovitis; suppurative arthritis, by a prominent neutrophilic inflammation; and osteoarthritis, by cartilaginous and subchondral bone changes. *(Cotran, pp 1255–1258)*

146. (D) Mesothelioma is the most common malignant tumor of the pleura. It is a highly invasive lesion and has been linked to inhalation of asbestos fibers, especially by persons in the shipbuilding and insulation industries. A history of smoking dramatically increases the risk of developing a mesothelioma. Histologically, the tumor may be either sarcomatous (composed of mesenchymal stromal cells), carcinomatous (resembling tubular or papillary structures), or a combination of these two types. These tumors are highly malignant, and most patients die within a year of diagnosis. (*Chandrasoma and Taylor, pp 531–532*)

147. **(A)** The photograph that accompanies the question demonstrates severe hydronephrosis, which is due to obstruction of the flow of urine. The obstruction may be located at any site along the urinary outflow tract and may be partial or total, unilateral or bilateral. Because glomerular filtration may continue for some time after the development of the obstruction, the renal pelvis and calices become dilated by continued urine production. The resultant back-pressure produces atrophy of the renal parenchyma with obliteration of the pyramids. The degree of hydronephrosis depends on the extent and rapidity of the obstructive process. (*Rubin and Farber, pp 858–859*)

148. **(C)** Down syndrome is the most common chromosome abnormality, occurring in 1 out of 800 live births. It is characterized by a trisomy 21 karyotype with an extra G group chromosome (chromosome 21), making 47 total chromosomes. In the majority of cases, the parents are phenotypically and genetically normal, and Down syndrome is secondary to a meiotic error in the ovum. The risk of having a Down syndrome child is proportional to increasing maternal age. The clinical features of Down syndrome include fat facies, epicanthic folds, oblique palpebral fissures, and mental retardation. The majority of affected individuals die early from cardiac or infectious complications. Thirty percent have a ventricular septal defect.

Trisomy 13 is also called Patau's syndrome, and affected children have microcephaly and severe mental retardation with absence of a portion of the forebrain. These children die soon after birth. Trisomy 18, or

Edwards' syndrome, is also a very severe genetic defect, and the average life-span is 10 weeks. Affected children have severe mental retardation and cardiac anomalies, including ventricular septal defect. Persons with an XO karyotype have Turner's syndrome and are phenotypically females. Only 3% of affected fetuses survive to birth; fetuses that do survive have severe edema of the hands, feet, and neck. Affected persons have a webbed neck, short stature, and congenital heart disease. At puberty there is failure to develop normal secondary sex characteristics, so their genitalia remain immature. Klinefelter's syndrome, or testicular dysgenesis, is characterized by an XXY karyotype. It occurs in 1 out of 600 live births. Affected individuals usually are diagnosed after puberty and have eunuchoid habitus, long legs, small atrophic testes and penis, and, often, low IQ. (*Chandrasoma and Taylor, pp 226–229*)

149. **(C)** Infarction of any organ is produced by occlusion of the main arterial blood supply. The common feature is ischemic change. The secondary events that take place in the tissue are to some extent determined by the nature of the tissue and whether or not the blood supply is extensive and whether there is more than one blood supply. An organ suffering infarction that has a rich vascular network and in which there is more than one blood supply with a considerable overlapping and anastomotic potential will suffer the consequences of infarction quite differently from one in which the vessels are end arteries.

Particularly, in the kidney and the brain the end arterial system is well developed and, therefore, localized forms of infarction will occur. These infarcts tend to become ischemic and pale in appearance and wedge-shaped. This is also true to some extent in the spleen.

In the heart, there is more possibility of anastomotic overlap, but the tissue is also firm in consistency and rigid, thus also producing more pallor in the infarcted area.

The lung exhibits the difference that allows for a hemorrhagic or red infarct. The lung tissue is spongelike and blood seeps into the ischemic area very easily from the adjacent lung tissue, producing a large amount of hemorrhage into the infarcted or ischemic area. In addition, there is a dual blood supply to the lung that allows the tissues to be still permeated although ischemic by blood from adjacent area. *(Cotran, pp 114–116)*

150. **(A)** Neoplastic transformation is a phenotypic change in cells that characterizes the malignant state and is passed on to progeny. These transformed cells show anaplasia and transplantability. They also show decreased sensitivity to contact inhibition and to density-dependent inhibition for growth. Thus, these tumor cells are more mobile and do not cease to grow when in contact with other cells or when more than a monolayer of confluent cells is present; instead, they continue to replicate and pile up. Unlike normal cells, these tumor cells also can grow and divide on fluid media and have lost the need for anchorage to grow. Malignant transformed cells have an infinite ability to replicate and survive under appropriate conditions. These transformed cells are capable of tumorigenesis, so they are able to produce a neoplasm when placed within a synergistic host. *(Cotran, pp 245–250)*

151. **(D)** Although pulmonary tuberculosis is worldwide, changes in public health awareness and treatments have reduced the incidence of the disease in many of the developed Western countries, although sporadic cases still occur, particularly in the poorer areas of these countries. Blacks in the United States have a higher rate of tuberculosis than US whites. The disease is very much reduced in modern times in Scandinavians and in Japanese. However, Black Africa is certainly the area where tuberculosis still remains one of the major causes of morbidity and mortality. It has been said that tuberculosis is the great tropical disease of Africa and still represents a major life-threatening disease to its inhabitants. *(Chandrasoma and Taylor, pp 184–185)*

152. **(B)** Toxemia of pregnancy occurs in about 6% of pregnant women, usually in the third trimester. Hypertension, proteinuria, and edema characterize the less severe form of the disease, preeclampsia. Women who also develop convulsions, disseminated intravascular coagulation (DIC), and coma have eclampsia. Anatomic lesions associated with eclampsia include acute atherosis in placental vessels, accentuated aging of the placenta with epithelial atrophy, hepatic hemorrhage, and fibrin thrombi in the small vessels of the liver, kidney, and brain.

The two most important factors in the pathogenesis of toxemia of pregnancy appear to be hypertension and DIC. Hypertension seems to be caused by both a hypersensitivity to angiotensin and a decreased production of prostaglandins by the placenta following an ill-defined immunologic insult to the uterine vasculature. Further organ damage develops as a result of hypertension-induced vascular changes. The pathogenesis of DIC is uncertain. Among the several theories explaining the occurrence of DIC is increased release of thromboplastin substances from an ischemic placenta. *(Cotran, pp 1079–1081)*

153. **(B)** Polyarteritis nodosa (PAN) typically involves medium-size muscular arteries. In contrast, large arteries and the aorta are involved in Takayasu's arteritis, and small arteries and arterioles are involved in a number of other diseases, including systemic lupus erythematosus. Active lesions in PAN demonstrate a neutrophilic infiltration of the involved vessel wall with thrombosis and segmental, fibrinoid necrosis. Intermittent healing produces fibrosis of the arterial wall and intimal thickening, which may lead to obstruction and infarction. Aneurysmal dilations may arise as a result of asymmetrical involvement. Although the lesions in PAN resemble other immune-mediated vascular lesions, the exact etiology of the disorder has not been elucidated. PAN generally affects middle-aged men and has a poor prognosis, although steroids may be beneficial. *(Chandrasoma and Taylor, pp 322–323)*

154. (A) Amyloidosis is caused by the deposition of an abnormal proteinaceous material between cells. The majority of the cases are idiopathic, but a small percentage are secondary to chronic infection or inflammation, plasma cell dyscrasias, or immune diseases. One of the characteristic presentations of amyloidosis is splenic infiltration and splenomegaly caused by deposition of amyloid in the follicular regions. Grossly, the spleen has a diffuse, pink, glassy, waxy appearance with obliteration of the white pulp. Amyloid infiltration also can affect the kidneys, liver, and heart. Clinical symptoms are usually due to functional impairment of the diseased organ. The diagnosis of amyloidosis is made by tissue biopsy or, more recently, by fat-pad biopsy looking for amyloid deposits. With Congo red stain, amyloid appears red; with polarization, it shows an apple-green birefringence, which is diagnostic of amyloid. *(Rubin and Farber, pp 1164–1174)*

155. (B) Toxoplasmosis is caused by *Toxoplasma gondii*, which is an obligate intracellular protozoan parasite. It is widely distributed among domestic animals and humans throughout the world. All the other examples quoted are forms of fungal disease. Aspergillosis and candidiasis are fungal diseases in which the fungal hyphae are very prominent features. Histoplasmosis and cryptococcosis produce their disease largely through the production of spores that are often engulfed by phagocytic cells, producing granulomatous types of reaction. *(Rubin and Farber, pp 410–426)*

156. (A) The p53 gene is a negative regulator of cell division. When a cell's DNA is damaged, the p53 gene senses this abnormality and holds the aberrant cell in S phase of the cell cycle to allow enzymatic repair of the damaged DNA to occur. Thus, mutations of the gene encourage replication of cells with abnormal DNA and increase the cell's propensity for malignant transformation. Mutations of the p53 gene are found in about 75% of human colon carcinomas, and in a significant percentage of breast carcinomas, hepatomas,

and small cell carcinomas of the lung. *(Rubin and Farber, p 182)*

157. (A) Kernicterus (bilirubin encephalopathy) is the morphologic term that describes toxic yellow discoloration seen in brains of severely jaundiced neonates. The pigment is especially prominent in the basal ganglia, pontine nuclei, and cerebellar dentate nuclei. Premature infants are more susceptible to developing kernicterus at lower levels of hyperbilirubinemia than are term infants. Surviving infants all experience some degree of neurologic impairment. *(Rubin and Farber, p 257)*

158. (D) About 1 in 11 women in the United States will have breast cancer during her lifetime. The incidence of breast cancer is much higher in the USA than in Japan. Other factors that have been associated with an increased risk of developing breast cancer include a family history of breast cancer, a high-fat diet, early menarche, late menopause, and atypical ductal or lobular hyperplasia. *(Chandrasoma and Taylor, p 812)*

159. (D) Germ cell tumors of the testis arise from the germinal epithelium of the seminiferous tubules. Although these tumors overall are rare, they are common in young men in the third decade of life. Germ cell tumors include the following: seminoma, which arises from the germinal epithelium of the maturing testis and accounts for 93% of germ cell tumors; choriocarcinoma, which is composed of trophoblastic elements; embryonal carcinoma, which consists of primitive immature cells without differentiation; teratoma, which is composed of cells differentiated into embryonic structures of endodermal, ectodermal, and mesodermal origin; and yolk sac tumors, which contain cells of extraembryonic endodermal and mesodermal derivation. These five tumors all represent attempts to imitate normal embryogenesis; thus, they all show some stage of differentiation toward normal embryonic structures. All these tumors except seminomas secrete serum tumor markers, primarily human chorionic gonadotropins and alpha-fetoprotein, which are useful for diagnosing and monitoring these tumors.

Leydig's cell tumors arise from interstitial cells situated between the seminiferous tubules. These tumors occur in adults and are often associated with the production of androgens, estrogens, or both. (*Chandrasoma and Taylor, pp 740–744*)

160. **(D)** Pheochromocytoma. Although many tumors can produce systemic effects by means of products of the tumor cells, the pheochromocytoma is by far the best choice of the ones listed because characteristically, in a high proportion of cases, it produces adrenalin and noradrenalinelike substances and, therefore, dramatic changes in the vasculature and in the blood pressure. It is often the symptoms produced by these substances, the by-products of which can also be measured in the urine, that first bring to light the presence of the tumor. Osteogenic sarcoma does not produce such effects and neither does anaplastic carcinoma of the thyroid. Follicular adenoma of the thyroid may occasionally be associated with increased uptake of radioactive iodine but does not produce the thyrotoxicosis characteristically seen in some cases of follicular thyroid carcinoma. Papillary carcinoma of the thyroid rarely produces such effects. (*Chandrasoma and Taylor, pp 288–291*)

161. **(D)** The photomicrograph accompanying the question shows bone and marrow spaces replaced by a well-differentiated adenocarcinoma. The normal bone trabeculae are eroded and replaced by poorly formed glands with cellular anaplasia. The presence of an adenocarcinoma in bone that shows erosion is diagnostic of a metastatic lesion. (*Rubin and Farber, pp 1095–1096*)

162. **(C)** Burkitt's lymphoma is a neoplasm of B-cell lymphocytes that is classified as a high-grade lymphoma of the small, noncleaved cell type, according to the National Cancer Institute's new working formulation classification system for non-Hodgkin's lymphomas. The search for the cause of Burkitt's lymphoma has revealed an association with the Epstein–Barr virus (EBV) in many cases. In endemic African Burkitt's lymphoma, 80 to 90% of tumors contain copies of the EBV DNA genome. However, in the sporadic and less frequent nonendemic cases of Burkitt's lymphoma, there has been an infrequent association with EBV (15 to 20% of cases). The search for a chromosomal abnormality has revealed an 8–14q translocation in many cases. However, this translocation is not apparent in 10 to 20% of cases; nor is it identified in all tumor cells in any given Burkitt's lymphoma. Despite many hypotheses, the cause of Burkitt's lymphoma remains unclear. (*Rubin and Farber, pp 1083–1084*)

163. **(B)** Hydropic swelling is a form of reversible cell injury due to the accumulation of fluid within the cisternae of the endoplasmic reticulum. Various reversible insults to the plasma membrane or its active sodium exchange pump may be responsible for these intracellular fluid shifts within organelles which are perceived microscopically as hydropic swelling. The other listed choices are all examples of irreversible cell injury. (*Rubin and Farber, p 3*)

164. **(B)** An increased risk of coronary artery disease is associated with elevated LDL cholesterol, elevated LDL/HDL ratio, diabetes, hypertension, sedentary lifestyle, type A personality, cigarette smoking, and male gender. Elevated HDL cholesterol levels confer a protective benefit against the development of coronary artery disease. (*Cotran, pp 473–476*)

165. **(A)** Fibrocystic disease is a common benign disease of the breast that usually affects women between the ages of 25 and 45 years. It is thought to be related to hormone levels. The process is usually bilateral, but one breast is often more affected than the other. The microscopic appearance of fibrocystic disease varies; changes may include duct dilatation with cyst formation, apocrine metaplasia (an eosinophilic glandular change), fibrosis, chronic inflammation, duct hyperplasia, and lobular distortion. Although hyperplastic epithelial cells may show atypical

changes and many pathologists believe there is a continuous spectrum between these dysplastic changes and breast cancer, studies have shown that there is only a slightly increased risk of cancer among patients with fibrocystic disease. Therefore, prophylactic mastectomy currently is not indicated for affected women. (*Chandrasoma and Taylor, pp 808–810*)

166–169. (166-B, 167-D, 168-E, 169-A) Hypertrophy is an amitotic increase in size of a cell. Hyperplasia is defined as an increase in the number of cells present without regard to the size of the individual cells. Dysplasia is an atypical potentially precancerous alteration usually characterized by nuclear enlargement and hyperchromatism. Metaplasia is the replacement of one adult cell type by another. Atrophy refers to loss of cell volume due to senescence, lack of trophic stimuli, or inactivity. (*Chandrasoma and Taylor, pp 245–254*)

170–172. (170-B, 171-C, 172-D) The most common congenital cardiac defect is a ventricular septal defect. Defects usually occur near the base of the heart and vary in size from small holes to nearly complete absence of the muscular septum. In the Ebstein's anomaly one or more of the tricuspid valve leaflets are abnormal. Heart failure, right ventricular dilation, arrhythmias, and sudden death may complicate the anomaly. A patent ductus arteriosus is an abnormal persistence of the channel between the aorta and pulmonary artery (ductus arteriosus). This channel usually closes shortly after birth. Persistent patency can result in heart failure, cardiac hypertrophy, and pulmonary vascular sclerosis. (*Rubin and Farber, pp 511–521*)

173–176. (173-E, 174-B, 175-A, 176-D) Rocky Mountain spotted fever is caused by *Rickettsia rickettsii*. Rash, fever, headache, and myalgia are systemic components of the disease. The organism is particularly well demonstrated in endothelial cells sampled by skin biopsy. Syphilis is a systemic infectious disorder with protean clinical findings. The etiologic agent is *Treponema pallidum*. Bubonic plague is caused by *Yersinia pestis*. Wild rodents and some domesticated animals serve as reservoirs. Fleas transmit the disease to humans. An enlarged, painful lymph node (bubo) arises in the area drained by the flea bite. Massive terminal ecchymoses give rise to the appellation "black death." Whooping cough (pertussis) is caused by *Bordetella pertussis*. Upper respiratory symptoms characterize the disease. Forced inspiratory stridor may produce a "whooping" sound, for which the disease is named. (*Rubin and Farber, pp 353–408*)

177–180. (177-E, 178-D, 179-B, 180-A) Pernicious anemia is due to a lack of vitamin B_{12}. Autoimmune destruction of gastric parietal cells or immune inactivation of intrinsic factor leads to inadequate absorption of the vitamin. Megaloblastic anemia, leukopenia, thrombocytopenia, and demyelination of the posterolateral spinal cord columns are seen in the fully developed disease. Pemphigus is a bullous skin disorder caused by autoantibodies to surface antigens on keratinocytes. Primary biliary cirrhosis is an autoimmune disorder characterized by chronic destructive cholangitis in the early stages and micronodular cirrhosis in the late stages of the disease. Antimitochondrial antibodies are seen in more than 90% of affected individuals. Systemic lupus erythematosis is an autoimmune disease with high titers of antinuclear antibodies. Facial rash, renal insufficiency, serositis, and pneumonitis are features of the disorder. (*Rubin and Farber, pp 740–743,1017–1018,1193–1197,1204–1206*)

181–184. (181-E, 182-A, 183-C, 184-B) Folate deficiency is usually seen with inadequate dietary intake. A megaloblastic anemia may result. Unlike the megaloblastic anemia seen with pernicious anemia, folate deficiency does not produce concomitant neurologic disease. Hemophilia A is a hereditary disorder characterized by spontaneous hemorrhage. The disorder is inherited in an X-linked manner, and abnormally low factor VIII activity is present. Myeloma is a malignant disease caused by an uncontrolled proliferation of plasma cells. The plasmacytes usually produce a monoclonal immunoglobulin molecule that can be detected in the serum, in urine, or in both serum and urine. Thalassemia is a hereditary disorder of discordant globin chain synthesis. Anemia is the most common clinical feature. *(Cotran, pp 596–601,608–610,622–623)*

185–187.   (185-F, 186-E, 187-C) Hodgkin's disease is a malignancy of lymphoreticular tissue. Adenopathy is a common clinical finding. The diagnostic Reed–Sternberg cell is large and binucleated, with prominent multiple eosinophilic nucleoli. The surrounding cellular population is composed variably of lymphocytes, histiocytes, plasma cells, eosinophils, neutrophils, and fibrocytes. Metastatic melanoma is usually seen in lymph nodes draining a primary cutaneous melanoma. The melanoma cells are noncohesive spindle or epithelioid cells with prominent nucleoli and usually display cytoplasmic melanin. Metastatic carcinoma may be seen in surgically removed lymph nodes. The presence of estrogen and progesterone receptors, the adenocarcinomatous architecture, and the axillary location all suggest that the metastatic tumor is mammary in origin. *(Rubin and Farber, pp 1086–1092)*

REFERENCES

Chandrasoma P, Taylor CR. *Concise Pathology.* 2nd ed. Norwalk, Conn: Appleton and Lange; 1995.

Cotran RS, Kumar V, Robbins SL. *Robbins Pathologic Basis of Disease.* 5th ed. Philadelphia: WB Saunders Company; 1994.

Rubin E, Farber JL. *Pathology.* 2nd ed. Philadelphia, Pa: JB Lippincott; 1994.

SUBSPECIALTY LIST: PATHOLOGY

Question Number and Subspecialty
140. Cardiovascular system
141. Circulatory disorders
142. Respiratory system
143. Nongenetic syndromes
144. Alimentary system
145. Cutaneous, osseous, and muscle systems
146. Respiratory system
147. Kidney and urinary systems
148. Genetic syndromes and metabolic diseases
149. Circulatory system
150. Neoplasia
151. Respiratory system
152. Abnormal growth and development
153. Nongenetic syndromes
154. Genetic and metabolic syndromes
155. Processes of infection
156. Neoplasia
157. Nervous system
158. Breast
159. Genital system
160. Neoplasia
161. Neoplasia
162. Blood and lymphatics
163. Cellular injury and response
164. Circulatory system
165. Breast
166. Cellular injury and response
167. Cellular injury and response
168. Cellular injury and response
169. Cellular injury and response
170. Cardiovascular system
171. Cardiovascular system
172. Cardiovascular system
173. Infectious diseases
174. Infectious diseases
175. Infectious diseases
176. Infectious diseases
177. Immunologic diseases
178. Immunologic diseases
179. Immunologic diseases
180. Immunologic diseases
181. Blood and lymphatics
182. Blood and lymphatics
183. Blood and lymphatics
184. Blood and lymphatics
185. Neoplasia
186. Neoplasia
187. Neoplasia

Pharmacology

David A. Johnson, PhD

DIRECTIONS (Questions 188 through 205): Each of the numbered items or incomplete statements in this section is followed by answers or by completions of the statement. Select the ONE lettered answer or completion that is BEST in each case.

188. The mechanism of action for propylthiouracil in treating hyperthyroidism is:

    (A) interference with the incorporation of iodine into thyroglobulin
    (B) interference with the concentration of iodide by the thyroid gland
    (C) inhibition of inositol phosphate signaling pathways within the thyrocyte
    (D) destruction of thyroid tissue
    (E) antagonism of thyroid hormones at receptor sites

189. Beta-lactam antibiotics are thought to act by

    (A) interfering with protein synthesis at the ribosome
    (B) attaching to sterols in cell membranes
    (C) inhibiting bacterial cell wall synthesis
    (D) inhibiting the transport of amino acids into bacteria
    (E) inhibiting dehydrofolate reductase

190. In persons suffering from severe anaphylactic shock, the drug of choice for restoring circulation and relaxing bronchial smooth muscle is

    (A) epinephrine
    (B) norepinephrine
    (C) isoproterenol
    (D) phenylephrine
    (E) dopamine

191. Primidone is metabolized to

    (A) phenobarbital
    (B) phenytoin
    (C) butabarbital
    (D) valproate
    (E) diazepam

192. Acyclovir-induced nephrotoxicity is caused by

    (A) the formation of toxic metabolites
    (B) decreased glomerular filtration rate
    (C) the precipitation of acyclovir in renal tubules
    (D) direct tubular cytotoxic injury
    (E) hypersensitivity interstitial nephritis

193. Which of the following is utilized primarily as a supplement to maintain general anesthesia?

    (A) halothane
    (B) enflurane
    (C) nitrous oxide
    (D) cyclopropane
    (E) d-tubocurarine

194. Which of the following statements about the hypnotic effects of the benzodiazepines is true?

    (A) only flurazepam has true sedative-hypnotic properties
    (B) they have no effect on rapid-eye movement (REM) patterns
    (C) they are all absorbed rapidly and thus can be taken at bedtime
    (D) the accumulation of metabolites enhances the hypnotic activity of some drugs
    (E) none of the above

195. Which of the following antiviral agents has as its primary mechanism of action, inhibition of reverse transcriptase?

    (A) gangciclovir
    (B) penciclovir
    (C) amantadine
    (D) zidovudine
    (E) alpha-interferon

196. The uricosuric agent probenecid has as its mechanism of action

    (A) the inhibition of xanthine oxidase
    (B) the inhibition of cyclooxygenase
    (C) the facilitation of urea metabolism
    (D) the inhibition of renal urate reabsorption
    (E) the facilitation of hepatic urate reabsorption

197. Which of the following can produce a potentially lethal drug interaction when administered with thiazide diuretics?

    (A) uricosuric agents
    (B) quinidine
    (C) insulin
    (D) vitamin D
    (E) sulfonylureas

198. Which of the following drugs is a potent inducer of cytochrome P-450 drug-metabolizing enzymes?

    (A) chloramphenicol
    (B) hydrochlorothiazide
    (C) phenobarbital
    (D) penicillin G
    (E) digoxin

199. During therapy for angina, reflex tachycardia and exacerbation of symptoms are concerns most closely associated with the use of

    (A) propranolol
    (B) nitroglycerin
    (C) verapamil
    (D) dobutamine
    (E) isoproterenol

200. Which of the following agents would be most appropriate for long-term control of ventricular arrhythmias in a patient with congestive heart failure?

    (A) propranolol
    (B) lidocaine
    (C) quinidine
    (D) disopyramide
    (E) verapamil

201. The biological half-life of a drug is generally related to

    (A) the time for a drug to be absorbed into the blood
    (B) the time for a drug to take effect following administration
    (C) the time for the body burden of a drug to be reduced by 50%
    (D) the serum concentration of a drug that is 50% of the toxic level
    (E) a value that is half the duration of action of a drug

202. Which of the following, concerning digoxin, is NOT true?

    (A) has a high margin of safety
    (B) has a number of effects on cardiac electrophysiology
    (C) inhibits the sodium/potassium ATPase pump
    (D) has positive inotropic effects
    (E) enhances vagal tone

203. Antineoplastic drugs that are alkylating agents have as their primary mechanism of action

    (A) inhibition of purine and pyrimidine synthesis
    (B) binding of tubulin
    (C) cross-linking of DNA
    (D) intercalation into DNA
    (E) inhibition of dihydrofolate reductase

204. The mechanism of heparin requires

    (A) blockade of prothrombin synthesis
    (B) inhibition of the action of thrombin on fibrinogen
    (C) inhibition of the synthesis of factors IX, X, XI, and XII
    (D) the presence of synthesis factor II
    (E) the antagonism of vitamin K

205. Epinephrine is often administered along with local anesthetics because it

    (A) prolongs and increases the depth of local anesthesia
    (B) neutralizes the irritant action of the local anesthetic agent
    (C) increases the rate of systemic absorption and therefore hastens the onset of action of the anesthetic agent
    (D) increases the pH of the anesthetic so that less anesthetic is required to produce nerve block
    (E) blocks neurotransmitter release (thus decreasing pain perception) via stimulation of presynaptic β_2 receptors

DIRECTIONS (Questions 206 through 213): Each group of items in this section consists of lettered headings followed by a set of numbered words or phrases. For each numbered word or phrase, select the ONE lettered heading that is most closely associated with it. Each lettered heading may be selected once, more than once, or not at all.

Questions 206 through 209

For each side effect listed below, select the antineoplastic agent with which it has been associated.

    (A) bleomycin
    (B) cisplatin
    (C) cytarabine
    (D) vincristine
    (E) doxorubicin

206. Peripheral neuropathy

207. Cardiotoxicity

208. Renal failure

209. Pulmonary toxicity

Questions 210 and 211

For each insulin preparation below, select the appropriate duration of action.

    (A) 2 to 4 hours
    (B) 6 to 8 hours
    (C) 12 to 24 hours
    (D) 20 to 24 hours
    (E) 24 to 36 hours

210. Lente

211. Protamine zinc

Questions 212 and 213

For each combination of electrophysiologic effects listed below, select an antiarrhythmic drug most closely associated with it.

(A) quinidine
(B) lidocaine
(C) encainide
(D) phenytoin
(E) amiodarone

212. Marked depression in the rate of rise of membrane action potential and minimal effects on the duration of membrane action potential and effective refractory period of the ventricle.

213. Depressed rate of the rise of membrane action potential and prolonged effective refractory period.

DIRECTIONS (Questions 214 through 234): Each of the numbered items or incomplete statements in this section is followed by answers or completions of the statement. Select the ONE lettered answer or completion that is BEST in each case.

214. The mechanism of action of theophylline is related to

(A) the stimulation of adenylate cyclase
(B) the stimulation of β_2 receptors
(C) inhibition of histamine H_1 receptors
(D) the stimulation of presynaptic α_2 receptors
(E) the inhibition of presynaptic adenosine receptors

215. Which of the following would not be effective in treating asthma?

(A) terbutaline
(B) beclomethasone dipropionate
(C) cromolyn sodium
(D) methacholine
(E) theophylline

216. With which drug(s) does phenylbutazone interact?

(A) warfarin
(B) penicillin
(C) acyclovir
(D) A and B are correct
(E) A, B, and C are correct

217. Which drug can be used as a treatment for warfarin toxicity?

(A) heparin
(B) allopurinol
(C) coumarin
(D) vitamin E
(E) vitamin K

218. Vitamin D supplementation can be helpful in treating which disease(s)?

(A) hyperparathyroidism
(B) hypoparathyroidism
(C) rickets
(D) B and C are correct
(E) none of the above is correct

219. Overdose with tricyclic antidepressants can result in lethal toxicity associated with

(A) coma
(B) respiratory depression
(C) paralysis
(D) hyperthermia
(E) cardiac arrhythmias

220. Which antidepressant drug has the least anticholinergic side effect?

(A) imipramine
(B) fluoxetine
(C) nortriptyline
(D) amitriptyline
(E) doxepin

221. Which of the following arrhythmias may occur in association with digitalis toxicity?

   (A) sinus bradycardia
   (B) complete sinoatrial block
   (C) atrioventricular junctional tachycardia
   (D) ventricular tachycardia
   (E) all of the above

222. The immunosuppressive properties of tacrolimus include

   (A) myelosuppression
   (B) inhibition of activation of helper T-cells
   (C) inhibition of B-cell formation
   (D) impairment of leukocyte chemotaxis
   (E) macrophage destruction

223. The mechanism of action of lithium in manic depression is related to

   (A) inhibition of reuptake of norepinephrine
   (B) inhibition of reuptake of serotonin
   (C) blockade of dopamine receptors
   (D) down-regulation of β receptors
   (E) none of the above

224. Pharmacologic agents that are useful in treating acute pulmonary edema associated with congestive heart failure include

   (A) propranolol
   (B) diltiazem
   (C) furosemide
   (D) mannitol
   (E) spironolactone

225. Diuretic agents that reduce potassium loss by an aldosterone-independent mechanism include

   (A) chlorothiazide
   (B) spironolactone
   (C) acetazolamide
   (D) ethacrynic acid
   (E) triamterene

226. A patient who has experienced a severe hypersensitivity reaction to penicillin in the past should NOT be given

   (A) tetracycline
   (B) cefotaxime
   (C) sulfamethoxazole
   (D) erythromycin
   (E) trimethoprim

227. Estrogen replacement therapy, without progestin, in postmenopausal women, is most frequently associated with an increased risk of which type of cancer?

   (A) Breast
   (B) Endometrial
   (C) Ovarian
   (D) Hepatic
   (E) Lung

228. In treating patients for gout, which of the following is effective in reducing the synthesis of uric acid?

   (A) indomethacin
   (B) colchicine
   (C) allopurinol
   (D) probenecid
   (E) sulfinpyrazone

229. The drug-metabolizing capability of the liver may be inhibited by

   (A) cimetidine
   (B) phenobarbital
   (C) ethyl alcohol
   (D) methylcholanthrene
   (E) penicillin

230. Rapid reversal of the anticoagulant effect of heparin is produced by administration of

   (A) cimetidine
   (B) heparinase
   (C) clofibrate
   (D) protamine sulfate
   (E) vitamin K

231. Which antidepressant drug is linked to alterations in plasma membrane phosphatidylinositides as a possible mechanism of action?

    (A) fluoxetine
    (B) amitriptyline
    (C) phenelzine
    (D) maprotiline
    (E) lithium

232. Aminoglycoside toxicity may be characterized by the following untoward effects EXCEPT

    (A) ototoxicity
    (B) depression
    (C) nephrotoxicity
    (D) neuromuscular blockade
    (E) optic nerve damage

233. Cholestyramine adversely affects the absorption of all the following EXCEPT

    (A) lipid-soluble vitamins
    (B) anticoagulants
    (C) digitalis glycosides
    (D) phenobarbital
    (E) water-soluble vitamins

234. Bupivacaine is a local anesthetic agent that is much more potent and whose duration of action is considerably longer than procaine. Possible reasons for this difference include all of the following EXCEPT

    (A) higher partition coefficient for bupivacaine than for procaine
    (B) higher protein binding of bupivacaine than procaine
    (C) decreased rate of metabolism of procaine compared to bupivacaine
    (D) pKa of bupivacaine is closer to 7.4 pH

ANSWERS AND EXPLANATIONS

188. **(A)** Drugs used to treat hyperthyroidism can be divided into 4 categories: (1) antithyroid drugs which interfere directly with thyroid hormone synthesis, such as propylthiouracil; (2) ionic inhibitors such as thiocyanate which block iodide transport mechanisms; (3) high dose iodide administration, which decreases the release of thyroid hormones; and (4) radioactive iodide which destroys thyroid tissue via γ-radiation. In particular, propylthiouracil inhibits the incorporation of iodine into tyrosyl residues of thyroglobulin and also inhibits the coupling of iodotyrosyl residues to form iodothyronines. These effects are the result of inactivation of the enzyme peroxidase, which occurs when the heme moiety is in the oxidized state. *(Hardman et al, pp 1397–1406)*

189. **(C)** Cephalosporin and penicillin antibiotics act by interfering with the late stages of bacterial cell wall synthesis, although the precise biochemical reactions are not entirely understood. Peptidoglycan provides mechanical stability to the cell wall because of its high degree of cross-linking with alternating amino pyranoside sugar residues (*N*-acetylglucosamine and *N*-acetylmuramic acid). The completion of the cross-linking occurs by the action of the enzyme transpeptidase. This transpeptidase reaction, in which the terminal glycine residue of the pentaglycine bridge is joined to the fourth residue of the pentapeptide (D-alanine) thereby releasing the fifth residue (D-alanine), is inhibited by β-lactams. *(Hardman et al, pp 1074–1075)*

190. **(A)** Epinephrine is the drug of choice for treating severe anaphylactic shock, because it has both α and β effects. The α and β effects constrict the smaller arterioles and precapillary sphincters, thereby markedly reducing cutaneous blood flow. Veins and large arteries also respond to epinephrine. The β effects of epinephrine cause relaxation of the bronchial smooth muscle and induce a powerful bronchodilation, which is most evident when the bronchial muscle is contracted, as in anaphylactic shock. Neither norepinephrine nor dopamine would be the drug of choice, since neither has action on the β$_2$ receptors and therefore would not cause the

bronchodilation needed for treating anaphylactic shock. Isoproterenol has a powerful action on all β receptors but almost no action on the α receptors, so vasodilation instead of vasoconstriction would be produced. Phenylephrine would be a poor drug of choice for anaphylactic shock because it has little effect on the β receptors and causes no bronchodilation. *(Gilman et al, pp 192–198)*

191. **(A)** Primidone is an anticonvulsant used to treat epilepsy. It is metabolized to both phenobarbital and phenylethylmalonamide. Both of these compounds contribute to the overall anticonvulsant activity of primidone. *(Katzung, pp 368–369)*

192. **(C)** Acyclovir is a useful antiviral drug. When used intravenously, acyclovir can precipitate in renal tubules, resulting in nephrotoxicity. This adverse effect especially occurs in dehydrated individuals. *(Hardman et al, p 1197)*

193. **(C)** Nitrous oxide is primarily used during surgery as an adjuvant to more potent anesthetic gasses. This is because when administered in combination with halogenated anesthetics such as enflurane, lower concentrations of the more potent agents may be administered to achieve surgical anesthesia. Therefore, the incidence of respiratory and circulatory depression is reduced and recovery is more rapid. As a single agent, nitrous oxide is an effective analgesic, however, it can not reliably induce surgical anesthesia without being administered under hyperbaric pressures. Cyclopropane is no longer utilized because of its flammability. d-Tubocurarine is not an anesthetic, but a neuromuscular blocker which has no anesthetic properties. *(Hardman et al, pp 319–321)*

194. **(D)** All benzodiazepines have hypnotic effects at appropriate doses. Although these agents may decrease the time required for a person to fall asleep, they have been shown to alter REM sleep patterns. The onset and duration of action of these agents depend on their absorption, metabolism to inactive or active products, and extent of accumulation

in the body. Some agents (eg, temazepam) are absorbed slowly from the gastrointestinal tract; peak plasma levels may not be obtained for 2 hours or more after a dose. Therefore, these agents should be administered well before bedtime. Flurazepam is extensively metabolized to active metabolites; one of these metabolites is excreted very slowly from the body. The accumulation of this metabolite appears to enhance the sedative-hypnotic effects of flurazepam by approximately the second or third night of administration. *(Berlin, p 398)*

195. **(D)** Zidovudine (AZT) is the prototype antiviral agent utilized against retroviruses such as human immunodeficiency virus (HIV). AZT is sequentially phosphorylated to the triphosphate which then can competitively inhibit reverse transcriptase by substituting for thymidine triphosphate. Ultimately, zidovudine is incorporated into DNA and causes inhibition of viral DNA polymerase. Amantadine inhibits viral uncoating and also viral assembly. Alpha-interferon contributes to viral resistance by stimulating the synthesis of a number of proteins which ultimately have antiviral action. *(Hardman et al, pp 1204–1205)*

196. **(D)** Probenecid is used in the management of hyperuricemia. Its mechanism of action is related to its ability to enhance the excretion of uric acid by inhibiting urate reabsorption from the renal tubule fluid. Small doses of the drug, however, may actually raise blood urate levels. *(Craig and Stitzel, p 505)*

197. **(B)** Quinidine can prolong the QT-interval resulting in the development of polymorphic ventricular tachycardia (torsades de points). Hypokalemia, a side-effect of thiazide diuretics increases the risk of torsades de points, which can then degenerate into fatal ventricular fibrillation. Thiazide diuretics may decrease the effectiveness of uricosuric agents, insulin and sulfonylureas and may increase the effects of vitamin D. However, these effects tend not to be life-threatening. *(Hardman et al, p 704)*

198. (C) The cytochrome P-450 enzyme is an important component of the mixed-function oxidase primarily located in the smooth endoplasmic reticulum of the liver. This enzyme and others are important in catalyzing drug inactivation by oxidation, reduction, and conjugation. Phenobarbital is a potent stimulator of cytochrome P-450 and causes enhanced metabolism of this agent as well as other drugs (eg, warfarin). Chloramphenicol is capable of inhibiting this enzyme; penicillin, hydrochlorothiazide, and digoxin have no known effects on cytochrome P-450. *(Hardman et al, p 16)*

199. (B) The goal of treatment of angina is to relieve symptoms and prolong exercise capacity by improving the relationship of oxygen demand and supply. Nitroglycerin is a smooth-muscle relaxant that produces both venodilation (reduced preload) and arteriolar dilation (reduced afterload). Although the combined effect is to reduce myocardial oxygen demands, the potential exists for reflex tachycardia and increased contractility. These reflexes tend to increase oxygen demands as well as potentially reduce coronary blood flow and should be avoided. Avoidance can be accomplished by carefully titrating the dose of nitroglycerin or the concurrent use of a beta blocker such as propranolol. Verap-amil is a calcium channel blocker that is particularly useful in primary angina. It has minimal ability to reduce afterload and thus is usually not associated with reflex tachycardia. This is in contrast to nifedipine, which has disadvantages similar to those of nitroglycerin. Isoproterenol would be contraindicated in angina because by itself it may increase myocardial oxygen demands. Similarly, dobutamine, an analogue of dopamine, is a β_1 adrenoreceptor agonist and would not be used to treat angina. *(Craig and Stitzel, pp 267–271)*

200. (C) Both propranolol and disopyramide may cause severe impairment of left ventricular function, particularly in persons with preexisting heart failure. Quinidine has less of an adverse effect on ventricular performance and would be the drug of choice for controlling ventricular arrhythmias in patients with congestive heart failure. Verapamil is not as effective in treating purely ventricular arrhythmias as quinidine. Because it must be given intravenously, lidocaine is inappropriate for long-term use. *(Hardman et al, pp 856–871)*

201. (C) The biological half-life of a drug is the time required for 50% of the dose to be eliminated. This value is useful in determining the duration of a drug's effect and therefore proper drug dose regimens. Half-life can be described mathematically by the formula $t_{1/2} = 0.692/k$, where k is the rate constant factor for drug elimination. *(Brody et al, p 38)*

202. (A) Digoxin has a relatively low therapeutic index. However, the incidence and severity of digoxin toxicity has diminished substantially in response to the development of drug alternatives to treat supra-ventricular arrhythmias, as well as an increase in the understanding of the pharmacokinetics of digoxin. Moreover, in recent years, a specific antidote for digoxin overdose has been developed which utilizes antibody fragments to bind to the digoxin molecule. Nonetheless, vigilance for conduction defects associated with digoxin therapy, remains critically important. *(Hardman et al, pp 819–820)*

203. (C) The antineoplastic alkylating agents work by covalently binding to DNA strands, linking them together. The result is strand breakage leading to inhibition of cell replication. The drugs of this class tend to be nonspecific and relatively toxic, but there is little cross resistance with other anticancer medications. Thus, alkylating agents are frequently administered in combination therapies with other classes of antineoplastic drugs. *(Hardman et al, pp 1233–1238)*

204. (B) Heparin acts by binding to a cofactor, antithrombin III. Antithrombin III is a normally circulating α_2-globulin that has the potential to bind to enzymes in the coagulation cascade. In combination with antithrombin

III, heparin inactivates clotting factors IXa, Xa, XIa, XIIa, kallikrein, and thrombin, therefore inhibiting conversion of fibrinogen to fibrin. The synthesis of prothrombin and the clotting factors is not affected by heparin. Oral anticoagulants such as warfarin, not heparin, antagonize vitamin K. *(Hardman et al, pp 1344–1345)*

205. **(A)** The duration of action of a local anesthetic is proportional to its contact time with the nerves. Therefore, if the drug can be localized at the nerve, the period of analgesia should be prolonged. Using a vasoconstrictor such as epinephrine decreases the systemic absorption of the local anesthetic. Once the absorption is decreased, the anesthetic remains longer at the desired site and is systemically absorbed at a slower rate, which allows destruction by enzymes and less systemic toxicity. *(Hardman et al, pp 336–337)*

206–209. **(206-D, 207-E, 208-B, 209-A)** The clinical toxicity of vincristine is mostly neurologic. Paresthesia, loss of deep-tendon reflexes, foot drop, and other adverse effects may occur. Doxorubicin use may result in dose-related cardiotoxicity, which manifests as a cardiomyopathy resulting in intractable congestive heart failure. Dose-related renal failure is associated with cisplatin therapy. The pulmonary toxicity of bleomycin is also dose related. The antimetabolite cytarabine causes severe myelosuppression. *(Hardman et al, pp 1257–1273)*

210–211. **(210-B, 211-C)** Preparations of insulin are divided into three categories according to their onset and duration of action after subcutaneous administration. The short-acting preparations include crystalline zinc (regular) insulin as well as semilente. The two long-acting insulins, protamine zinc and ultralente, have a duration of action that extends beyond 24 hours. Intermediate-acting insulins (NPH and lente) have an onset and a duration of action intermediate between those of regular and protamine zinc insulins. These preparations are most often used for diabetic persons whose insulin requirements

can be met with a single daily injection of insulin. *(Hardman et al, pp 1498–1500)*

212–213. **(212-C, 213-A)** Although it is difficult to assign categories of antiarrhythmic drugs according to their mechanism of action, certain generalities have proven useful, especially as new drugs are developed. Class I antiarrhythmic drugs are characterized by their ability to affect sodium entry during cardiac membrane depolarization and affect the required membrane potential to be achieved before the membrane becomes excitable and can propagate an action potential. Typical of class IA compounds is quinidine, which decreases V_{max} of phase 0 and prolongs cardiac action potential duration. Lidocaine and phenytoin are typical of type IB agents, which do not affect phase 0 and shorten cardiac action potential duration. Encainide is a newly developed drug that is unique (type IC) in markedly decreasing V_{max} of phase 0 and not significantly affecting cardiac action potential duration. In contrast, amiodarone is a class III-type agent and does not affect phase 0 of depolarization while prolonging the duration of the action potential. Other classes not discussed included class II (propranolol) and class IV (calcium channel blockers such as verapamil). *(Craig and Stitzel, pp 283–284)*

214. **(E)** Theophylline and other methylxanthines are known to alter intracellular calcium availability and also inhibit cyclic nucleotide phosphodiesterases; however at therapeutic levels the main effect of these drugs seems to be inhibition of adenosine receptors. The role of adenosine in asthma is not well understood; however, inhalation of adenosine can precipitate bronchoconstriction in asthma patients yet have no effect in normal individuals. *(Hardman et al, pp 673–677)*

215. **(D)** Methacholine, a cholinergic agonist stimulates bronchoconstriction, and so would exacerbate asthma. In fact, methacholine is used diagnostically to test for bronchial reactivity. Terbutaline is a β_2-agonist which stimulates bronchodilation. Beclomethasone

dipropionate is a glucocorticoid antiinflammatory. Cromolyn inhibits pulmonary mast cell degranulation. Theophylline is a methylxanthine which relaxes bronchial smooth muscle via a mechanism which is not well understood, but may involve adenosine antagonism. *(Hardman et al, pp 145, 660–678)*

216. (A) Phenylbutazone has a well-known interaction with warfarin that results in increased bleeding time. This effect is mediated in part by the displacement of warfarin by phenylbutazone from plasma proteins, thus increasing warfarin's availability for binding with its target. In addition, phenylbutazone potentiates the effects of warfarin by inhibiting the renal elimination of its more active enantiomer. *(Hardman et al, p 643)*

217. (E) Warfarin acts as a vitamin K antagonist by blocking the regeneration of the reduced form of the vitamin. The result is a decrease in clotting factors II, VII, IX, and X, leading to an increase in bleeding time. Warfarin toxicity can be alleviated by increasing the availability of vitamin K. *(Hardman et al, pp 1346–1349)*

218. (D) Vitamin D is actually a hormone that, along with parathyroid hormone and calcitonin, regulates plasma calcium concentration. One action of vitamin D is to increase plasma Ca^{2+}, which can be reduced in hypoparathyroidism. Rickets is a bone disease caused by either a diet deficient in vitamin D or inadequate exposure to sunlight. *(Hardman et al, pp 1529–1532)*

219. (E) Some of the more serious symptoms of toxicity associated with tricyclic antidepressant overdose include anticholinergic symptoms, coma, seizure, and cardiac arrhythmias. Cardiac toxicity characterized by supraventricular tachycardia and/ or QRS widening can be especially difficult to manage. Children may be especially vulnerable to overdose resulting in death. *(Hardman et al, pp 442–443)*

220. (B) Fluoxetine is an atypical antidepressant with little anticholinergic activity. Because of its high specificity as a serotonin uptake inhibitor, fluoxetine does not have many of the symptoms linked to muscarinic blockade such as dry mouth, tachycardia, and drowsiness, which are typical of tricyclic antidepressants. *(Hardman et al, pp 258–259)*

221. (E) Although the likelihood of cardiac toxicity from digitalis glycosides is related to the presence of underlying heart disease, almost any arrhythmia may be associated. Sinoatrial block and sinus bradycardia probably result from the combinations of vagal effects and diminished sympathetic influence, as well as direct effects of the drug. Enhanced phase 4 depolarization can result in atrioventricular junctional tachycardia. Ventricular tachycardia occurs as a consequence of increased automaticity of Purkinje fibers. *(Hardman et al, pp 819–820)*

222. (B) Tacrolimus (FK506), inhibits T-cell activation by binding to a specific protein FKBP. The result is inhibition of calcinekurin-dependent activation of lympokine gene expression, apoptosis, and degranulation. Cyclosporin has a similar mechanism, but binds to a different cytoplasmic protein (cyclophilin). *(Hardman et al, p 1299)*

223. (E) The mechanism of action for lithium effects in bipolar depression is not well understood. It may, however, inhibit the phosphatase responsible for the intracellular release of inositol; however, the connection to manic behavior remains uncertain. Lithium is useful in treating acute manic episodes but is also utilized prophylactically to decrease the occurrences of mania and to decrease the intensity of the depression phase. *(Brody et al, pp 336–337)*

224. (C) Furosemide is effective in treating the acute pulmonary edema associated with congestive heart failure by virtue of its potent diuretic action, which rapidly eliminates excess body fluid volume. Both propranolol and verapamil may decrease cardiac output and thus exacerbate congestion. Mannitol tends to increase vascular fluid volume, which can result in increased congestion. Spironolactone is not potent enough as a diuretic to be effective in treating this condition. *(Hardman et al, pp 697–701)*

225. **(E)** Triamterene interferes with the transport of sodium in the collecting ducts of the nephron, which results in a modest increase in Na$^+$ excretion. Since Na$^+$ is normally exchanged for K$^+$ in this segment of the nephron, decreased sodium transport results in decreased potassium excretion. The actions of this diuretic are similar to those of spironolactone but do not involve aldosterone receptor blockade. *(Hardman et al, pp 704–706)*

226. **(B)** Cross-sensitivity between penicillin and cephalosporins ranges from 5% to 20%. Cephalosporins all have a β-lactam ring, which is the major determinant of penicillin allergy. All these agents should be avoided by persons with severe previous hypersensitivity reactions. Since none of the other agents are structurally related to penicillin, cross-reactivity would not be a concern with their use. *(Hardman et al, pp 1095–1096)*

227. **(B)** The administration of estrogens alone is associated with an increase in endometrial cancer of 1.7 to 15 fold. The risk varies with both the dose administered and the duration of treatment. The co-administration of progestins with estrogen reduces the risk of endometrial cancer even below that of nonusers. Most studies report no increase in the risk of breast cancer for women who take estrogen alone or in combination with progestin, although continued use for longer than 10 years may be associated with a slight increase in risk. Oral contraceptive use appears to slightly lessen the risk of ovarian cancer. Hepatocellular carcinoma is a rare complication of oral contraceptives. *(Craig and Stitzel, p 756)*

228. **(C)** All of the drug choices in the question are useful in the management of gout, a condition resulting from hyperuricemia. Allo-purinol reduces the synthesis of uric acid by blocking the metabolism of xanthine and hypoxanthine to uric acid via xanthine oxidase inhibition. Probenecid and sulfinpyrazone enhance urate excretion by blocking the reabsorption of urate from the proximal tubule. Colchicine is effective in treating acute gout attacks by inhibiting leukocyte migration and phagocytosis. Indomethacin and other NSAIDs can be effective in treating acute gout attacks by inhibiting urate crystal phagocytosis, however, low dose aspirin may actually increase the risk of acute gout. *(Katzung, pp 552–556)*

229. **(A)** Cimetidine inhibits the metabolism of other drugs by affecting hepatic microsomal enzyme activity. Therefore, serum levels should be monitored when cimetidine is used concomitantly with drugs with a low therapeutic index, such as warfarin, phenytoin, and theophylline. Phenobarbital, ethyl alcohol, and methylcholanthrene induce liver enzymes. *(Brody et al, p 812)*

230. **(D)** Protamine sulfate is a strongly basic molecule that is thought to inhibit acidic heparin electrostatically. It may not, however, affect heparin-induced platelet aggregation. Cimetidine is an H$_2$-antagonist that *increases* the anticoagulant response by an as yet unknown mechanism. Clofibrate is an agent used to reduce plasma lipid levels. Vitamin K is used to reverse the effect of warfarin. Heparinase is not used clinically. *(Brody et al, pp 287)*

231. **(E)** The mechanism of action for lithium is somewhat uncertain but may be related to inhibition of the phosphatase that converts inositol monophosphate to inositol. Fluoxetine, amitriptyline, and maprotiline inhibit the reuptake of norepinephrine, serotonin, or both neurotransmitters. Phenelzine is an inhibitor of monoamine oxidase. *(Brody et al, pp 336–337)*

232. **(B)** Aminoglycosides can induce ototoxicity distinguished by both vestibular and auditory dysfunction. Moreover, aminoglycosides accumulate in the proximal tubular cells of

the kidney, resulting in a defect in renal concentrating ability and reduced glomerular filtration after several days. Impairment of renal function is almost always reversible. Aminoglycosides can inhibit prejunctional release of acetylcholine and reduce postsynaptic sensitivity to the transmitter, resulting in neuromuscular blockade when administered intraperitoneally or intrapleurally. Streptomycin, in particular, may damage the optic nerve. *(Hardman et al, pp 1110–1113)*

233. (E) Cholestyramine, a bile acid sequestrant, reduces plasma cholesterol levels by decreasing concentrations of low-density lipoproteins. Orally administered drugs (especially those that are lipid soluble) may be bound by cholestyramine as well. This problem may be avoided to a large extent by administering other drugs at least 1 hour before or 4 hours after cholestyramine. Steatorrhea may be another side effect, impairing absorption of fat-soluble vitamins. If this condition develops, vitamin supplementation is recommended. *(Hardman et al, p 889)*

234. (C) Local anesthetics exist in solution in uncharged base and charged cationic forms. The base diffuses across the nerve sheath and membrane and then reequilibrates within the axoplasm. It is intracellular penetration of the cation into and attachment to a receptor at a site within the sodium channel that leads to inhibition of sodium conductance and ultimate conduction blockade. Bupivacaine is typical of amide-linked local anesthetics with high anesthetic potency and long duration of action (class III). Procaine is typical of class I agents that are ester-linked and have low anesthetic potency and short duration of action. Important features of group III compounds include: (1) high degree of lipid solubility or high partition coefficient that aid in penetration of the drug, (2) high degree of protein binding that aids in attachment of the drug once it has penetrated the cell, and (3) pKa closer to pH = 7.4 so that more of the drug is in the un-ionized form and is free to penetrate the membrane. Ester-linked anesthetics, such as procaine, are rapidly metabolized by

pseudocholinesterases, whereas bupivacaine is slowly degraded by hepatic enzymes. *(Craig and Stitzel, pp 361–368)*

REFERENCES

Berlin RM. Management of insomnia in hospitalized patients. *Ann Intern Med.* 1984;100:398.

Brody TM, Larner JL, Minneman KP, Neu HC eds. *Human Pharmacology Molecular to Clinical.* 2nd ed. St Louis: Mosby; 1994.

Craig CR, Stitzel RE, eds. *Modern Pharmacology.* 4th ed. Boston: Little, Brown & Co Inc; 1994.

Gilman AG, Goodman RW, Nies AS, et al, eds. *The Pharmacological Basis of Therapeutics.* 8th ed. New York: Pergamon Press Inc; 1990.

Hardman JG, Limbird LE, Molinoff PB, Ruddon RW, Gilman AG eds. *Goodman & Gilman's The Pharmacological Basis of Therapeutics.* 9th ed. New York: McGraw-Hill; 1996.

Katzung ed. *Basic & Clinical Pharmacology.* 6th ed. Norwalk, Conn: Appleton & Lange; 1995.

SUBSPECIALTY LIST: PHARMACOLOGY

Question Number and Subspecialty

188. Endocrine system
189. Chemotherapeutic agents
190. Cardiovascular and respiratory systems
191. Central and peripheral nervous systems
    Anticonvulsants
192. Chemotherapeutic agents (topical and systemic)
    Antiviral drugs
193. Central and peripheral nervous systems
    Anesthetic agents
194. Central nervous system drugs
195. Antibiotics
196. Kidneys, bladder, fluids, and electrolytes
197. Kidneys, bladder, fluids, and electrolytes
    Diuretics
198. General principles
199. Cardiovascular and respiratory systems
200. Kidney, bladder, fluids, and electrolytes
    Diuretics

201. General principles
202. Cardiovascular and respiratory systems
203. Chemotherapeutic agents
204. Blood and blood-forming organs
205. Central and peripheral nervous systems
206. Antineoplastic and immunosuppressive agents
207. Antineoplastic and immunosuppressive agents
208. Antineoplastic and immunosuppressive agents
209. Antineoplastic and immunosuppressive agents
210. Endocrine system
211. Endocrine system
212. Endocrine system
213. Endocrine system
214. Endocrine system
215. Cardiovascular and respiratory systems
216. Analgesics, nonnarcotics
217. Anticoagulants
218. Endocrine system
219. Central nervous system drugs
220. Central nervous system drugs
221. Cardiovascular and respiratory systems
222. Immunosuppressive drugs
223. Central and peripheral nervous systems (mood and behavior)
224. Cardiovascular and respiratory systems
225. Kidney, bladder, fluids, and electrolytes Diuretics
226. Chemotherapeutic agents, Antibacterial drugs
227. Endocrine system
228. Chemotherapeutic agents
229. General principles
230. Blood and blood-forming organs
231. Central nervous system drugs
232. Chemotherapeutic agents, Antibacterial drugs
233. Cardiovascular and respiratory systems
234. Central and peripheral nervous system, local anesthetics

Physiology

Andreas Carl, MD, PhD

DIRECTIONS (Questions 235 through 252): Each of the numbered items or incomplete statements in this section is followed by answers or by completions of the statement. Select the ONE lettered answer or completion that is BEST in each case.

235. All of the following are important mechanisms for body temperature regulation in persons exposed to extreme cold EXCEPT

    (A) vasodilation of the skin
    (B) conscious behavioral adjustments
    (C) increased heat production resulting from circulating epinephrine and norepinephrine
    (D) increased heat production resulting from thyroxine production
    (E) hypothalamic-stimulated shivering

236. Stimulation of the sympathetic fibers to the heart most likely will

    (A) increase myocardial blood flow through an increase in local metabolism
    (B) decrease myocardial blood flow by vasoconstriction of endocardial arteries
    (C) decrease myocardial blood flow because of increased afterload
    (D) not affect myocardial blood flow, since there is little innervation of the blood vessels of the heart
    (E) not affect myocardial blood flow because of autoregulatory mechanisms

237. If systolic pressure is 120 mm Hg, diastolic pressure is 90 mm Hg, right atrial pressure is 0 mm Hg, cardiac output is 5 L/min, and stroke volume is 50 mL, then which of the following values is correct?

    (A) mean systemic arterial pressure is 110 mm Hg
    (B) total peripheral vascular resistance is 20 mm Hg/L per min
    (C) pulse pressure is 100 mm Hg
    (D) heart rate is 72/bpm
    (E) stroke work is 6000 mm Hg/mL

238. A local anesthetic causes transmission to first become depressed in the nerve's

    (A) A α fibers
    (B) A β fibers
    (C) A δ fibers
    (D) B fibers
    (E) C fibers

239. The action potential recorded at the soma of a spinal motor neuron after stimulation of a ventral root is

    (A) preceded by an excitatory postsynaptic potential (EPSP)
    (B) preceded by an inhibiting postsynaptic potential (IPSP)
    (C) evoked only after multiple stimuli
    (D) unaffected by blockage of synaptic transmission
    (E) graded in amplitude

240. Primary adrenal insufficiency (Addison's disease) is frequently associated with hyperpigmentation of the skin. This is most likely due to

(A) increased photosensitivity associated with decreased cortisol

(B) increased melanin deposition secondary to hyperkalemia

(C) pleotropic effects of ACTH

(D) increased levels of serum tyrosine in the low cortisol state

(E) none of the above

241. Patients suffering with Graves' disease have circulating autoimmune antibodies that mimic the effects of TSH. Symptoms of this condition would be expected to include all of the following EXCEPT

(A) obesity

(B) heat intolerance

(C) hyperreflexia

(D) tachycardia

(E) diarrhea

242. In the figure below, two nondistensible tubes (tube 1 and tube 2) are arranged in parallel. Flow in (Q_{in}) equals flow out (Q_{out}). The pressure in (P_{in}) is initially higher than the pressure out (P_{out}). The resistance in tube 1 (R_1) is greater than the resistance in tube 2 (R_2). The resistance of the entire system (R_T) is represented as follows:

$$R_T = (P_{in} - P_{out})/\dot{Q}_{in}$$

$\dot{Q}_1$ and $\dot{Q}_2$ are flows in tubes 1 and 2, respectively. Which of the following statements is true?

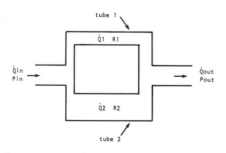

(A) $\dot{Q}_{in} = (\dot{Q}_1 + \dot{Q}_2)$

(B) $R_T = R_1 + R_2$

(C) P_{in} in tube 1 is greater than P_{in} in tube 2

(D) $\dot{Q}_1 = \dot{Q}_2$

(E) flow will continue through tube 1 only when P_{out} equals P_{in}

243. The figure below is a schematic representation of force developed during isometric contraction of cat papillary muscle. Which pair of drugs would most likely elicit this response?

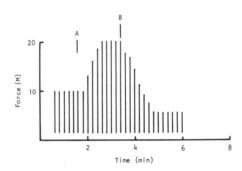

	Drug A	Drug B
(A)	norepinephrine	propranolol
(B)	epinephrine	phenoxybenzamine
(C)	isoproterenol	phenoxybenzamine
(D)	acetylcholine	atropine
(E)	atropine	epinephrine

244. Pontogeniculooccipital spikes are most closely associated with

(A) arousal

(B) slow-wave sleep

(C) paradoxical sleep

(D) epileptic seizures

(E) painful stimuli

245. In a normal individual, 15 mg of Evans blue (a substance that rapidly binds to plasma proteins) is injected intravenously, and a blood sample is drawn 10 minutes later. The concentration of dye in plasma of this sample is 5 µg/mL, and the hematocrit (corrected for trapped plasma and whole body differences) is 40%. The person's blood volume is

    (A) 1.25 L
    (B) 3.00 L
    (C) 5.00 L
    (D) 10.00 L
    (E) 12.50 L

246. The structure and effects of which of the following substances most closely resemble those of growth hormone?

    (A) somatomedin C
    (B) epidermal growth factor
    (C) thyroid-stimulating hormone
    (D) human chorionic gonadotropin
    (E) human chorionic somatomammotropin

247. All of the following are important compensatory mechanisms in hemorrhagic shock EXCEPT

    (A) tachycardia
    (B) venoconstriction
    (C) decreased peripheral vascular resistance
    (D) absorption of fluid from the interstitial space
    (E) formation of angiotensin II

248. Temporary occlusion of both common carotid arteries is promptly accompanied by

    (A) vasodilation throughout the peripheral circulation
    (B) an increase in the number of impulses from the carotid sinus nerve
    (C) an increase in venous capacity
    (D) an increase in arterial pressure
    (E) a decrease in heart rate

249. In normal adult men, the major source of circulating estradiol is provided by

    (A) secretion from Leydig's cells in the testes
    (B) secretion from Sertoli's cells in the testes
    (C) the action of aromatase on circulating androgens
    (D) the action of aromatase on circulating estrone
    (E) release from the inner layers of the adrenal cortex

250. Tumors of acidophilic cells in the anterior pituitary of adults are most likely to lead to

    (A) dwarfism
    (B) acromegaly
    (C) Cushing's syndrome
    (D) gigantism
    (E) adrenogenital syndrome

251. The most active form of thyroid hormone in the stimulation of oxygen use is

    (A) thyroxine
    (B) thyroglobulin
    (C) triiodothyronine
    (D) reverse triiodothyronine
    (E) monoiodotyrosine

252. In the normal heart, the major source of energy for oxidative metabolism is

    (A) glucose
    (B) lactate
    (C) fatty acids
    (D) pyruvate
    (E) amino acids

DIRECTIONS (Questions 253 through 259): Each group of items in this section consists of lettered headings followed by a set of numbered words or phrases. For each numbered word or phrase, select the ONE lettered heading that is most closely associated with it. Each lettered heading may be selected once, more than once, or not at all.

Questions 253 through 255

For each of the functions listed below, choose the region of the hypothalamus or pituitary gland that animal studies have shown to be involved in its control.

(A) ventromedial nucleus of the hypothalamus
(B) suprachiasmatic nucleus of the hypothalamus
(C) posterior lobe of the pituitary gland
(D) intermediate lobe of the pituitary gland
(E) anterior lobe of the pituitary gland

253. Circadian rhythms

254. Satiety

255. Milk-ejection reflex

Questions 256 through 259

For each of the numbered alterations listed below, identify the determinant of cardiac performance (A–E) on which it exerts its most profound influence:

(A) end-diastolic volume
(B) heart rate
(C) aortic pressure
(D) inotropic state
(E) pulmonary artery diastolic pressure

256. Parasympathetic discharge

257. Peripheral vasoconstriction

258. Ventricular noncompliance

259. Increased venous return

DIRECTIONS (Questions 260 through 268): Different regions of a juxtamedullary nephron are indicated by letter choices (A through G) on the illustration below. Following the illustration are several numbered descriptions or statements. For each numbered description or statement select the ONE lettered item that is most closely associated with it. For this set of questions, letter choices may be used once, more than once, or not at all.

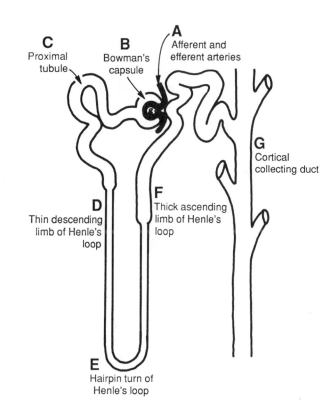

260. Principal site of aldosterone action on sodium reabsorption

261. Site of action at which autoregulation mediates its effect

262. Principal site of potassium secretion

263. Primary location of D-glucose reabsorption

264. Primary site of action of antidiuretic hormone (ADH, vasopressin) on water permeability

265. Location of most intercalated cells with proton-secreting ATPase activity for acidification of the urine

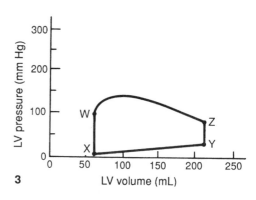

266. Location with maximal osmolality

267. Location with very low permeability to water at all times in a normal, healthy adult

268. Site of reabsorption of 65% of filtered sodium

DIRECTIONS (Questions 269 through 273): Lettered headings (A through I) are followed by a set of five numbered descriptions or conditions. For each numbered condition select the ONE lettered heading that is most closely associated with it. Lettered headings may be used once, more than once, or not at all.

(A) increased exchange vessel hydrostatic pressure ($\uparrow P_c$)

(B) decreased exchange vessel hydrostatic pressure ($\downarrow P_c$)

(C) increased interstitial hydrostatic pressure ($\uparrow P_{isf}$)

(D) decreased interstitial hydrostatic pressure ($\downarrow P_{isf}$)

(E) increased plasma colloidal osmotic pressure ($\uparrow \pi_{pl}$)

(F) decreased plasma colloidal osmotic pressure ($\downarrow \pi_{pl}$)

(G) increased interstitial colloidal osmotic pressure ($\uparrow \pi_{isf}$)

(H) decreased interstitial colloidal osmotic pressure ($\downarrow \pi_{isf}$)

(I) decreased lymphatic flow ($\downarrow J_{lymph}$)

269. Responsible for local edema secondary to venous occlusion or obstruction

270. Responsible for mobilization of some of the interstitial fluid into blood in victims of severe hemorrhage

271. Responsible for edema in individuals on a protein-deficient diet

272. Responsible for edema following prolonged infection with filarial worms *Wuchereria bancrofti* or *Brugia malayi*

273. Responsible for the myxedema of hypothyroidism

DIRECTIONS (Questions 274 through 283): Each of the numbered items or incomplete statements in this section is followed by answers or by completions of the statement. Select the ONE lettered answer or completion that is BEST in each case.

Questions 274 and 275

Above are illustrated three left-ventricular pressure-volume loops. PV loop 1 represents a normal, healthy adult at rest. PV loop 2 develops a mean arterial pressure (MAP) that is twice as high as that in PV loop 1 but with the same stroke volume (SV). PV loop 3 has the same MAP as PV loop 1 but has twice the SV.

274. Which of the following statements about the external work of the left ventricle with each beat (stroke work) is correct?

(A) the stroke work performed in either PV loop 2 or 3 is double that in PV loop 1

(B) the stroke work performed in PV loop 2 is twice that in PV loop 1 but three times that in PV loop 3

(C) the stroke work performed in PV loop 2 is twice that in PV loop 3

(D) the stroke work performed in PV loop 2 is one half that of PV loop 3

(E) the stroke work performed in all three PV loops is the same

275. Which of the following statements about the left-ventricular myocardial oxygen consumption (LVMV_{O_2}) or myocardial efficiency is correct?

(A) the LVMV_{O_2} for PV loop 2 is greater than that for PV loop 3

(B) the LVMV_{O_2} for PV loop 1 is greater than that for PV loop 3

(C) the LVMV_{O_2} for PV loops 2 and 3 is the same

(D) the LVMV_{O_2} for all three PV loops is the same

(E) the myocardial efficiency for all three PV loops is the same

Questions 276 through 283

276. In myelinated nerve fibers, action potentials are not conducted continuously down the axon but "jump" from node to node. This process of saltatory conduction has each of the following advantages EXCEPT

(A) conduction is considerably faster than that in unmyelinated fibers

(B) the decreased capacitance of myelinated fibers results in more rapid repolarization

(C) depolarization at nodes only results in a much smaller expenditure of metabolic energy in reestablishing sodium and potassium gradients

(D) saltatory conduction is more efficient, as it carries with it no requirement for ion flow through axoplasm or extracellular fluid

(E) conduction of the nerve impulse is accomplished almost entirely by sequential changes in voltage-gated sodium channels

277. Choreiform movements in humans are most likely to be associated with degeneration of the

(A) subthalamic nuclei

(B) nigrostriatal tracts

(C) cerebellum

(D) lateral spinothalamic tracts

(E) caudate nucleus

278. The stimulation of electrodes implanted in the medial forebrain bundle of experimental animals is most likely to lead to

(A) repeated self-stimulation

(B) rage reactions

(C) avoidance reactions

(D) temporary paralysis

(E) repeated turning movements

279. Insulin deficiency leads to which of the following phenomena?

(A) decreased glucose uptake by the brain

(B) inhibition of exercise-mediated increase in glucose uptake by skeletal muscle

(C) decreased catabolism of proteins

(D) increased glucagon secretion

(E) increased entry of potassium into cells

280. Many neurons in the basal ganglia are observed to begin to discharge

(A) in association with somatosensory stimulation

(B) at the onset of acoustic stimulation

(C) before the onset of slow movements

(D) at a low rate that is independent of motor activity

(E) during visual accommodation

281. The introduction of cold water into one ear may cause giddiness and nausea. The primary cause of this effect of temperature is

(A) temporary immobilization of otoliths

(B) decreased movement of ampullar cristae

(C) increased discharge rate in vestibular afferents

(D) decreased discharge rate in vestibular afferents

(E) convection currents in endolymph

282. Reflex sneezing is most likely to be initiated by

(A) inhibition of olfactory receptor neurons

(B) stimulation of olfactory receptor neurons

(C) stimulation of nasal trigeminal nerve endings

(D) stimulation of gustatory receptors

(E) stimulation of efferent fibers from olfactory striae

283. A patient comes to your office stating that he has difficulty hearing, especially with his right ear. You perform the Weber test by placing a vibrating tuning fork on top of the patient's skull. With a surprised look the patient states that he hears the sound more clearly with his right ear. You conclude:

(A) the patient has conductive hearing loss on the left side

(B) the patient has conductive hearing loss on the right side

(C) the patient has sensory hearing loss on the left side

(D) the patient has sensory hearing loss on the right side

(E) no conclusion can be drawn unless a Rinne test is performed

ANSWERS AND EXPLANATIONS

235. **(A)** Persons exposed to cold exhibit increased production of heat as well as decreased heat loss. Heat production is augmented by activation of the primary motor center for shivering in the dorsomedial portion of the hypothalamus, by chemical thermogenesis resulting from norepinephrine and epinephrine stimulation of brown fat and other tissues, and by increased thyroxine production from the thyroid as a result of centrally mediated thyrotropin-releasing factor and thyrotropin production. Heat conservation is primarily achieved through release of hypothalamic sympathetic inhibition, with resultant **vasoconstriction** of skin vessels. When exposed to cold, humans make significant behavioral adjustments, such as dressing

more warmly and seeking external heat sources. *(Guyton, pp 911–922)*

236. **(A)** Stimulation of the sympathetic nerves to the heart will most likely increase heart rate and contractility and thus increase myocardial metabolism. Through mechanisms as yet unknown, changes in myocardial blood flow appear to parallel closely those changes in local metabolism. Thus, even though sympathetic stimulation may tend to cause direct vasoconstriction as a result of α effects in the myocardial blood vessels, the indirect vasodilation accompanying increased metabolism is dominant. This effect is independent of afterload and overrides any autoregulatory mechanisms. *(Berne and Levy, pp 513–514)*

237. **(B)** Mean systemic arterial pressure (P_a) is the time-averaged pressure in a cardiac cycle. It is the area under the arterial pressure curve divided by the time of the cardiac cycle and may be estimated as follows: $P_a = P_d + \frac{1}{3}(P_s - P_d)$, where P_d is diastolic and P_s is systolic pressure. Thus, in the example given in the question, $P_a = 90 + \frac{1}{3}(120 - 90) = 100$ mm Hg, not 110 mm Hg. Total peripheral vascular resistance = $(P_a - P_{ra})/Q$, where P_{ra} is right atrial pressure and Q is cardiac output. Resistance = $(100 - 0)/5 = 20$ mm Hg/L per minute. The pulse pressure = $(P_s - P_d) = 120 - 90 = 30$ mm Hg. Heart rate equals cardiac output/stroke volume = (5 L/min)/50 mL = 100/min. Stroke work is the product of stroke volume times P_a, or 50 mL × 100 mm Hg = 500 mm Hg mL. *(Berne and Levy, pp 457–461)*

238. **(E)** Different types of nerve fibers may be classified according to their conduction velocities. This classification is readily accomplished by extracellular recording of compound action potentials from, for example, the dorsal root fibers. The slowest conducting fibers are the C fibers, which have a conduction velocity of about 0.5 to 2.0 m/sec. These fibers are the most sensitive to local anesthetics but are the least sensitive to pressure or hypoxia. *(Ganong, pp 52–53)*

239. (D) Motor neurons in the anterior horn of the spinal cord send their axons into the ventral roots. Stimulation of the ventral roots produces an action potential that is propagated both orthodromically toward the neuromuscular junction and antidromically toward the anterior horn. The earliest response recorded at the soma of the motor neuron is therefore the all-or-none antidromically propagated action potential, which is not affected by a blockage of synaptic transmission. *(Ganong, p 49)*

240. (C) A portion of the sequence of ACTH is homologous to the hormone α-melanocyte stimulating factor (α-MSH). It is hypothesized, therefore, that the extremely high levels of ACTH achieved in primary adrenal insufficiency exert a direct pigmenting effect through the action of this hormone's α-MSH portion on melanocytes. Thus, hyperpigmentation appears to be due to a pleotropic effect of ACTH. *(Guyton, pp 967–968)*

241. (A) Hyperthyroidism (from Graves' disease or any other cause) is associated with an elevated state of metabolic activity. Its symptoms, therefore, include weight loss, sleep loss, heat intolerance, diarrhea, tachycardia, and hyperreflexia, among others. *(Guyton, pp 948,953)*

242. (A) In the example given in the question, flow through the system occurs when P_{in} exceeds P_{out} and stops when P_{out} is equal to or greater than P_{in}. Since $\dot{Q}_{in}$ equals $\dot{Q}_{out}$, then $\dot{Q}_{in} = \dot{Q}_1 + \dot{Q}_2$. R_T in a parallel system is equal to

$$\frac{1}{R_T} = \frac{1}{R_1} + \frac{1}{R_2}$$

Thus R_T is always less than the resistance in any individual segment of a parallel array. Although the pressure drop is by definition identical in each tube, if the resistance in one tube is higher than that in another, then $\dot{Q}$ will be lower in that respective tube. Accordingly, since $R_2 < R_1$, then $\dot{Q}_1 < \dot{Q}_2$. *(Berne and Levy, pp 444–445)*

243. (A) Myocardial contractility is under the influence of neural control. This fact can be demonstrated in isolated papillary muscle undergoing isometric contraction, as illustrated in the figure that accompanies the question. The sympathetic nervous system can increase contractility, predominantly by the action of β receptors on the myocardial muscle. Parasympathetic input is minimal and, if anything, may decrease contractility. In the figure, norepinephrine (drug A), by its β-receptor-mediated effects, increases contractility and propranolol (drug B), a β blocker, antagonizes this effect. Epinephrine or isoproterenol would also increase contractility, but phenoxybenzamine, an α blocker, would not be expected to antagonize the β effect of either agent. Cholinergic effects of acetylcholine either would not affect this preparation or would decrease contractility. Atropine, in itself, might increase contractility very slightly; however, epinephrine (drug B), even in the presence of atropine, would increase rather than decrease contractility. *(Berne and Levy, pp 513–514)*

244. (C) Pontogeniculooccipital (PGO) spikes are phasic electrical potentials, usually occurring in groups of three to five, that may be recorded in the brain. The potentials originate in the pons and are propagated to the occipital cortex through the lateral geniculate bodies. Under normal circumstances the onset of PGO spikes is closely associated with the onset of paradoxical rapid-eye-movement sleep. The role of PGO spikes in the various physiologic changes that occur during paradoxical sleep has, however, not been fully elucidated. Although the other choices listed in the question may be associated with specific changes in the electrical activity of the nervous system, they are not closely associated with PGO spikes. *(Ganong, p 177)*

245. (C) The dye generally used for measuring plasma volume is Evans blue. By the dilution principle, blood volume equals the quantity of dye injected divided by the concentration of dye dispersed in the fluid drawn. In the individual described in the question, this would be represented as 15 mg/(5µg/mL) =

3L. Because the dye binds to plasma proteins and thus defines plasma volume, whole blood volume for the person described is represented as follows:

$$\frac{\text{plasma volume}}{(1-\text{hematocrit})} = \frac{3\,\text{L}}{1-0.4} = 5\,\text{L}$$

The rate of loss of Evans blue was ignored. (*Guyton, p 302*)

246. **(E)** The structure of human growth hormone closely resembles that of human chorionic somatomammotropin (hCS). Both have a peptide chain of 191 amino acids, of which only 29 differ in the two proteins. Both proteins also resemble prolactin, and it is generally assumed that these proteins evolved from a single ancestral protein. During pregnancy, hCS is secreted in large amounts, and its effects are generally similar to those of growth hormone. (*Ganong, pp 413–414*)

247. **(C)** Although metabolic acidosis may occur and hydrogen ion concentration increase, the initial compensatory response to hemorrhage results in a large increase in total peripheral vascular sympathetic drive causing vasoconstriction. Thus, vascular resistance increases, heart rate increases, and blood pressure returns toward normal. Slightly later the kidneys may secrete renin, and the production of angiotensin II by converting enzyme activity ultimately ensues. Fluid also will shift from the interstitial compartments to the vascular space, helping to restore cardiac output. Other humoral agents, including epinephrine, vasopressin, and glucocorticoids, may also be released to further compensate for the cardiovascular effects of hemorrhage. (*Guyton, pp 286–288*)

248. **(D)** Temporary occlusion of both common carotid arteries will decrease vascular pressure within the carotid sinus area. This important peripheral baroreceptor reflex is significant in maintaining relatively constant arterial pressure on a short-term basis. A decrease in pressure will **depress** the number of impulses that travel from the carotid sinus nerve. Because these impulses normally inhibit the central vasoconstrictor area and excite the vagal center, a decrease in impulses will reflexively cause arterial pressure to rise and heart rate and contractility to increase. Virtually the entire circulation will be stimulated to constrict. Venoconstriction will also occur, thus reducing venous capacitance. (*Guyton, pp 213–215*)

249. **(C)** Aromatase is the enzyme that controls the conversion of testosterone to estradiol. It also catalyzes the formation of estrone from androstenedione. The major proportion of circulating estradiol in adult men is formed directly by aromatization of these circulating androgens. Lesser amounts may be secreted by Leydig and Sertoli cells in the testes and by the adrenal cortex. (*Ganong, pp 393,405*)

250. **(B)** Acidophilic cells of the anterior pituitary are those cells that stain with acidic dyes. The major peptide hormones found in cells of this type are growth hormones and prolactin. Tumors of acidophilic cells may lead to excessive secretion of growth hormone, causing gigantism in children and acromegaly in adults. Acromegaly is associated with changes in facial features and enlargement of the hands and feet. Dwarfism may be the result of deficiencies in growth hormone or of growth factors. Cushing's syndrome is caused by excess secretion of glucocorticoids and may result from tumors of ACTH-containing cells in the pituitary. In contrast to the growth-hormone–containing cells, the cells that synthesize ACTH may be chromophobic or basophilic. Adrenogenital syndrome results from excessive adrenal secretion of androgens. (*Ganong, pp 366–367*)

251. **(C)** The thyroid gland synthesizes and secretes thyroxine (3,5,3′,5′,-tetraiodothyronine, T_4) and 3,5,3′-triiodothyronine (T_3) as well as lesser amounts of reverse triiodothyronine (3,3′,5′-triiodothyronine, RT_3) and monoiodotyrosine. Of these, T_3 is most active in stimulating oxygen consumption in the body, being three to five times as potent as T_4, although it is secreted in smaller amounts. RT_3 and monoiodotyrosine are not active. Thyroglobulin is a glycoprotein of the thyroid gland that plays a major role in the syn-

thesis of thyroid hormones. It is not, however, believed to play a role in the actions of the thyroid hormones. *(Ganong, pp 291–293,295)*

252. (C) Although the heart is versatile in its use of substrates, more than 60% of myocardial oxygen consumption is derived from free fatty acids. Glucose and lactate are the major carbohydrate sources but make up only 30% to 35% of the total sources for myocardial energy. In the normal heart, pyruvate uptake is very low and oxidation of amino acids provides little input to myocardial energy expenditure. In general, the heart uses the substrate in greatest supply—for example, ketone bodies may be used during diabetic acidosis. However, under normal conditions free fatty acids are the major substrate. *(Berne and Levy, p 517)*

253–255. (253–B, 254–A, 255–C) The suprachiasmatic nuclei in the hypothalamus play a central role in the control of the circadian rhythms. Lesions in these nuclei disrupt the approximately 24-hour cycle that can be measured in the circulating concentrations of hormones and in the activity patterns of animals. Input to cells in the suprachiasmatic nuclei from the retina serves to entrain the endogenous circadian rhythm to the daily light–dark cycle.

Stimulation of ventromedial nuclei in the hypothalamus prevents feeding behavior in experimental animals. Lesions in this region result in obesity. For these reasons this region has been denoted as a "satiety center," and evidence suggests that the center may function by inhibiting the activity of neurons in the nearby hypothalamic feeding center. How peripheral and central mechanisms interact to control feeding behavior has yet to be elucidated, however.

The milk-ejection reflex is under the control of oxytocin, a neurohormone that is secreted within the posterior pituitary. The firing rate of oxytocin-containing neurons may be markedly enhanced by various stimuli, including the stimulation of touch receptors on the breasts. In lactating women, released oxytocin acts on myoepithelial cells in the ducts of the breasts, resulting in milk ejection. Oxy-

tocin also has effects on uterine smooth muscle. *(Ganong, pp 215,224)*

256–259. (256–B, 257–C, 258–A, 259–A) Parasympathetic discharge (mediated by acetylcholine) exerts a profound slowing effect on the heart by hyperpolarizing cells of the S-A node. A small effect on atrial contraction is also noted. Peripheral vasoconstriction will increase aortic pressure—ie, left ventricular afterload. A noncompliant ventricle is unable to fill completely, and end-diastolic volume will be decreased. Increased venous return results in increased ventricular filling, ie, increased end-diastolic volume. *(Berne and Levy, pp 403–404,433,459)*

260. (G) Most of sodium reabsorption occurs in the proximal tubule (about two thirds of filtered load) by an aldosterone-independent mechanism. Similarly, all the remaining sodium filtered, except for a few percent, is reabsorbed by an aldosterone-independent mechanism as well in the thick, ascending limb of Henle's loop and in the initial part of the distal tubule. The last few percent of filtered sodium left is subject to control by aldosterone acting on principal cells ("light" cells) of the last third of the distal tubule and in the collecting ducts. Aldosterone increases sodium reabsorption by principal cells both through an increase in luminal (apical) permeability to sodium and through an increase in the basolateral membrane sodium, potassium-ATPase activity. *(Guyton, pp 344–345)*

261. (A) The term autoregulation as applied to most organs refers to a regulatory system that attempts to maintain a normal or near-normal rate of blood flow despite changes in perfusion pressure (eg, a change in arterial blood pressure). This is also true for the kidney; however, in addition there is a second kind of autoregulation, namely autoregulation of the glomerular filtration rate. Both are flow rates and both are regulated at the same site: the afferent arterioles of the glomeruli. If arterial blood pressure increases, one might expect to find an increase in blood flow and glomerular filtration. However, because of autoregulation, the afferent arteriolar resistance is increased, which tends to keep both the blood flow and filtration at normal levels. Similarly, if arterial blood pressure decreases, there is a decrease in afferent arteriolar resistance to minimize a fall in blood flow and glomerular filtration. *(Vander, pp 33–37)*

262. **(G)** The average diet contains a substantial amount of potassium. Normally the amount of potassium excreted each day equals the amount taken in. Most of the potassium that is filtered by the glomeruli is reabsorbed. Indeed, the majority of the potassium excreted is not merely potassium that failed to be reabsorbed but is what was secreted into the tubular lumen, particularly by the collecting ducts. This potassium secretion is mainly from principal cells ("light" cells) located in the late part of the distal tubule and particularly in the cortical collecting ducts, where these cells make up about two thirds of the total epithelial cell population. Thus, most potassium in the urine comes mainly from cortical collecting duct principal cells by secretion. *(Guyton, pp 375–377)*

263. **(C)** D-glucose and L-amino acids are nutrients that are normally completely reabsorbed by sodium-dependent cotransport systems in the proximal tubule. The uptake of the glucose (even against a concentration gradient) is coupled with the uptake of sodium (moving down its concentration gradient). Thus, both are transported across the luminal (apical) border into the proximal tubule cells. Once inside the cell, the glucose must cross the basolateral membrane before it can be reabsorbed into the blood of the peritubular capillaries. This latter transport across the basolateral membrane involves facilitated diffusion by a different carrier protein. In the normal individual, essentially all the glucose is reabsorbed proximally. In diabetics with hyperglycemia, the filtered load of glucose may be so great as to saturate the transport capacity of the glucose reabsorptive system (exceeds the transport maximum, or T_{max}). Once the transport system is saturated, continued filtration of glucose results in glycosuria. *(Guyton, pp 337–338)*

264. **(G)** The juxtamedullary nephrons generate a medullary hyperosmolality (by a mechanism involving countercurrent flow in Henle's loop). In the presence of medullary hyperosmolality, all that is necessary to regulate water reabsorption is to control the permeability of the collecting ducts to water. With increased permeability, more water is reabsorbed (by osmosis) into the medullary interstitial fluid space. With decreased permeability, less water can cross (and is excreted). Antidiuretic hormone (ADH, vasopressin) is a peptide hormone that increases collecting duct (both cortical and medullary collecting ducts) permeability to water. The mechanism is thought to involve the insertion of water channels into the luminal (apical) border of the collecting duct cells. Thus, as more water is reabsorbed, less is excreted (hence the term "antidiuretic" hormone). On the other hand, when the body needs to increase water excretion (a water diuresis), all that is needed is a fall in ADH secretion. In the absence of ADH, or the presence of low levels, the water channels detach from the membrane and become internalized into the cytoplasm. *(Guyton, pp 356–358)*

265. **(G)** For a normal individual on an average diet (that contains meat), the body has a daily net gain of about 70 milliequivalents of acid. To counter this continuous tendency toward metabolic acidosis, it is essential to maintain a normal extracellular fluid pH by acidification of the urine (so that net acid production equals net acid excretion). Beginning in the late distal tubule and particularly in the collecting ducts are intercalated cells ("brown" or "dark" cells) that secrete H^+ by primary active transport. This secretion utilizes an electrogenic proton-secreting ATPase located in the luminal (apical) border. Intercalated cells are capable of transporting H^+ against a considerable concentration gradient (up to 900:1). The source of the H^+ is from hydration of CO_2 to carbonic acid (catalyzed by carbonic anhydrase), which dissociates into HCO_3^- and H^+. For each H^+ secreted the body gains a HCO_3^-. *(Guyton, pp 393–395)*

266. (E) An important requisite condition that allows antidiuretic hormone (ADH) to regulate renal reabsorption of water in the collecting ducts is the establishment of a high medullary interstitial osmolality (hyperosmolality) relative to plasma entering the kidney. The descending and ascending limbs of Henle's loop participate in a countercurrent multiplier system that increases tubular and interstitial osmolality as the loop descends deeper into the renal medulla. The hairpin turn of the loop in juxtamedullary nephrons has the deepest penetration and the highest osmolality (maximum of 1200 to 1400 mOsm/L). About one half of the hyperosmolality is due to increased accumulation of NaCl and the remainder is due to increased urea. *(Guyton, pp 352–356)*

267. (F) Areas of the nephron that always have low or no permeability to water independently of antidiuretic hormone (ADH) presence or absence are: the thin ascending limb of Henle's loop, the thick ascending limb, and the distal convoluted tubule. Since, of these, only the thick ascending limb is offered as a choice, this is the correct answer. The thick ascending limb of Henle's loop is impermeable to water, but permeable to NaCl (responsible for about 25% of reabsorption of the total filtered load). The impermeability of this segment to water is a constant condition in any normally functioning nephron under all circumstances. Unlike the collecting ducts, this lack of permeability to water is not altered by hormones (ADH has no effect here) or by any other physiological mechanisms; it is always impermeable to water. *(Guyton, pp 356–357)*

268. (C) The proximal tubule reabsorbs the bulk (about two thirds) of filtered NaCl and water by a virtually completely isoosmotic mechanism. That is, both the NaCl concentration and the osmolality remain at the normal levels (same as in plasma arriving by renal arterial flow) throughout the length of the proximal tubule. That the proximal tubule can reabsorb so much sodium with no change in tubular fluid osmolality indicates that reabsorption of water there must easily follow sodium and in proportion (the reabsorption of water there is dependent on and coupled with the active reabsorption of sodium salts and other solutes). Proximal tubule cells are relatively thick and contain numerous mitochondria. They have the appearance of highly metabolic cells able to support large and rapid active transport systems. *(Guyton, pp 337–338)*

269. (A) The four Starling forces (actually pressures) are: capillary hydrostatic pressure (P_c), capillary colloidal osmotic pressure (π_{pl}), interstitial hydrostatic pressure (P_{isf}), and interstitial colloidal osmotic pressure (π_{isf}). Fluid movements associated with these forces in the microcirculation are filtration, absorption, and lymph flow. There is normally a kind of balance operating across the endothelium of exchange vessels (capillaries and venules). In some parts of the microcirculation the forces for filtration predominate (usually considered to be the case at the arteriolar ends of exchange vessels). In other parts, the forces for absorption of fluid back into the blood predominate (probably at the venular ends). Generally filtration is slightly greater than absorption, and fluid usually does not continuously accumulate in the interstitial fluid (ISF) space because of lymphatic flow. Hence, in normal circumstances, filtration rate equals absorption rate plus lymphatic flow rate. Changes in lymphatic function or in P_c, π_{pl}, or π_{isf} can result in considerable shifts in fluid volume between plasma and ISF. Primary changes in P_{isf} are minor and rarely have much effect. An increase in exchange vessel hydrostatic pressure ($\uparrow P_c$) is a common cause of edema. Venous occlusion from outside pressures or venous obstruction within a vein (eg, from thrombophlebitis) raises the hydrostatic pressures in the blood upstream from the resistance. This increase in P_c causes an increase in filtration of fluid into the ISF. If the increased rate of filtration is greater than the maximal lymphatic flow rate possible for that tissue or organ, edema results. *(Guyton, pp 187–192, 309–313)*

270. (B) In hemorrhage there is a loss of blood volume and a decrease in cardiac output. In an attempt to maintain as much arterial blood pressure as possible (for brain and heart function) following hemorrhage, there is a generalized vasoconstriction of pre-capillary resistance vessels in many tissues (particularly in skin, skeletal muscle, and splanchnic circulations). This increase in total peripheral resistance helps to prevent a drastic fall in arterial blood pressure and also mobilizes some of the interstitial fluid into the plasma to help minimize vascular volume loss. This mobilization comes about because of the decrease in exchange vessel hydrostatic pressure ($\downarrow P_c$) on the downstream side of the vasoconstriction. This diminishes filtration so that now absorption predominates. The increased shift of protein-free, cell-free fluid into the blood accounts for the drop in plasma colloidal osmotic pressure and drop in hematocrit that follows hemorrhage. *(Berne and Levy, pp 537–540)*

271. **(F)** Hypoproteinemia resulting from a protein-deficient diet lowers the plasma colloidal osmotic pressure. This favors greater filtration and lower absorption across the micro-circulatory exchange vessels. If the greater rate of filtration is more than can be handled by the lymphatics, interstitial fluid volume will increase (edema). *(Guyton, p 309)*

272. **(I)** Obstruction of lymphatic vessels by adult filarial nematodes (eg, *Wuchereria bancrofti* or *Brugia malayi*) interferes with the volume of fluid indirectly returned to the blood by the lymphatics. As a result, a considerable edema can ensue. Occasionally, in chronic infections with filarial worms, affected limbs can become so swollen as to be elephantine in size ("elephantiasis"). *(Guyton, p 309)*

273. **(G)** In patients with a severe reduction in thyroid function there is an increase in interstitial protein and glycosaminoglycans (eg, hyaluronic acid). This raises the π_{isf} and produces the characteristic nonpitting edema of myxedema of severe hypothyroidism. *(Guyton, p 955)*

274. **(A)** For each beat, the stroke work performed by the left ventricle could be accurately measured from the area within the pressure-volume loop. A more convenient estimate can be made by multiplying the mean arterial pressure (MAP) developed by the stroke volume (SV) ejected (pressure times volume is equivalent to force times distance, the physical definition of work). It should be evident that by this estimate, or by visual inspection of the areas illustrated, that there is a twofold increase in stroke work if MAP is doubled while SV remains the same (PV loop 2) or if MAP is the same but SV is doubled (PV loop 3). *(Guyton, pp 113–115; West, p 256)*

275. **(A)** Although external left ventricular work for each beat (stroke work) is doubled in both PV loops 2 and 3 compared to that in PV loop 1, their rates of left-ventricular myocardial oxygen consumption ($LVM\dot{V}_{O_2}$) are not increased equally. The myocardial efficiency of pressure work (PV loop 2) is not as high as that for volume work (PV loop 3), and therefore the $LVM\dot{V}_{O_2}$ is higher for PV loop 2 than it is for PV loop 3. *(Guyton, pp 113–115; West, p 256)*

276. **(D)** Saltatory conduction does have ion movements through axoplasm and extracellular fluid (otherwise no current flow would be possible). Saltatory conduction is 5 to 50 times faster than conduction in unmyelinated fibers. The fact that depolarization occurs only at nodes results in a much smaller net movement of ions for a given transmission distance. Thus, less metabolic energy is required to reestablish ion gradients between action potentials. Myelination provides excellent insulation and greatly diminishes the total membrane capacitance. Fewer ions have to move in order to produce a depolarization. Repolarization occurs as soon as the sodium channels close and before the bulk of the potassium channels have had time to open. Therefore, propagation is accomplished almost entirely by sequential changes in sodium conduction, with little need for contribution by potassium channels. *(Guyton, pp 68–70)*

277. **(E)** Huntington's disease in humans is characterized by the degeneration of the caudate nuclei. This is associated with the appearance of disorganized, choreiform movements.

Damage to other regions of the nervous system involved in the control of movements may produce other forms of movement disorders. For example, damage to the subthalamic nuclei may result in sudden, intense, and involuntary movements, termed ballistic movements. Degeneration of the nigrostriatal dopaminergic system characterizes Parkinson's disease, which is associated with akinesia and tremor. Lesions of the cerebellum may result in the incoordination of voluntary movements, termed ataxia. The spinothalamic tracts convey sensory information to the thalamus, and their loss does not produce choreiform movements. (*Ganong, pp 196–197*)

278. **(A)** Experiments have been performed in which stimulating electrodes were implanted in certain regions of the nervous system of rats and the animals were allowed to control the stimulus by pressing a bar that triggered the application of the stimulating current. Electrodes implanted in the medial forebrain bundle, as well as in areas of the frontal cortex, caudate nucleus, ventral tegmentum, and the septal nuclei, frequently led to repeated self-stimulation by the animals. The neural circuits that subserve this self-stimulation behavior have been considered to constitute an endogenous reward system within the brain. Rage reactions and avoidance reactions may be induced by stimulation of other parts of the CNS, such as regions of the hypothalamus. Temporary paralysis or repeated turning movements are not normally observed on stimulation of the medial forebrain bundle. (*Ganong, pp 238–239*)

279. **(D)** One of the effects of insulin is to inhibit the secretion of glucagon from the α cells in pancreatic islets. Thus, a deficiency of insulin, such as occurs in diabetes mellitus, is associated with increased secretion of glucagon, which contributes to the observed hyperglycemia. The increased levels of glucagon are also apparently due to increased glucagon release by cells in the gastrointestinal tract. Although insulin deficiency may cause coma from a variety of causes, insulin does not control glucose uptake in the brain. In insulin deficiency, an increase in the rate

of uptake of glucose into skeletal muscle may still be observed with exercise, and the rate of catabolism of proteins is increased. The latter effect contributes to increased gluconeogenesis in the liver. (*Ganong, pp 312–316,321*)

280. **(C)** The basal ganglia constitute part of the extrapyramidal system concerned with the control of movement. Many neurobiologists believe that the basal ganglia play an important role in the initiation of voluntary movement. Consistent with such a notion is the experimental observation that unit activity in the basal ganglia is associated with movements and that many units start to fire before the onset of slow, sustained movements. Basal ganglia units are less likely to discharge during rapid movements. The discharge of units in basal ganglia has not been linked to somatosensory stimulation, acoustic stimulation, or visual accommodation. (*Ganong, pp 194–197*)

281. **(E)** Water that is either higher or lower than body temperature and that is introduced into the external auditory meatus may set up convection currents within the endolymph of the inner ear. These currents may result in the stimulation of the semicircular canals by causing movements of the ampullar cristae. Conflicting, different information from the right and left sides, in turn, may result in vertigo and nausea. Decreased movement or immobilization of the otoliths or of the ampullar cristae are not caused by such changes in temperature. Furthermore, changes in the discharge rate of vestibular afferents, which must occur with caloric stimulation, are most likely to be caused by the changes in the activity of the receptors rather than being a direct response of the afferents to changes in temperature. (*Ganong, p 166*)

282. **(C)** The olfactory mucous membranes are rich in trigeminal nerve endings, which may respond to nasal irritants and initiate a variety of reflex reactions that include sneezing and lacrimation. Neither olfactory nor gustatory receptors nor the efferent pathways to the olfactory bulb are believed to be involved in the initiation of such reflex responses. The

activation of trigeminal nerve endings by certain olfactory stimuli may, however, contribute to the characteristics of certain odors. *(Ganong, pp 167–170)*

283. **(B)** Conduction deafness and nerve deafness (sensory hearing loss) can be distinguished by simple tests using a tuning fork. The Weber test is performed by placing a vibrating tuning fork on top of the patient's skull. If conductive hearing loss is present, the sound will be perceived louder on the deaf side due to the masking effect of environmental noise and nerve cell sensitization. If sensory hearing loss is present, the sound will be perceived louder on the healthy side. The Rinne test is performed by placing a vibrating tuning fork on the patient's mastoid process until the sound cannot be heard anymore. Normal subjects and patients with partial sensory hearing loss will hear the sound again if the still vibrating tuning fork is held in the air next to the ear (air conduction is better than bone conduction). However, patients with conductive hearing loss will not be able to hear this sound. *(Ganong, pp 164–165).*

REFERENCES

Berne RM, Levy MN. *Physiology.* 3rd ed. St. Louis, Mo: Mosby Year Book, Inc; 1993.

Ganong WF. *Review of Medical Physiology.* 17th ed. Stamford, Conn: Appleton & Lange; 1995.

Guyton AC. *Textbook of Physiology.* 9th ed. Philadelphia, Pa: WB Saunders Co; 1996.

Vander AJ. *Renal Physiology.* 5th ed. New York, NY: McGraw-Hill Book Co; 1995.

West JB. *Physiological Basis of Medical Practice.* 12th ed. Baltimore, Md: Williams & Wilkins; 1991.

SUBSPECIALTY LIST: PHYSIOLOGY

Question Number and Subspecialty

235. Temperature
236. Circulation in specific organs
237. Hemodynamics
238. Nervous system
239. Nervous system
240. Endocrinology
241. Endocrinology
242. Hemodynamics
243. Cardiovascular regulation
244. Nervous system
245. Body fluids
246. Endocrinology
247. Cardiovascular regulation
248. Cardiovascular regulation
249. Endocrinology
250. Endocrinology
251. Endocrinology
252. Circulation in specific organs
253. Endocrinology
254. Endocrinology
255. Endocrinology
256. Cardiac cycle
257. Cardiac cycle
258. Cardiac cycle
259. Cardiac cycle
260. Renal physiology
261. Renal physiology
262. Renal physiology
263. Renal physiology
264. Renal physiology
265. Renal physiology
266. Renal physiology
267. Renal physiology
268. Renal physiology
269. Microcirculation
270. Microcirculation
271. Microcirculation
272. Microcirculation
273. Microcirculation
274. Cardiac physiology
275. Cardiac physiology
276. Neurophysiology
277. Nervous system
278. Nervous system
279. Endocrinology
280. Nervous system
281. Nervous system
282. Nervous system
283. Sensory physiology

Behavioral Sciences

Hoyle Leigh, MD

DIRECTIONS (Questions 284 through 301): Each of the numbered items or incomplete statements in this section is followed by answers or by completions of the statement. Select the ONE lettered answer or completion that is BEST in each case.

284. A middle-aged man complains of insomnia. Further history reveals that he has been unable to sleep through the night for the past 2 to 3 months and has early morning awakening, unable to go back to sleep. He lost approximately 12 lb during the past 2 months. He also complains of vague aches and pains and the feeling that he has committed serious sins for which he is going to be punished. The most likely diagnosis is

    (A) schizophrenia
    (B) somatization disorder
    (C) major depression
    (D) dysthymic disorder
    (E) organic brain syndrome

285. Insight-oriented psychotherapy is an example of which of the following models of doctor–patient relationship?

    (A) activity–passivity
    (B) exploitive
    (C) guidance–cooperation
    (D) mutual participation
    (E) authoritarian

286. All the following factors have been clearly associated with poor adherence to medical regimens EXCEPT

    (A) field dependence
    (B) very old age
    (C) male sex
    (D) socially marginal status
    (E) severe physical illness

287. Concerning major depression, which of the following statements is true?

    (A) may occur as a part of hypothyroidism
    (B) average age of onset is in the 20's
    (C) about 25% of women may be afflicted with it
    (D) about 10% of men may be afflicted with it
    (E) all of the above

288. If in a medical school department it is observed that most of the junior faculty and residents dress and speak like the department's chairperson, this phenomenon may be an example of

    (A) sublimation
    (B) projection
    (C) denial
    (D) reaction formation
    (E) identification

289. All the following are common examples of society's "sick role" expectations EXCEPT

   (A) individuals are responsible for maintenance of health
   (B) individuals who are sick are exempt from normal responsibilities
   (C) individuals who are sick should seek help from a competent professional
   (D) individuals who are sick cannot be expected to get well by "pulling themselves together"
   (E) being sick is an undesirable state

290. Salivary secretion is increased in many people when they think of biting into a sour apple. This is an example of

   (A) operant conditioning
   (B) classical conditioning
   (C) cognitive learning
   (D) shaping
   (E) instinctual behavior

291. The part of the brain that seems most intimately related to emotions is the

   (A) frontal cortex
   (B) limbic system
   (C) pineal body
   (D) locus ceruleus
   (E) ventricular system

292. According to the Holmes and Rahe social adjustment rating scale, the highest degree of adjustment is required after which of the following changes?

   (A) marital separation
   (B) detention in jail
   (C) loss of a job
   (D) marriage
   (E) death of spouse

293. All the following sexual behaviors are usually considered pathologic in nature EXCEPT

   (A) frigidity
   (B) masturbation
   (C) premature ejaculation

   (D) fetishism
   (E) transsexualism

294. Clinical indications for brain imaging studies such as CT and MRI include all of the following EXCEPT

   (A) change in personality after 50
   (B) history of seizures
   (C) a depressive episode at age 20
   (D) first episode of psychosis
   (E) eating disorder

295. All of the following statements about adoption are true EXCEPT

   (A) emotional and behavior disorders are more common among adopted children than among nonadopted children
   (B) the later the age of adoption, the higher the incidence of behavioral problems
   (C) children often have fantasies of having two sets of parents
   (D) adopted children, in general, do not wish to know their biological parents
   (E) meeting biological parents tends to be a positive experience for the adopted child in adolescence or early adulthood

296. Generally speaking, Erikson's developmental stage in which basic trust is the major developmental task corresponds with the Freudian

   (A) oral stage
   (B) anal stage
   (C) oedipal stage
   (D) latency
   (E) genital stage

297. A 30-year-old woman complains of episodic faintness, tingling sensation in her hands, shortness of breath, and severe anxiety. Thorough medical work-up reveals no pathologic condition. During an episode of these symptoms, chemical analysis of her serum would probably reveal

   (A) decreased chloride concentration
   (B) increased blood urea nitrogen concentration

(C) increased ammonia concentration

(D) increased pH

(E) decreased protein concentration

298. A 42-year-old widow complains of persistent burning pain in her right forearm. She has a history of recurrent depression, and her husband died of a myocardial infarction within the past year. She says she has difficulty falling asleep and frequently awakens from sleep because of the pain. All of the following statements are true EXCEPT

(A) depression is a possible diagnosis

(B) causalgia is a possible diagnosis

(C) the symptoms are indicative of anxiety

(D) the pain is unlikely to be due to an organic cause

(E) the pain may be a manifestation of distorted grief reaction

299. The following statements concerning early adolescence are true EXCEPT

(A) may be completely self-centered

(B) may be completely altruistic and giving

(C) rebellious, rejecting of parental control

(D) very conforming to peer norms and fads

(E) consistent in behavior and mood

300. A five-year-old girl secretly believes that she was a princess who was stolen by the people who call themselves her parents. This is an example of

(A) delusional psychosis

(B) family romance

(C) childhood autism

(D) childhood mania

(E) all of the above

301. A transitional object is

(A) a stress-induced physiologic reaction

(B) an instability in object relations

(C) a mother substitute

(D) a hallucinated object usually seen in schizophrenia

(E) all of the above

DIRECTIONS (Questions 302 through 312): Each group of items in this section consists of lettered headings followed by a set of numbered words or phrases. For each numbered word or phrase, select the ONE lettered heading that is most closely associated with it. Each lettered heading may be selected once, more than once, or not at all.

Questions 302 through 304

(A) Skinner

(B) Pavlov

(C) fixed interval schedule

(D) fixed ratio schedule

(E) variable interval reinforcement

(F) reciprocal inhibition

(G) negative reinforcement

(H) shaping

(I) biofeedback

302. The father of classical conditioning

303. A steady rate of performance occurs

304. When a rat jumps five times, food is delivered

Questions 305 through 308

For each age listed below, select the pattern that, according to Bender, a child of that age should be able to copy accurately.

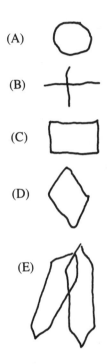

(A)

(B)

(C)

(D)

(E)

305. 2 years

306. 3 years

307. 5 years

308. 7 years

Questions 309 through 312

For each stage of life listed below, select the type of sleep–wake cycle with which it is most likely to be associated.

(A) continuous sleep
(B) cycle frequency of every 3 or 4 hours
(C) increased daytime wakeful periods and nighttime sleep
(D) true diurnal rhythm
(E) variable nocturnal–diurnal states

309. Neonate

310. First year

311. Fourth year

312. Eighth year

DIRECTIONS (Questions 313 through 330): Each of the numbered items or incomplete statements in this section is followed by answers or by completions of the statement. Select the ONE lettered answer or completion that is BEST in each case.

313. All of the following statements concerning the epidemiology of mental health are correct EXCEPT

(A) the Chicago study (Faris & Dunham) showed that mental illness was associated with higher socioeconomic class

(B) the Midtown Manhattan study (Rennie & Srole) showed 81% of persons from 20 to 59 years of age had emotional symptoms that were mild to severely incapacitating

(C) the New Haven Study (Hollingshead & Redlich) showed that psychosis was more prevalent among the lower socioeconomic classes and neurosis more prevalent among the upper socioeconomic classes

(D) the "drift hypothesis" posits that impaired persons slide down the social scale because of their illness

(E) the "segregation hypothesis" posits that schizophrenic persons actively seek city areas where anonymity and isolation protect them from societal demands

314. Factors that may contribute to secondary orgasmic dysfunction in women include

(A) substance abuse
(B) dyspareunia
(C) depression
(D) extramarital relationships
(E) all of the above

315. Types of psychotherapy include all of the following EXCEPT

   (A) hypnotherapy
   (B) behavior modification
   (C) cognitive-behavioral therapy
   (D) psychoanalysis
   (E) hydrotherapy

316. Depression in children and adolescents may be manifest by

   (A) excessive clinging
   (B) poor school performance
   (C) antisocial behavior
   (D) sexual promiscuity
   (E) all of the above

317. In a 1983 editorial, Rothenberg concluded that children who witness violence on television may

   (A) learn new forms of aggressive behavior from the violence they see on TV
   (B) experience a decrease in sensitivity to violence seen on TV
   (C) feel themselves becoming more aggressive when they are watching aggression on TV
   (D) sometimes undergo an inhibition of aggression when they become aware of the consequences of aggression that are revealed on TV
   (E) all of the above are true statements

318. The study of the development of a sense of self as an integrated, dependably competent, and strong person is called

   (A) psychoanalysis
   (B) self-psychology
   (C) ego-psychology
   (D) object-relations theory
   (E) cognitive psychology

319. According to Piaget, infants in the sensorimotor stage of cognitive development can do all of the following EXCEPT

   (A) use familiar means to obtain ends
   (B) repeat actions
   (C) generalize actions
   (D) concrete operations
   (E) use available means to obtain particular goals

320. The following are benzodiazepines EXCEPT

   (A) buspirone
   (B) chlordiazepoxide
   (C) triazolam
   (D) diazepam
   (E) clorazepate

321. Which of the following statements is most helpful in differentiating schizophrenia from organic psychosis?

   (A) visual hallucinations are more likely in organic psychosis
   (B) in schizophrenia, sensorium is generally impaired
   (C) delusions are common in both conditions
   (D) auditory hallucinations are unlikely in schizophrenia
   (E) all of the above are true statements

322. All the following statements about technical language, such as medical jargon, are true EXCEPT

   (A) it's more specific than nontechnical language
   (B) it's useful to define the context of meaning
   (C) it's less emotionally laden than nontechnical language
   (D) it's more likely to be understood by patients than nontechnical language
   (E) it may imply acceptance to a group

323. Concerning adolescent sexuality, all of the following are correct EXCEPT

(A) masturbation is common

(B) a significant portion have heterosexual intercourse

(C) overt homosexual behavior is uncommon

(D) the first sexual partner may have marked similarity or dissimilarity with the opposite-sex parent

(E) true mutuality and love is impossible in this stage

324. Concerning placebo, all of the following statements are true EXCEPT

(A) its analgesic effect may be blocked by naloxone

(B) it is effective in the differential diagnosis of psychogenic pain

(C) it may produce side effects

(D) its effect may be a conditioned response

(E) its effect may be different from that of hypnosis

325. Acute grief reaction can be described as

(A) waves of somatic distress

(B) a precursor of major depression

(C) never associated with hallucinations

(D) symptomatology indistinguishable from posttraumatic stress disorder

(E) all of the above are correct statements

326. Factors that may increase the likelihood of medical help-seeking include

(A) the symptom is a familiar one

(B) the symptom is a common one

(C) the symptom is a threatening one

(D) the symptom is unlikely to cause disability

(E) all of the above

327. Concerning anxiety, all the following statements are correct EXCEPT

(A) it may be unconscious

(B) it may be a conditioned response

(C) it always reduces performance

(D) it may be caused by psychological conflicts

(E) it may be caused by a brain dysfunction

328. The cognitive functions include all of the following EXCEPT

(A) memory

(B) orientation

(C) abstraction

(D) affect

(E) judgment

329. Concerning primary degenerative dementia (Alzheimer's disease), all the following statements are correct EXCEPT

(A) it is the most common dementing disease in the elderly

(B) it is associated with Down syndrome

(C) neurofibrillary tangles, senile plaques, and granulovacuolar bodies are found in the brain of patients

(D) cholinergic neurons are especially affected

(E) it is an autosomal dominant trait caused by an abnormality in chromosome 21

330. Physicians, as compared with the general population, have a higher prevalence of all of the following EXCEPT

(A) drug addiction

(B) suicide

(C) alcoholism

(D) homicide

(E) troubled marriage

ANSWERS AND EXPLANATIONS

284. **(C)** Early morning awakening, weight loss, and feelings of guilt as well as vague pains and aches are common and rather characteristic symptoms of major depression. Additional symptoms to look for would be anhedonia, suicidal ideations, diurnal variation of mood, psychomotor agitation, or retardation. *(Leigh and Reiser, pp 101–144)*

285. (D) The three basic models of the doctor–patient relationship are activity–passivity, guidance–cooperation, and mutual participation models. Activity–passivity model is the traditional model, in which the patient is a passive recipient of treatment. Guidance–cooperation model implies patient cooperation with the treatment regimen. Mutual participation, which characterizes insight-oriented psychotherapy, implies a model of doctor–patient relationship in which the physician aids the patient in self-help. *(Simons, p 21)*

286. (C) There is controversy concerning the factors influencing adherence to medical regimens. Among the demographic factors, female sex has clearly been associated with poor adherence. Field dependence has been associated with poor adherence among individuals suffering from alcoholism. Severe physical illness, contrary to what one would suspect, has also been associated with poor adherence, as have old age and marginal social status. *(Simons, pp 38–47)*

287. (E) Almost any endocrinopathy and metabolic disorder may be associated with major depression. Hypothyroidism is one of the common medical conditions causing depressive symptoms. The average age of onset is in the mid-twenties and there is indication that the age of onset is decreasing more recently. The lifetime risk for major depression is 10 to 25% in women and 5 to 12% in men. *(DSM IV p 341)*

288. (E) Identification is the psychological defense mechanism by which an individual becomes like an admired (or otherwise psychologically important) person. Identification is an important phenomenon in personality development. *(Leigh and Reiser, pp 79–100)*

289. (A) Society's "sick role," as described by Parsons, includes exemption from normal social role expectations. Sick individuals are not responsible for being sick and cannot be expected to get well simply by wanting to get well. Being sick is an undesirable state, and sick individuals should try to get well and seek competent help to get well. The idea that individuals are responsible for the maintenance of health is contrary to the second expectation described above. *(Leigh and Reiser, pp 18–24)*

290. (B) Temporal pairing of a neutral stimulus with a stimulus that produces an inherent response characterizes classical or Pavlovian conditioning. In this case, the thought of biting into an apple would be a neutral stimulus, until the person associates it with the sour taste that causes salivation. *(Leigh and Reiser, pp 45–47)*

291. (B) The limbic system, the inner brain tissue that surrounds the brain stem, which includes the amygdala, hippocampus, cingulate gyrus, fornix, hypothalamus, and mammillary body, is considered to be directly involved in the emotional experiences including anxiety, fear, and anger. The evidence for this comes from studies of animals and persons who had ablations of certain parts of the limbic brain, as well as by stimulation of specific parts, either artificially, or in seizure states. *(Leigh and Reiser, pp 52–61)*

292. (E) Holmes and Rahe found that of all major life changes, death of a spouse was rated across population samples as requiring the most adjustment. The second highest rating was given to divorce, the third to marital separation. Detention in jail and loss of a job also are serious life changes that produce stress and require adjustment. *(Leigh and Reiser, pp 341–349)*

293. (B) Frigidity is a common orgasmic dysfunction in women, and premature ejaculation is a common orgasmic dysfunction in men. Fetishism is classified as a paraphilia (disorder in sexual objects) in current psychiatric classification, and transsexualism is a gender identity disorder. Masturbation is a normal phenomenon. *(Simons, pp 338–390)*

294. (C) Personality change over 50, seizure disorders, eating disorders, and first episode of psychosis may be associated with intracranial mass lesions and/or focal brain diseases. Changes consistent with generalized neuronal loss in dementia may be demonstrated. First episode of affective syndrome after age 50 is also an indication for imaging studies, but the onset of depression at a young age generally does not require imaging studies. *(Kaplan and Sadock, p 115)*

295. **(D)** Adopted parents often tell their children of their adoption around the ages of 2 and 4. Emotional and behavioral problems have been reported to be higher among adopted children than nonadopted children including aggressive behavior, stealing, and learning disturbances. The later the age of adoption, the higher the incidence of behavioral problems. Children, adopted or not, often have fantasies of having two sets of parents, one good and one bad. Adopted children usually have a desire to know their biological parents. Meetings between sought-out parents and adopted children seem to be positive, especially in late adolescence and early adulthood. *(Kaplan and Sadock, pp 49–50)*

296. **(A)** According to Erikson, during the first year of life, corresponding to the Freudian oral stage, the child experiences a trusting relationship with the family and thus society in the form of feeding and comfort. An unsuccessful outcome during this stage results in a basic sense of mistrust. *(Leigh and Reiser, pp 361–362)*

297. **(D)** Faintness, tingling of the hands, shortness of breath, and severe anxiety are indicative of the hyperventilation syndrome, which causes respiratory alkalosis as a result of the loss of carbon dioxide. Vasoconstriction then develops and causes dizziness and decreased ionization of calcium, which may produce paresthesia and, in some cases, tetany. *(Leigh and Reiser, p 64)*

298. **(D)** Difficulty falling asleep may be caused by anxiety, depression, and pain. Pain that awakens a person from sleep is more likely to be organic than psychogenic in origin. Depression may contribute to the pain, and vice versa. Causalgia is a burning pain in the arm; its cause is unknown. In distorted grief reaction, the bereaved may take on the symptoms of the deceased. The husband had a myocardial infarction, may have had anginal pains. The patient may be unaware that anginal pain is usually in the left arm. *(Leigh and Reiser, pp 106–112,211–243)*

299. **(E)** Changeability and contradiction are characteristic of early adolescence. They may be completely self-centered and materialistic one moment, then extremely altruistic the next. They may be rebellious to parents, but often quite conforming to peers. Consistency of behavior and mood is totally lacking in this period. *(Simons, p 260)*

300. **(B)** First described by Freud, family romance is a fantasy of an Oedipal child that he/she cannot possibly belong to the disappointing parents. These parental disappointments are inevitable because of the aggression inherent in the Oedipal situation, as well as the inevitable frustrations and disappointments of growing up. Family romance is a normal part of growing up for many children. The other diagnoses listed can only be considered if there is other evidence of serious psychopathology. *(Simons, p 287)*

301. **(C)** Toward the end of the first year of life, many infants become attached to a specific article, such as a piece of clothing, called a transitional object. Linus' blanket in the *Peanuts* cartoon is an example of this. A teddy bear, a doll, or a bottle might also serve as transitional objects. Transitional objects are symbolic of the mother. This is a normal phase-limited phenomenon. *(Simons, pp 176–178)*

302. **(B)** Ivan Pavlov and his coworkers in Russia developed the theory of classical conditioning through carefully designed experiments. Classical conditioning (respondent conditioning) results from the repeated pairing of a neutral (conditional) stimulus with another stimulus that evokes a response (unconditional stimulus). Eventually, the neutral

stimulus evokes the response. *(Kaplan and Sadock, pp 165–166)*

303. **(E)** A fixed interval reinforcement schedule results in an increase in performance (response) as the time of reinforcement (reward) approaches during the interval. By varying the delivery of reinforcement randomly around a particular interval of time, the response behavior stabilizes at a stable rate. This schedule is useful in clinical situations to increase the rate of performance of a desired behavior. *(Kaplan and Sadock, pp 166–168)*

304. **(D)** On fixed ratio schedule of reinforcement, a low rate of behavior occurs immediately after reinforcement, followed by very high rates of responding. A smoother pattern is found with a variable ratio schedule, in which reinforcement is delivered on a schedule randomly changing around a given ratio. *(Kaplan and Sadock, pp 166–168)*

305–308. **(305-A, 306-B, 307-C, 308-D)** The patterns that accompany the question are simplified designs drawn from the more formal patterns used by Bender in her Visual Motor Gestalt Test. In her more formal test, Bender created eight figures and established age norms at which each could be reproduced by the child. The formal test and this clinical application are useful in assessing the maturation of visuomotor coordination. *(Bender [1938], p 200; [1952], p 335)*

309–312. **(309-B, 310-C, 311-D, 312-D)** Full-term infants change from active rapid-eye-movement (REM) sleep to quiet REM sleep about every 50 to 60 minutes, and neonates have a sleep–wake cycle of approximately 3 to 4 hours. During the first year of life, prolongations of daytime wakefulness and nighttime sleep occur, usually settling into a true diurnal rhythm by about 4 years of age. In general, sleep–wake rhythm seems to be more culturally determined, whereas REM–nonREM rhythms seem to be more genetically determined. *(Anders, pp 421–432)*

313. **(A)** The Chicago study by Faris and Dunham showed that first hospital admissions for schizophrenia were higher among the city's lowest socioeconomic group. Faris and Dunham postulated the "drift hypothesis," that posits that the schizophrenic patients tend to drift downward in the socioeconomic scale. The "segregation hypothesis," in contrast, holds that schizophrenic patients actively seek the lower class areas where they may be protected from the stresses of more organized society. All epidemiologic studies tend to confirm that mental illness is more prevalent among the lower socioeconomic classes. *(Kaplan and Sadock, pp 192–195)*

314. **(E)** Secondary orgasmic dysfunction is defined as the absence of orgasm in a woman who in the past had orgasms with some regularity. Substance abuse, particularly opiate abuse, lowers sexual desire and enjoyment. Dyspareunia (pain during intercourse) often prevents orgasm. Depression also causes loss of libido and, hence, lack of orgasm. Extramarital relationships may cause a lack of orgasm with the woman's husband or with the extramarital partner because of guilt feelings. Many women who complain of the absence of orgasm during intercourse can and do achieve orgasm with clitoral stimulation. *(Leigh, pp 311–336)*

315. **(E)** While there may be psychotherapeutic value in physical therapy, including hydrotherapy, it is usually not considered to be a type of formal psychotherapy. Formal psychotherapies may be classified according to theoretical orientations, eg, psychodynamic psychotherapy including psychoanalysis, cognitive-behavioral therapy, learning-theory–based therapy (behavior modification), or by the specialized techniques used, eg, hypnotherapy, narcosynthesis, biofeedback, or on the number or types of patients involved, eg, group, family, couples therapy, etc. *(Leigh and Reiser, pp 421–436)*

316. **(E)** In addition to the symptoms listed, school phobia, truancy, running away from home, and substance abuse may often be

symptomatic of depression in children and adolescents. *(Kaplan and Sadock, pp 531–532)*

317. **(E)** By the time a child who watches TV has finished high school, he or she will have seen depicted on television approximately 8000 murders and countless beatings, robberies, and other forms of violence. The research conducted since 1975 has led to several conclusions, including the belief that TV violence can have both an excitatory and inhibitory effect on children. *(Rothenberg, pp 86–87)*

318. **(B)** Kohut emphasized the development of a sense of self as an important aspect of psychopathology and psychotherapy. Psychoanalysis is a broader term referring to both the psychodynamic theories and their practices. Ego psychology is concerned with ego structures, mechanisms of defense, and coping. Object relations theory deals with enduring internal psychic representations of influential people of infancy and childhood and the effects of those on patterning of relationships in later life. Cognitive psychology is a broad field that deals with thinking processes (cognition). *(Leigh and Reiser, pp 351–367)*

319. **(D)** The sensorimotor period, encompassing the ages of 0 to 1½ years, is divided into six stages that are characterized by: (1) inborn motor and sensory reflexes; (2) primary circular reaction and first habits; (3) secondary circular reaction; (4) use of familiar means to obtain ends; (5) tertiary circular reaction and discovery through active experimentation; (6) insight and object permanence. Concrete operation is performed during the period of the same name, which occurs during ages 7 to 11. *(Kaplan and Sadock, pp 40–42)*

320. **(A)** While all the drugs listed are antianxiety agents, buspirone is a nonbenzodiazepine substance. Benzodiazepines bind to benzodiazepine receptors and act synergistically with the GABA system. Buspirone enhances dopaminergic transmission and antagonizes GABA transmission. Its antianxiety effect may be through specific serotonergic inhibition. *(Kaplan and Sadock, pp 906–915, 921–922)*

321. **(A)** Visual hallucinations are more likely in organic psychosis, whereas auditory hallucinations are more common in schizophrenia. While delusions are common in both conditions, this does not help in differentiating the two conditions. *(Leigh and Reiser, pp 145–209)*

322. **(D)** Technical language has the advantages of being more specific, more easily defines the context (eg, cancer of the cervix rather than a growth in the womb), and is less emotion-laden. It is, however, often not understood by the lay person who is a patient. *(Leigh and Reiser, pp 25–38)*

323. **(E)** The series of relationships in adolescence often leads to a final relationship that shows true mutuality and mature love. At least 10% of adolescents have sexual intercourse by the end of junior high school. At least in one study of 103 boys, no one admitted to overt homosexual behavior. *(Simons, pp 255–270)*

324. **(B)** The placebo effect may be endorphinergically mediated; it often has side effects such as flushing and vomiting. Some placebo effect may be a conditioned response to a previous pill-taking behavior. Some studies have shown naloxone blockade of placebo analgesia, but not of hypoanalgesia. *(Leigh and Reiser, pp 211–243)*

325. **(A)** While acute grief may precipitate a major depression, it does not do so in a majority of cases. Acute grief may be associated with hallucinations and illusions, such as feeling or seeing the deceased. The symptomatology has some similarities to posttraumatic stress disorder (PTSD), but they are distinguishable in that flashbacks and nightmares are more common and vivid in PTSD, and avoidance of situations or items that remind the person of the trauma does not usually occur in acute grief. *(Leigh and Reiser, pp 101–144)*

326. **(C)** Mechanic described the factors that influence how a person perceives a symptom: commonality, familiarity, predictability of outcome, and degree of threat. In the exam-

ples given, only the degree of threat is in the positive direction. *(Leigh and Reiser, pp 3–15)*

327. **(C)** The relationship between performance and anxiety seems to be an inverted U-shaped curve. For optimal performance, a moderate degree of anxiety may be necessary. Severe anxiety reduces performance. *(Leigh and Reiser, pp 41–78)*

328. **(D)** The cognitive, or thinking, function includes orientation, memory, abstraction, calculation, and judgment. These functions are generally associated with the functions of the cerebral cortex, as opposed to affect and emotions, which are limbic system functions. *(Leigh and Reiser, pp 325–340)*

329. **(E)** While a familial form of Alzheimer's disease is an autosomal dominant trait with abnormality in chromosome 21, this is only a subset of Alzheimer's disease. Although both are located in chromosome 21, the gene coding for the amyloid protein precursor, which may be involved in sporadic Alzheimer's disease, is not the same as the one implicated in familial form of the disease. *(Leigh and Reiser, pp 183–188)*

330. **(D)** The incidence of narcotic addiction in physicians is estimated to be 30 to 100 times greater than general population. One in 10 physicians will become dependent on alcohol or drugs sufficiently to impair their careers and 1 in 10 physician addicts or alcoholics will commit suicide. Male physicians have 1.15 times greater and female physicians 3 times greater rate of suicide than the expected rate for the general population of respective gender. According to one study, 47% of physicians had bad marriages. There is, so far, no report of increased incidence of homicide among physicians. *(Scheiber and Doyle, pp 3–10)*

REFERENCES

American Psychiatric Association: *Diagnostic and Statistical Manual of Mental Disorders.* 4th ed. (DSM IV), Washington, DC: American Psychiatric Association; 1994.

Anders T. Home-recorded sleep in 2- and 9-month-old infants. *J Am Acad Child Psychiatry.* 1978;17: 421–432.

Bender L. *A Visual Motor Gestalt Test and its Clinical Use.* New York: American Orthopsychiatric Association; 1938. Research Monograph No. 3.

Kaplan HI, Sadock BJ, Grebb JA. *Kaplan and Sadock's Synopsis of Psychiatry, Behavioral Sciences, Clinical Psychiatry.* 7th ed. Baltimore: Williams & Wilkins; 1994.

Leigh H, ed. *Psychiatry in the Practice of Medicine.* Menlo Park, Calif: Addison-Wesley; 1983.

Leigh H, Reiser MF. *The Patient: Biological, Psychological, and Social Dimensions of Medical Practice.* 3rd ed. New York: Plenum Press; 1992.

Rothenberg MB, ed. The role of television is shaping the attitudes of children. *J Am Acad Child Psychiatry.* 1983;22:86–87.

Scheiber SC, Doyle BB, eds. *The Impaired Physician.* New York: Plenum Publishing Corp; 1983.

Simons RC. *Understanding Human Behavior in Health and Illness.* 3rd ed. Baltimore, Md: Williams & Wilkins; 1985.

SUBSPECIALTY LIST: BEHAVIORAL SCIENCES

Question Number and Subspecialty

284. Depression, sleep and dreaming, pain
285. Doctor–patient relationship
286. Medical sociology
287. Depression, psychiatric epidemiology
288. Individual dynamics
289. Medical sociology
290. Learning theory
291. Neurobiology, emotions
292. Stress

293. Human sexuality
294. Psychiatric imaging
295. Life cycle, social psychiatry
296. Individual dynamics
297. Physiologic correlates of behavior, emotions, and anxiety
298. Pain, emotions, and mood disorders
299. Life cycles, child psychology
300. Life cycle, psychodynamics, psychological assessment
301. Life cycle, psychodynamics
302. Learning theory
303. Learning theory
304. Learning theory
305. Child psychology
306. Child psychology
307. Child psychology
308. Child psychology
309. Child psychology
310. Child psychology
311. Child psychology
312. Child psychology
313. Psychiatric epidemiology, social psychiatry
314. Sexual development and behavior
315. Learning theory, personality and psychodynamics
316. Depression, life cycle, child psychiatry
317. Life cycle, child development, aggression
318. Personality and psychodynamics
319. Life cycle, perception and cognition
320. Biochemical correlates of behavior, pharmacologic correlates of behavior
321. Psychosis, organic mental syndromes, psychological assessment
322. Communication
323. Life cycle, human sexuality
324. Pharmacologic correlates of behavior, pain, emotions
325. Stress and adaptation, emotions, mood disorder, anxiety disorder
326. Ethics, beliefs, norms, values
327. Emotions, cognition
328. Psychological assessment, cognition, emotions
329. Genetics and behavior, organic mental syndromes, degenerative disease of the nervous system
330. Medical sociology, substance abuse, physician stress

Clinical Sciences Review

Obstetrics and Gynecology

Samuel L. Jacobs, MD

DIRECTIONS (Questions 331 through 355): Each of the numbered items or incomplete statements in this section is followed by answers or by completions of the statement. Select the ONE lettered answer or completion that is BEST in each case.

331. Primary dysmenorrhea is thought to arise from uterine contractions originated by prostaglandin release from the endometrium. Pharmacologic measures to control the pain include all of the following EXCEPT

    (A) ibuprofen
    (B) ethinyl estradiol and norethindrone
    (C) bromocriptine
    (D) indomethacin
    (E) mefenamic acid

332. Herpes genitalis, a widespread venereal disease, can be described by all of the following statements EXCEPT

    (A) acyclovir administration shortens symptomatic periods and viral shedding during primary infections
    (B) acyclovir administration may decrease the incidence of recurrences
    (C) a lesion on the perineum at 32 weeks' gestation should preclude vaginal delivery at term
    (D) 50% of patients affected with a primary lesion never experience a recurrence
    (E) viral shedding may occur even when patients have no active lesions

333. Which of the following findings on colposcopic examination of the cervix would be considered normal and not merit biopsy?

    (A) white areas with red stippling (punctation)
    (B) sharp-bordered areas with a mosaic vascular pattern
    (C) a sharply demarcated squamocolumnar junction in a 24-year-old woman
    (D) a small area of white tissue with sharply demarcated borders at the squamocolumnar junction
    (E) an area with a clearly delineated tortuous, irregular vessel

334. A 35-year-old woman has a history of fibrocystic breast disease with symptomatic mastalgia. All of the following agents have been used in the treatment EXCEPT

    (A) tamoxifen
    (B) danazol
    (C) clomiphene
    (D) bromocriptine
    (E) oral contraceptives

335. Oxytocin is a drug widely used in obstetrics. Potential adverse side effects of oxytocin include all of the following EXCEPT

    (A) hypotension
    (B) uterine tetany
    (C) water intoxication
    (D) hypertension
    (E) fetal distress

336. To be most effective in contraception, a diaphragm coated with a spermicidal agent should be left in place at least how many hours after intercourse?

(A) 1 hour
(B) 4 hours
(C) 6 to 8 hours
(D) 12 to 24 hours
(E) 48 to 72 hours

337. Which of the following modalities is not used as a diagnostic aid to help identify lesions on the vulva?

(A) Pap smear
(B) colposcopy
(C) toluidine blue dye
(D) acetic acid
(E) podophyllin

338. The type of obstetric forceps most appropriate for use on an aftercoming head in a breach presentation is

(A) Kjelland's forceps
(B) Barton's forceps
(C) Tucker–McLean forceps
(D) Dewees' forceps
(E) Piper's forceps

339. In a noninflammatory, postmenopausal Pap smear, what percentage of the cells in the maturation index are superficial cells?

(A) 0%
(B) 25%
(C) 50%
(D) 75%
(E) 100%

340. When a euthyroid woman becomes pregnant, which of the following thyroid function tests would be most likely to decrease?

(A) total serum triiodothyronine (T_3) concentration
(B) total serum thyroxine concentration
(C) free thyroxine index

(D) resin T_3 uptake
(E) serum thyroid-stimulating hormone (TSH) concentration

341. At one minute of life, a newborn has the following characteristics: heart rate, 90 beats per min; respiratory rate, good (crying); body color, pink with blue extremities; muscle tone, some flexion of the extremities; and reflex irritability, grimace response. This baby's Apgar score is

(A) 5
(B) 6
(C) 7
(D) 8
(E) 9

342. Which of the following findings on histologic examination of the endometrial biopsy specimen is most characteristic of postmenstrual, preovulatory endometrium?

(A) subnuclear glycogen vacuoles
(B) stromal edema and predecidualization
(C) marked leukocytic infiltration
(D) marked glandular growth and mitoses
(E) prominent coiled spiral arterioles

343. "Protracted active phase" labor is said to occur when the rate of cervical dilation per hour in a primigravid woman is less than

(A) 1.2 cm
(B) 1.5 cm
(C) 1.7 cm
(D) 2.0 cm
(E) 2.5 cm

344. Abnormal maternal serum alpha-fetoprotein levels have been found to be associated with all of the following conditions EXCEPT

(A) maternal liver disease
(B) multiple gestation
(C) intrauterine fetal death
(D) fetal congenital nephrosis
(E) fetal hydrocephalus

345. All the following risk factors are associated with an increased incidence of breast cancer in women EXCEPT

   (A) family history of breast cancer
   (B) obesity
   (C) early menarche
   (D) early natural menopause
   (E) first pregnancy after the age of 35 years

346. At what age should a female with primary amenorrhea be evaluated, regardless of normal growth and development and the presence of secondary sex characteristics?

   (A) 12 years of age
   (B) 14 years of age
   (C) 16 years of age
   (D) 18 years of age
   (E) 20 years of age

347. The most common extrauterine site of endometriosis is the

   (A) uterosacral ligaments
   (B) round ligaments
   (C) ovaries
   (D) rectovaginal septum
   (E) sigmoid colon

348. Cancer of the cervix has been found to have infiltrated the upper two thirds of a patient's vagina and parametrium but not to extend to the pelvic sidewall. The correct International Federation of Obstetricians and Gynecologists (FIGO) staging classification of this carcinoma is

   (A) stage IB
   (B) stage IIA
   (C) stage IIB
   (D) stage IIIA
   (E) stage IIIB

349. All the following statements are true concerning epidural anesthesia used during obstetric procedure EXCEPT

   (A) for abdominal deliveries the epidural block should extend no higher than the T-10 level
   (B) a common complication is maternal hypotension resulting from sympathetic blockage
   (C) convulsions are a significant complication
   (D) actual or anticipated maternal hemorrhage may be a contraindication
   (E) the tip of the catheter should lie between the ligamentum flavum and the dura mater

350. Clomiphene citrate (Clomid) is best described as a

   (A) synthetic preparation of luteinizing hormone (LH)
   (B) weak nonsteroidal estrogen
   (C) progestin of the 19-nortestosterone class
   (D) methylated androgen
   (E) none of the above

351. At her first prenatal visit, a woman says she has no idea of the date of her last menstrual period and that she has not felt any fetal motion. The fetal heartbeat is audible with Doppler technique but not with a stethoscope. At her second visit, a month later, she says she has felt fetal quickening; the fetal heartbeat is audible with a stethoscope. This woman is probably now in what stage of her pregnancy?

   (A) 10 to 12 weeks
   (B) 12 to 14 weeks
   (C) 16 to 20 weeks
   (D) 21 to 23 weeks
   (E) 24 to 26 weeks

352. Which of the following conditions would be the LEAST relevant in determining whether to provide tocolysis to a patient presenting with preterm labor?

(A) a precise determination of gestational age

(B) ruptured placental membranes

(C) fetal lung maturity status

(D) maternal age

(E) etiology of the preterm labor

353. A 19-year-old nulliparous woman is found on routine pelvic examination to have a 5-cm mass. Ultrasonography is performed and shows the mass to be entirely fluid-filled. The proper procedure at this point would be

(A) observation and rechecking the mass after the next menses

(B) medroxyprogesterone therapy

(C) a 10-day course of oral antibiotics

(D) diagnostic therapy

(E) exploratory laparotomy and removal of the cyst

354. A 27-year-old woman has tried unsuccessfully for 5 months to become pregnant. At this point, the recommended evaluative procedure would be

(A) semen analysis

(B) hysterography

(C) endometrial biopsy

(D) diagnostic laparoscopy

(E) none of the above

355. A primigravid patient presents with the following labor curve. She asks how much longer it will be until her delivery. You answer:

(A) it is just impossible to know

(B) 2 hours or less

(C) from this point on her curve, it should be within the next 6 hours

(D) with some pitocin augmentation and the use of forceps, you should be able to reduce the time to 2 hours or less

(E) it looks as though a cesarean section may be necessary

Cervical Dilatation in Labor

DIRECTIONS (Questions 356 through 370): Each group of items in this section consists of lettered headings followed by a set of numbered words or phrases. For each numbered word or phrase, select the ONE lettered heading that is most closely associated with it. Each lettered heading may be selected once, more than once, or not at all.

Questions 356 through 359

For each description below, select the type of female genital cancer with which it is most closely associated.

(A) ovarian carcinoma

(B) cervical carcinoma

(C) tubal carcinoma

(D) vulvar carcinoma

(E) endometrial carcinoma

356. Causes more deaths than any other gynecologic malignancy

357. Precancerous states are often detected by routine screening tests

358. Presents with postcoital bleeding

359. Presents most often as postmenopausal bleeding

Questions 360 through 363

For each of the abnormalities listed below, select the corresponding finding or condition.

- (A) associated with known metabolic abnormality and resultant mental deficiency
- (B) lymphangiectatic edema of hands and feet at birth
- (C) cleft palate, cleft lip, eye defects, polydactyly
- (D) characteristic facial findings often not recognized at birth
- (E) cataracts, microcephalus, cardiac defects, deafness, mental retardation

A 360. Phenylketonuria

E 361. Rubella

B 362. Turner's syndrome

D 363. Down syndrome

Questions 364 through 366

For each statement below, select the disorder with which it is most likely to be associated.

- (A) retained placental fragments
- (B) bleeding from uterine myomas
- (C) uterine atony
- (D) coagulation disorders
- (E) amniotic fluid embolus

C 364. It is the most common cause of immediate postpartum hemorrhage (ie, hemorrhage occurring within the first 24 hours after delivery)

A 365. It is the most common cause of late postpartum hemorrhage (after the first 24 hours)

C 366. General anesthesia increases the incidence

Questions 367 through 370

For each condition below, select the clinical sign likely to be associated with that condition.

- (A) palpable breast mass
- (B) bloody nipple discharge
- (C) bilateral breast pain
- (D) eczema of the nipple

B 367. Intraductal papilloma

A 368. Fibroadenoma

D 369. Paget's disease

C 370. Fibrocystic breasts

DIRECTIONS (Questions 371 through 390): Each of the numbered items or incomplete statements in this section is followed by answers or completions of the statement. Select the ONE lettered answer or completion that is BEST in each case.

371. Vulvovaginal trichomonas can be described most accurately by which of the following statements?

- (A) caused by the overgrowth of bacteria native to some individuals
- (B) not associated with an alteration of normal vaginal pH
- (C) causes pelvic inflammatory disease
- (D) a sexually transmitted disease
- (E) diagnosis can be made by obtaining a wet smear and mixing with KOH (potassium hydroxide)

372. Regarding bacterial vaginosis, which of the following statements is FALSE?

- (A) referred to by many as nonspecific vaginitis
- (B) the offending organism has been referred to as *Haemophilus, Corynebacterium,* and *Gardnerella*
- (C) associated with characteristic diagnostic findings of clue cells and a vaginal pH of 5.0 to 6.0
- (D) treated equally effectively by metronidazole, ampicillin, tetracyclines, or sulfas
- (E) characterized by a fishy odor

373. The use of human $Rh_0(D)$ immune globulin (RhoGAM) as prophylaxis of potential Rh disease can be described by which of the following statements?

(A) the medication must be given within the first 24 hours postpartum

(B) administration of the medication carries with it a risk of hepatitis for the recipient

(C) the prophylaxis success rate is 85%

(D) pain at the site of injection can be a complication

(E) it should be given to Rh-positive women delivering Rh-negative babies

374. All of the following factors would increase the likelihood of a pregnant woman developing pregnancy-induced hypertension after the 24th week of pregnancy EXCEPT

(A) underlying essential hypertension

(B) primigravid status

(C) age, 14 years

(D) presence of multiple gestation

(E) refractoriness to angiotensin

375. Regarding precocious puberty, which of the following statements is true?

(A) precocious puberty is the initiation of sexual maturation occurring before 8 years of age in girls

(B) affected individuals are most often very tall with eunuchoid features

(C) the etiology of this problem is most commonly a central nervous system lesion

(D) the only reliable treatment of this problem in the female is the administration of high-dose estrogen

(E) it is more common in boys than girls

376. During normal pregnancy, tests of resting respiratory function that would likely be increased would include all of the following EXCEPT

(A) minute O_2 uptake

(B) tidal volume

(C) residual volume

(D) minute ventilation

(E) airway conductance

377. Phenytoin (Dilantin), when prescribed during pregnancy, can cause what has been called the hydantoin syndrome in the fetus. Characteristics of the hydantoin syndrome include all of the following EXCEPT

(A) craniofacial anomalies

(B) cardiac defects

(C) cleft lip

(D) kidney defects

(E) mental retardation

378. All the following drugs can appear in human breast milk. The agent associated with "gray baby syndrome" is

(A) propylthiouracil

(B) isoniazid

(C) chloramphenicol

(D) erythromycin

(E) propranolol

379. The mentum posterior presentation can be described by which of the following statements?

(A) spontaneous delivery can almost always occur

(B) it is an unstable lie

(C) mentum posterior must rotate anteriorly in order to be born vaginally

(D) the incidence is approximately 6% of all presentations

(E) forceps can be useful to effect delivery

380. Work-up of a couple who are habitual aborters should include all of the following EXCEPT

(A) maternal and paternal karyotype analysis

(B) hysterosalpingogram

(C) endometrial biopsy

(D) serum estradiol levels

(E) serum progesterone levels

381. A 32-year-old woman who has never been pregnant complains of increasing pelvic pain and dyspareunia. Diagnostic laparoscopy confirms the clinical impression of endometriosis. The medical therapy of choice is

    (A) bromocriptine
    (B) danazol
    (C) progesterone
    (D) oral contraceptives
    (E) gonadotropin-releasing hormone (GnRh) agonists

382. Risk factors for endometrial carcinoma exclude

    (A) obesity
    (B) hypertension
    (C) diabetes
    (D) renal disease
    (E) late menopause

383. Primary fallopian tube cancers are described by all of the following statements EXCEPT

    (A) most are adenocarcinomas
    (B) peak incidence is during the sixth decade
    (C) they constitute fewer than 2% of female genital tract cancers
    (D) they produce few or no symptoms early in their course
    (E) the diagnosis is usually made by ultrasound

384. A 46-year-old woman with five children has a discrete, painful breast mass that has persisted for 3 months. She is particularly frightened because her father's sister died of breast cancer. Factors that indicate the need for a biopsy include

    (A) her family history
    (B) her parity
    (C) pain
    (D) persistence after menstrual periods
    (E) history of breast-feeding

385. Disseminated intravascular coagulation (DIC) is a catastrophic obstetric event that may accompany all of the following EXCEPT

    (A) placental abruption
    (B) sepsis
    (C) amniotic fluid embolism
    (D) retention of a dead fetus
    (E) placenta previa

386. Midtrimester pregnancy termination may be achieved by all of the following EXCEPT

    (A) intrauterine instillation of saline
    (B) intrauterine instillation of prostaglandin F_2
    (C) intravenous administration of pitocin
    (D) oral antiprogesterone RU 486
    (E) dilatation and evacuation

387. Common sites of *early* spread from ovarian carcinoma include all of the following EXCEPT

    (A) spleen
    (B) diaphragm
    (C) uterus
    (D) omentum
    (E) contralateral ovary

388. Which of the following states is NOT associated with an elevated prolactin?

    (A) the first trimester of pregnancy
    (B) pituitary adenoma
    (C) familial hirsutism
    (D) the use of phenothiazines
    (E) herpes zoster

389. Sarcoma botryoides can be described by all of the following statements EXCEPT

    (A) it usually affects prepubertal girls
    (B) it is very uncommon
    (C) it usually is accompanied by a bloody vaginal discharge
    (D) it is highly malignant
    (E) chemotherapy is not an effective treatment modality

390. Risk factors for cervical carcinoma include all of the following EXCEPT

(A) multiple sex partners

(B) infection with human papillomavirus

(C) initiation of coital activity during adolescence

(D) early menarche

(E) early childbearing

Questions 391 through 394

A 34-year-old woman (gravida 7, para 5, spontaneous abortion 1) registers in a clinic for obstetric care when she learns she is pregnant. She had an uncomplicated dilatation and curettage (D&C) procedure performed between her second and third pregnancies for irregular bleeding. All deliveries have been vaginal and uncomplicated. Her blood pressure is 124/76 mm Hg. She is euthyroid.

391. The woman described above is at increased risk for all of the following obstetric complications EXCEPT

(A) placenta previa

(B) placenta accreta

(C) postpartum hemorrhage

(D) multifetal pregnancy

(E) ectopic pregnancy

392. After a first trimester complicated only by mild nausea and vomiting, the woman returns after 19 weeks of pregnancy. She says she has had vaginal spotting and increased vomiting for the past 2 weeks. Her blood pressure is 150/94 mm Hg. The fundus size is 22 weeks, and no fetal heart tones are heard by auscultation or Doppler. There is clinical evidence of hyperthyroidism. The most likely diagnosis is

(A) hydramnios

(B) missed abortion

(C) fibroid uterus

(D) urinary retention

(E) hydatidiform mole

393. The most useful diagnostic procedure to perform at this point in the case described would be

(A) urine pregnancy test

(B) clotting studies

(C) culdocentesis

(D) abdominal x-ray

(E) uterine ultrasound

394. After the pregnancy is ended, the woman described should have which of the following tests?

(A) chromosomal analysis

(B) chorionic gonadotropin titers

(C) thyroid function tests

(D) hysterography

(E) cystometrography

Questions 395 through 397

A 22-year-old woman (gravida 0) seeks a gynecologic examination. She has regular menstrual cycles, is sexually active, uses oral contraceptives, and has no dysmenorrhea or dyspareunia. She weighs 54.5 kg (120 lb). Her external genitalia are normal. On speculum examination, a red vaginal circumferential fold, looking like a concentric ring around the cervix, is noted.

395. The most likely diagnosis of the genital lesion described is

(A) contraceptive-induced metaplasia of the cervix

(B) hypertrophic vagina secondary to monilial vaginitis

(C) herpes simplex virus, type II, infection

(D) vaginal adenosis

(E) wolffian duct cyst

396. The most important next step in the evaluation of this woman's disorder would be

(A) cervical culture

(B) wet-mount (physiologic saline) microscopic examination

(C) aspiration of the tissue surrounding the cervix using a small-gauge needle

(D) gentian violet staining of the lesion

(E) visualization, palpation, and cytologic sampling of the entire cervix and vagina

397. Appropriate management of the woman's disorder would best include

(A) serial cytologic examinations

(B) serial cervical cultures

(C) VDRL testing

(D) blood viral antibody titers

(E) discontinuation of oral contraceptives

Questions 398 through 400

Results of clinical pelvimetry on a 27-year-old woman (gravida 1, para 0) are as follows: flat, forward-inclined sacrum; prominent ischial spines; convergent sidewalls; and a narrow, deep pubic arch.

398. The pelvimetric description given above is typical of which of the following pelvic types (by the Caldwell–Moloy classification)?

(A) gynecoid

(B) android

(C) anthropoid

(D) platypelloid

(E) gynecoid with platypelloid features

399. Which of the following statements is true regarding this type of pelvis?

(A) usually portends a good delivery prognosis

(B) occurs in less than 5% of gravidas

(C) increases the frequency of difficult forceps delivery

(D) is not associated with any increase in fetal morbidity or mortality

(E) is associated often with occiput anterior presentation

400. Which of the following conjugates is most important as a measure of the anteroposterior diameter of the pelvic inlet and cannot be measured directly by clinical pelvimetry?

(A) anatomic conjugate

(B) anterior conjugate

(C) diagonal conjugate

(D) obstetric conjugate

(E) sagittal conjugate

ANSWERS AND EXPLANATIONS

331. **(C)** Prostaglandin inhibition is the key to control of dysmenorrhea. Even the dysmenorrhea associated with endometriosis is thought to be secondary to excess prostaglandins. Ibuprofen, mefenamic acid, and indomethacin are potent prostaglandin inhibitors. Ethinyl estradiol and norethindrone are the most common components of birth control pills; they decrease prostaglandin synthesis by causing atrophy and decidualization of the endometrium. Bromocriptine suppresses production of prolactin and does not seem to affect dysmenorrhea. *(Gant, p 81)*

332. **(C)** Other than HIV disease, many experts consider herpes to be our most serious venereal disease. Unfortunately, no preventive medication exists. Topical application of acyclovir is only recommended for primary cases, and even then it does not prevent recurrences. The virus may be shed by asymptomatic carriers. On the brighter side, as many as 50% of patients who suffer an initial attack never experience recurrence. Regarding pregnancy management, most neonatologists agree that as long as a woman has no active lesions at the time of delivery, she may deliver vaginally. *(Cunningham, pp 1305–1309)*

333. **(C)** The colposcope provides the magnification and intensified light used to delineate abnormal areas of epithelium on the cervix, vagina, and vulva. On the cervix, areas that are whitish, thickened, or possess abnormal vascular patterns (punctation, mosaic, tortuosity) are abnormal and a biopsy specimen should be taken. The principle of colposcopy relies on the fact that all metaplastic change occurs at the squamocolumnar junction (SCJ) and, therefore, the visualization of a clearly demarcated SCJ is imperative to obtain a satisfactory examination. In a 24-year-old patient this zone should be readily visible. In an elderly woman, metaplasia of columnar to squamous epithelium may have moved this junction well up into the cervical canal where visualization is impossible with the colposcope. *(Gant, pp 222–223)*

334. **(C)** Breast discomfort is a major problem associated with fibrocystic breast disease. Simple palliative measures include administration of vitamin E, 600 units daily, and limiting methylxanthines by eliminating coffee and other caffeine-containing substances; the mechanics of action of these measures are not well understood. Danazol, in doses of 200 to 400 mg daily, does alleviate the problem. Other treatments include tamoxifen, OC's, and bromocriptine. Clomiphene would not be used because it raises estrogen levels, thereby exacerbating the problem. *(Gant, p 109)*

335. **(D)** The major prenatal complications with the use of oxytocin relate to overstimulation of the uterus, leading to tetany and possibly fetal distress. After delivery, an inadvertent bolus of oxytocin can cause a rapid fall in arterial blood pressure. Unlike ergonovine, oxytocin does not produce hypertension. With chronic administration, oxytocin can act like a similar peptide hormone, ADH, and produce reabsorption of free water; electrolytes must be carefully monitored in a woman receiving large doses of oxytocin to prevent hyponatremia and subsequent seizures. *(Cunningham, pp 337–340)*

336. **(C)** The use of a diaphragm coated with a spermicidal agent is an effective method of contraception. For the spermicidal agent to be most effective, the diaphragm should be left in place for at least 6 hours after intercourse. After 6 hours have elapsed, the diaphragm can be removed when it is most convenient to do so but should not be left in place for a prolonged period of time. *(Gant, p 201)*

337. **(E)** Cytology (Pap smear) or superficial scrapings can be helpful in the diagnosis of dysplastic and infectious lesions of the vulva. Colposcopy, just like the hand lens of the dermatologist, aids by providing magnification and good lighting, allowing lesions to be seen that would not be visible to the unaided eye. Toluidine blue is an acidophilic dye that is taken up by lesions with a high DNA content (neoplastic cells). Acetic acid is an astringent for cells with large glycogen content. When applied to areas of neoplasia, it makes them stand out because of the high nuclear to cytoplasmic ratio. These dense areas then appear as well-demarcated white lesions. Podophyllin is a form of chemical debrisant and not a diagnostic aid. *(Gant, pp 214–215)*

338. **(E)** Piper's forceps were expressly designed for use on the aftercoming head in a breech presentation. The forceps should be applied to an engaged head; the long shank and the double pelvic curve facilitate the long reach of the head. None of the other forceps listed has these features. *(Cunningham, p 583)*

339. **(A)** The maturation index is a measure of percentages of cell layers in cervical and vaginal cytology. It is typically written as $x/y/z$ with x as the percentage of parabasal cells, y as the percentage of intermediate cells, and z as the percentage of superficial cells. The percentages change under hormonal influence and are not useful in the presence of dysplastic cells.

In a noninflammatory, postmenopausal Pap smear, none of the cells in the maturation index are superficial cells. (Superficial cells occupy the topmost layer of the epithelium; the nucleus is small and lacks a chromatin pattern.) In the absence of extrinsic estrogens or inflammation, the presence of significant numbers of superficial cells is abnormal in the postmenopausal period. The number of superficial cells can increase as a result of infection, vaginal dermatoses, estrogen administration, certain neoplasms, and certain hormonal abnormalities. *(DeCherney, pp 625–626,1042)*

ABNORMAL LABOR PATTERNS, DIAGNOSTIC CRITERIA, AND METHODS OF TREATMENT.[1]

Labor Pattern	Diagnostic Criterion		Preferred Treatment	Exceptional Treatment
	Nulliparas	Multipara		
Prolongation disorder (Prolonged latent phase)	> 20 h	> 14 h	Therapeutic rest	Oxytocin or cesarean deliveries for urgent problems
Protraction disorders 1. Protracted active phase dilatation 2. Protracted descent	< 1.2 cm/h < 1.0 cm/h	< 1.5 cm/h < 2 cm/h	Expectant and supportive	Cesarean delivery for CPD
Arrest disorders 1. Prolonged deceleration rate 2. Secondary arrest of dilatation 3. Arrest of descent 4. Failure of descent	> 3 h > 2 h > 1 h No descent in deceleration phase or second stage of labor	> 1 h > 2 h > 1 h	Without CPD: oxytocin With CPD: cesarean delivery	Rest if exhausted Cesarean delivery

[1]Modified from Cohen W, Friedman EA (editors): *Management of Labor,* University Park Press, 1983.

340. (D) Total serum triiodothyronine (T_3) and thyroxine (T_4) levels both show a significant elevation during pregnancy. These levels begin to rise early in pregnancy and return to normal only after delivery. The concentration of thyroid-stimulating hormone (TSH) has been reported to be normal or slightly increased during the first half of pregnancy. Free thyroxine index remains in the normal range during pregnancy. Resin T_3 uptake decreases somewhat during pregnancy. *(DeCherney, p 481)*

341. (B) Apgar scores of newborn infants at 1 minute and 5 minutes of life judge five parameters: heart rate, respiratory function, body color, muscle tone, and reflex irritability. The maximum score is 10—ie, 2 points in each category. For the baby described in the question, heart rate below 100/min rates a score of 1; respiratory status, 2; body color, 1; muscle tone, 1; and reflex irritability, 1. (This last parameter is tested by inserting the tip of a catheter into the nostril; a score of 2 is given if the response to the stimulation is crying.) Thus, the Apgar score for this baby is 6. *(Gant, p 312)*

342. (D) Postmenstrual, preovulatory edometrium is described as proliferative: the endometrial layer proliferates and thickens under the hormonal influence of estrogen. His-

tologic examination of endometrial tissue at this stage shows marked glandular growth and much evidence of mitosis. All the other histologic findings listed in the question are characteristic of secretory or progestational (postovulatory, premenstrual) endometrium. *(Gant, p 10)*

343. (A) "Protracted active phase" labor occurs when cervical dilation is less than 1.2 cm/h in a primigravid woman and less than 1.5 cm/h in a multigravid woman. Friedman found several causes for protracted active phase labor, including cephalopelvic disproportion, excessive sedation or analgesia, and the use of conduction anesthesia. Protracted active phase labor can lead to secondary arrest of labor when dilation ceases to progress. *(Gant, pp 356–357)*

344. (E) The presence of alpha-fetoprotein (AFP) in maternal serum has been associated with a number of conditions, including multiple gestation, intrauterine fetal death, fetal congenital nephrosis, and maternal liver disease. Other problems that can produce abnormal AFP levels in maternal blood are other fetal defects, such as omphalocele, and fetus-to-mother bleeding (either spontaneous or caused by amniocentesis). By contrast, closed neural-tube defects, including those associated with hydrocephalus in the fetus, are not associated with abnormal AFP levels in maternal serum. *(Gant, pp 411–412)*

345. (D) A family history of breast cancer increases the risk of death from breast cancer by a factor of two to three. Obesity, early menarche, and first pregnancy after the age of 35 years also increase the risk. A late natural menopause also seems to increase the risk of breast cancer; in fact, women with natural menopause after 55 years of age have approximately twice the risk of women whose natural menopause occurred before the age of 45 years. *(Gant, pp 102–103)*

346. (C) Most girls experience menarche by 16 years of age. Therefore, absence of menses by that age suggests delayed puberty or abnormal ovarian function and should be evaluated. Because the median age of menarche in the United States is 12.8 years, evaluation of primary amenorrhea at 12 years of age would be inappropriate. Evaluation at 14 years of age is appropriate if the girl has not had menstrual periods nor development of secondary sexual characteristics. *(Gant, p 163)*

347. (C) The most common extrauterine location of endometriosis is the ovary. In many cases, ovarian involvement is bilateral. Other sites (in approximate order of decreasing frequency) include the peritoneum of the pouch of Douglas (including the uterosacral ligaments and the rectovaginal septum), other pelvic peritoneal surfaces, the round ligament, the oviduct, the intestines, and the pelvic lymph nodes. *(Gant, p 180)*

348. (C) See table in second column. By definition, this is stage IIB. *(Gant, p 226)*

349. (A) For abdominal deliveries an epidural block must extend from at least T-8 to S-1; the thoracic end of a block necessary for vaginal delivery would be T-10. Complications of epidural block include convulsions and hypotension secondary to sympathetic blockage. The presence or threat of maternal hemorrhage may be a contraindication to the use of epidural anesthesia during delivery. The

FIGO (1986) STAGING OF CANCER OF THE CERVIX.

Stage 0	Carcinoma in situ, intraepithelial carcinoma.
Stage I	Carcinoma strictly confined to the cervix (extension to the corpus should be disregarded).
Ia	Preclinical carcinomas of the cervix, ie, those diagnosed only by microscopy.
Ia 1	Minimal microscopically evident stromal invasion.
Ia 2	Lesions detected microscopically that can be measured. The upper limits of the measurement should not show a depth of invasion of > 5 mm taken from the base of the epithelium, either surface or glandular, from which it originates; and a second dimension, the horizontal spread, must not exceed 7 mm. Larger lesions should be staged as Ib.
Ib	Lesions of greater dimensions than stage Ia2, whether seen clinically or not. Preformed space involvement should not alter the staging but should be specifically recorded so as to determine whether it should affect treatment decisions in the future.
Stage II	Carcinoma extends beyond the cervix but has not extended onto the pelvic wall. Carcinoma involves the vagina, but not the lower third.
IIa	No obvious parametrial involvement. The vagina has been invaded, but not the lower third.
IIb	Obvious parametrial involvement.
Stage III	Carcinoma has extended onto the pelvic wall. On rectal examination, there is no cancer-free space between the tumor and the pelvic wall. The tumor involves the lower third of the vagina. All cases with hydronephrosis or nonfunctioning kidney should be included unless known to be due to other causes.
IIIa	No extension onto the pelvic wall but involvement of the lower third of the vagina.
IIIb	Extension onto the pelvic wall and/or hydronephrosis or nonfunctioning kidney.
Stage IV	Carcinoma extending beyond the true pelvis or clinically involving the mucosa of the bladder or rectum. Do not allow a case of bullous edema as such to be allotted to stage IV.
IVa	Spread to adjacent organs (ie, rectum or bladder, with positive biopsy from these organs).
IVb	Spread to distant organs.

epidural catheter should be placed between the ligamentum flavum peripherally and the dura mater centrally. *(Cunningham, pp 437–440)*

350. (B) Clomiphene citrate (Clomid) is a non-steroidal, weakly estrogenic agent distantly related to diethylstilbestrol. Clomiphene binds to estrogen receptors in the hypothalamus and perhaps in the pituitary gland as well. Endogenous production of follicle-stimulating hormone (FSH) rises during clomiphene therapy; because FSH stimulates ovarian follicles, clomiphene is used in ovulation induction. *(Gant, pp 187–188)*

351. (C) Most pregnant women become aware of fetal movement between 16 and 20 weeks of gestation. This is called "quickening." *(Cunningham, p 22)*

352. (D) Preterm labor and its management are often controversial areas in obstetrical management. There are certain situations or factors mitigating these conditions, however, that always need to be considered as relevant in decision making. First, a precise knowledge of both the gestational age and the status of fetal lung maturity are tremendous aids in management. Seldom will most obstetricians stop labor occurring after the 34th to 35th week of gestation or in gestations beyond the 33rd to 34th week of gestation with demonstrated fetal lung maturity. Ruptured membranes to many obstetricians would be a contraindication to stopping preterm labor, whereas to others it might be an indication for immediate tocolysis. Either way the status of the membranes is important in decision making. The etiology when one can be found is obviously important. If the etiology is infectious or a significant abruption, few caregivers would try to stop labor. The same is true for serious maternal disease, but disease is certainly not synonymous with age of the mother. Age by itself should have no bearing on the decision to provide tocolysis. *(Gant, pp 438–440)*

353. (A) A pelvic mass is an alarming finding in a woman. In prepubertal women, most lesions derive from germ cells, and nearly half of these tumors are malignant. In postmenopausal women, ovarian masses are frequently malignant, and many gynecologists believe that any palpable ovary in postmenopausal women should be removed. In women in their reproductive years, however, the majority of cysts are fluid-filled follicular cysts, which are completely benign. If such a mass is noted in a young woman, she should be observed for at least one menstrual cycle. At times, suppression of the cyst with oral contraceptive therapy to decrease stimulation may be attempted, but medroxyprogesterone is not routinely used for these purposes. If a mass persists for several months and is more than 8 cm in diameter, most gynecologists would advocate its removal. *(Gant, pp 29–30)*

354. (E) Infertility is defined as a year of unprotected coitus without conception. The incidence of conception in couples experiencing regular unprotected intercourse is 15 to 20% after 1 month, 50% after 6 months, and 80 to 90% after 1 year. Therefore, although many patients become disconcerted if they are not pregnant after 4 or 5 months of trying, such a situation is statistically not unlikely. After an unsuccessful year of attempted conception, extensive fertility testing procedures may be initiated if necessary. *(Gant, p 185)*

355. (C) Although labor is not an entirely predictable event, the work of Friedman has shown that plotting dilatation of the cervix and descent of the fetal head does allow easier recognition of abnormal labor and good predictability of the course of labor based on immediate past progress. This is a normal labor curve:

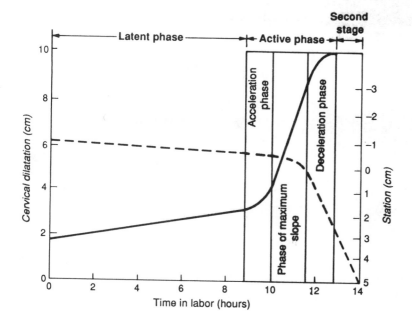

Question 355. Composite of cervical dilatation and fetal descent curves, illustrating their interrelationship and their component phases. (Courtesy of Cohen W, Friedman EA [editors]: Management of Labor. University Park Press, 1983.)

If it remains on this course (and you have no reason to believe it will not), delivery should occur in about 6 hours. Poor understanding of the labor process and lack of use of these invaluable graphic representations by those providing obstetrical care has contributed to the increased rates of cesarean section seen in the last 10 years. When used correctly, these curves are invaluable to the obstetric attendant. *(Gant, pp 356–357)*

356–359. (356-A, 357-B, 358-B, 359-E) Although cervical and endometrial carcinomas are more common than ovarian carcinoma, ovarian carcinoma causes more deaths than any other gynecologic malignancy because of its aggressiveness and lack of early symptoms. The Pap smear is a routine test that can detect dysplasia and carcinoma in situ of the cervix, both of which are treatable precursors of invasive carcinoma of the cervix. Carcinoma of the fallopian tube is a very rare malignancy, accounting for fewer than 2% of female genital tract neoplasms. Pruritus is the most common presenting symptom of vulvar cancer, although local irritation may have been present for many years. Occasionally a lump in the vulvar area is the presenting symptom. Although ovarian carcinoma classically gives no indication of its presence un-

til late in its course, the most common initial symptoms are an abdominal mass, ascites, and pain. Postcoital bleeding is the classic presentation of carcinoma of the cervix. Any episode of postmenopausal bleeding should be investigated, and carcinoma of the endometrium must be ruled out by a dilatation and curettage or an endometrial biopsy. Endometrial cancer usually presents with postmenopausal bleeding. *(Gant, pp 221,225,233, 239)*

360–363. (360-A, 361-E, 362-B, 363-D) Phenylketonuria is an autosomal recessive inborn error of metabolism resulting in a syndrome associated with mental retardation. Early recognition and a special diet can greatly alter the prognosis of this disease. The diet can then be discontinued later in life but must be restarted before pregnancy to avoid phenylalanine toxicity in the unborn offspring. Rubella is an infectious environmental teratogen and the most common cause of congenital deafness. Retardation, heart defects, and ophthalmologic abnormalities are also associated. Turner's syndrome is associated with abnormalities of the lymphatics. The webbing of the neck that occurs is from in utero lymphedema of the neck (cystic hygroma). Seeing a baby born with edema isolated to the hands and feet and no cardiac failure should automatically alert you to this diagnosis. Down syndrome, though very characteristic in the adult facies, can be completely unnoticed in the newborn. (*Cunningham, pp 921–922,925,927,1285–1287*)

364–366. (364-C, 365-A, 366-C) Of all the types of life-threatening hemorrhage associated with pregnancy, hemorrhage from uterine atony in the immediate postpartum period is the most common. General anesthesia using a halogenated anesthetic is associated with the development of uterine atony in the immediate postpartum period, as are prolonged labor, rapid delivery, and overdistention of the uterus from a large baby, multiple gestation, or hydramnios. Other, less common causes of hemorrhage in the immediate postpartum period include uterine myoma, retained placental fragments, coagulation disorders, and cervical or vaginal lacerations.

Late postpartum hemorrhage occurs less frequently than immediate hemorrhage. It is caused most frequently by retained placental fragments or subinvolution of the placental implantation site. (*Gant, p 383*)

367–370. (367-B, 368-A, 369-D, 370-C) The most common cause of bloody or serosanguineous nipple discharge is intraductal papilloma. It is a benign condition usually occurring in middle-aged women. Usually, a breast or nipple mass is not palpable, because tumor size is small (only 3 mm).

Fibroadenoma is a benign, slow-growing, well-circumscribed tumor that typically is palpable. The tumor may remain the same size for years or enlarge rapidly. Nipple discharge is not associated with fibroadenoma.

Paget's disease is a malignancy originating in the ductal system of the breast. The lesion often has an innocent appearance and should be suspected in a patient with a persistent eczematous eruption of the nipple.

Fibrocystic changes of the breasts are the most common of the benign breast diseases. They are an exaggerated response of breast tissue to the cyclic levels of ovarian hormones. The classic symptom is cyclic bi-

lateral breast pain. (*Gant, pp 108,109; DeCherney, p 1124*)

371. (D) Trichomonas is in most cases a sexually transmitted disease caused by a protozoan, not a bacteria. It is generally more common when the pH has become more alkaline than the normal vagina (postmenstruation, vaginosis, etc.). It may often be asymptomatic. Successful eradication requires treatment of all sexual partners. Trichomonads can be identified as pear-shaped motile organisms when a sample of vaginal discharge is mixed with normal saline. A KOH (potassium hydroxide) preparation is useful for identifying the hyphae associated with candidal vaginitis. (*Gant, pp 45–47*)

372. (D) Bacterial vaginosis (nonspecific vaginitis) is the most common type of vaginal infection and is associated with the overgrowth of anaerobic bacteria. It has been called by many names (both repeatable and nonrepeatable). It has a characteristic fishy odor from the release of amines when KOH (potassium hydroxide) is applied to a wet preparation. Its low pH is an excellent diagnostic sign, as is the characteristic appearance of clue cells using light microscopy. The anaerobic nature of the infection makes it very susceptible to metronidazole but less responsive to other agents used for treatment in the past. (*Gant, p 47*)

373. (D) Rh disease, caused by isoimmunization of an Rh-negative mother exposed to Rh-positive red blood cells, results in hemotologic and other consequences for the Rh-positive child. Postpartum administration of Rh immune globulin to Rh-negative mothers who have delivered an Rh-positive child has been standard care since the late 1960s. More recently, antepartum prophylaxis has been recommended. Human $Rh_0(D)$ immune globulin (RhoGAM) is an effective prophylaxis for Rh disease if given within the first 72 hours postpartum. The success rate is usually quoted as 98% to 99%. Pain at the injection site is a potential complication of RhoGAM therapy, but hepatitis is not because preparation of the γ-globulin by alcohol or ether extraction would destroy any hepatitis virus present. *(Gant, pp 415–417)*

374. **(E)** Preeclampsia is much more common in primigravid than in multigravid women, and the younger and older primigravidas are at greatest risk. For example, older primigravid women are more likely to have chronic hypertension, which predisposes to the development of preeclampsia. Hypertension induced during or aggravated by pregnancy is also one of the many complications that occur more commonly during "multifetal" pregnancies. Normal pregnant patients are refractory to the pressor effects of angiotensin, whereas many patients destined to manifest preeclampsia lose this refractoriness. *(Cunningham, pp 211–212,227–228)*

375. **(A)** Precocious puberty usually consists of the normal sequence of events of sexual maturation but occurring before the age of 8. Unfortunately, the increased production of sex steroid leads to premature epiphyseal closure with 50% of affected individuals less than 5 feet tall. When an etiology can be found, it is most commonly a central nervous system lesion or the sequelae of the same, but the greatest majority remain idiopathic as to cause. The treatment lies in suppression of gonadotropins either with injectable medroxyprogesterone acetate in a depot form or suppression with gonadotropin-releasing hormone agonists. Precocious puberty is seen five times more frequently in girls than in boys. *(Gant, p 100)*

376. **(C)** Tidal volume, minute ventilatory volume, and minute oxygen uptake increase appreciably during pregnancy. Airway conductance is increased, while total pulmonary resistance is reduced. Residual volume and functional residual capacity are decreased. *(Gant, p 286)*

377. **(D)** The administration of phenytoin (Dilantin) to pregnant women is associated with a relatively high risk of developmental defects. The fetal hydantoin syndrome, caused by maternal ingestion of phenytoin, is associ-

ated with a number of abnormalities. The syndrome consists of mild to moderate growth retardation, mental retardation, facial abnormalities (including cleft lip or palate), cardiac defects, limb dysmorphism, and coagulopathy. Kidney defects do not seem to be part of the syndrome. Pregnant women requiring phenytoin should receive the lowest dosage able to achieve seizure control. *(Cunningham, pp 967–968)*

378. **(C)** Chloramphenicol can be toxic to the breast-fed infant, potentially causing "gray baby syndrome" and death. Propylthiouracil (PTU) is excreted into breast milk in very low amounts and has not been found to cause fetal thyroid problems. Likewise, isoniazid, although it is secreted in breast milk, has not been found to be associated with fetal toxicity. Neither erythromycin nor propranolol are associated with adverse fetal reactions, although it is recommended that infants of nursing mothers on propranolol be closely observed for symptoms of beta-blockade. *(Cunningham, p 962)*

379. **(C)** The incidence of the mentum posterior presentation is less than 1 in 1200. Only 30% of mentum presentations are posterior, and two thirds of these rotate to the anterior. Those posterior mentum presentations that do not rotate anteriorly carry a potentially poor prognosis, because they do not deliver spontaneously. As such, forceps should not be applied to a mentum posterior position. A brow presentation is an unstable state of partial ob-flexion, and will usually convert to a mentum (ie, face) or occiput presentation. *(Gant, pp 364–365)*

380. **(D)** Habitual abortion is defined as three or more consecutive pregnancy losses before the 20th week of gestation. Many causes have been implicated; most cases are still diagnosed as idiopathic. Because as many as 60% of fetuses miscarried during the first trimester document some genetic anomaly, it is important to study parental chromosomes. In as many as 10% of cases a parental anomaly such as balanced translocation will be found.

Occasionally a uterine septum or fibroid can account for losses. A hysterogram will identify these patients, and surgical correction can be performed. Occasionally the mother may have an inadequate luteal phase and produces too little progesterone to achieve successful implantation of a fertilized ovum. Such cases may be diagnosed by endometrial biopsy and serum progesterone levels, and the women may receive treatment with supplemental progesterone. A serum estradiol level is not helpful in the work-up of this condition. (DeCherney, pp 311–314)

381. **(E)** Laparoscopy is the ideal test for confirming the presence of endometriosis. Women who clearly desire to remain fertile should receive conservative therapy rather than radical pelvic surgery such as hysterectomy. The most effective drug treatments for endometriosis are those that cause suppression of ovarian function and endometrial tissue with GnRH agonists. Although Danazol is also effective, its masculinizing side effects make it a less optimal choice. (Gant, pp 180–183)

382. **(D)** Obesity is a major risk factor for endometrial carcinoma, which is thought to be caused by excessive estrogen stimulation of the endometrium. Peripheral conversion of estrogen in fat cells makes obese women particularly susceptible to endometrial carcinoma. Other recognized risk factors associated with estrogen excess or imbalance include early menarche and late menopause, nulliparity, failure of ovulation in young women, estrogen-secreting tumors, and exogenous supplementation of estrogens. Ten percent of women with endometrial carcinoma have diabetes, and 50% have an abnormal response to a glucose tolerance test. More than half of all women with endometrial carcinoma are hypertensive. Renal disease is not associated with any type of endometrial malignancy. (Gant, pp 231–232)

383. **(E)** Primary tubal carcinomas are usually papillary adenocarcinomas, although squamous cell carcinomas occasionally occur. Although tubal carcinoma can occur at any time

during and after the reproductive years, the peak incidence is during the sixth decade of life. Tubal carcinoma is very rare, accounting for 0.1% to 0.5% of female genital tract cancers. Like ovarian cancer, tubal cancers produce few or no symptoms during their early phase. The most common presenting symptoms include vaginal discharge or bleeding, menstrual irregularities, and pain. The diagnosis of fallopian tube carcinoma is usually made at the time of surgery. (Gant, p 245)

384. **(D)** The only significant risk factor for the patient described in the question is the persistence of the mass after a period. Benign cysts vary with the menstrual cycle; painful masses are usually benign. Low parity, not high parity, is a risk factor of breast cancer. Although a family history is definitely a risk factor and warrants close observation, it is not, by itself, an indication for a biopsy. Breast feeding has not been found to impact positively or negatively on the incidence of breast cancer. (Gant, pp 102,103)

385. **(E)** Of all the cases of placental abruption resulting in fetal death, 30% are associated with hypofibrinogenemia at levels <150 mg/dl. These cases are characterized by significant coagulation retroplacentally as well as intravascularly. Sepsis, particularly with *Clostridium perfringens*, may cause significant hemolysis and disseminated intravascular coagulation (DIC). The cause of amniotic fluid embolism-induced DIC may be the mucus contained in the fluid, which may incite coagulation by activation of factor X. Thromboplastin activation from dead products of conception may trigger DIC, particularly if the fetus is retained for longer than 1 month. Placenta previa is not associated with DIC, since the thromboplastin produced with placental separation tends to escape out the cervix and not into the maternal circulation. (Gant, pp 432–437)

386. **(D)** Several methods have been used successfully, alone and in combination, to terminate midtrimester pregnancies. Current statistics available from the Centers for Disease Control show dilatation and evacuation to

have the lowest mortality rates; however, a very experienced operator must perform the procedure. Intra-amniotic injection of prostaglandin may result in a live-born fetus, whereas saline injection terminates fetal viability. Saline injection, however, can lead to hyperosmolar crisis and DIC. Pitocin administered intravenously acts slowly on the midtrimester cervix, which is not very receptive to oxytocics. The antiprogesterone RU 486 can effect abortion in early gestation but has not been approved for use in the United States and is not effective in midtrimester. *(Gant, pp 75–77)*

387. **(A)** Ovarian cancer spreads widely early in its course. Common sites of spread include the uterus, contralateral ovary, fallopian tubes, rectum, and bladder. Omental metastases occur very early in the course of the disease, as do metastases to the diaphragm, especially to the inferior aspect of the right hemidiaphragm. Metastases to the stomach and spleen may occur, but they are not common and develop relatively late. Even in patients with disease apparently limited to one ovary, biopsy of the contralateral ovary and the omentum is indicated at the time of laparotomy. *(Gant, p 241)*

388. **(C)** Elevated prolactin is associated with anything that may inhibit hypothalamic function (decreasing the secretion of prolactin inhibiting factor) or stimulate the breast. Destructive hypothalamic or pituitary tumors, central nervous system suppressants, and primary pituitary insufficiency are all examples. Any event or substance or local irritant that stimulates the breast, chest wall, or nipple may also stimulate prolactin secretion. Lactation is one sign of these, as are herpes zoster, scars on the chest wall, jogging, sexual activity, or even breast examination. *(DeCherney, p 144)*

389. **(E)** Sarcoma botryoides is a grapelike polypoid lesion that arises from the müllerian tubercle. It is a very uncommon and extremely aggressive neoplasm that occurs during the first decade of life. In most cases the present-ing symptom is a bloody vaginal discharge. Pelvic exenteration was, at one time, the only therapeutic approach but has now been replaced by a multimodality approach consisting of chemotherapy or radiotherapy followed by hysterectomy and vaginectomy. *(Gant, p 220)*

390. **(D)** The cause of cervical cancer appears to involve an increased susceptibility of the adolescent cervix to oncogenic stimuli. It is believed that there may be a factor that is sexually transmitted or acquired. Thus, adolescent girls who engage in promiscuous sexual activity are especially at risk. Infection with human papilloma virus also seems to increase the risk of cervical carcinoma. Jewish women have a lower incidence of cervical cancer than do women of most other ethnic groups, perhaps because of a preventive effect of penile circumcision. *(Gant, p 222)*

391–394. **(391-E, 392-E, 393-E, 394-B)** The woman described in the question is at risk for several disorders at the start of her pregnancy. Multiparity is associated with placenta previa, placenta accreta, and postpartum hemorrhage. (Placenta previa occurs when the placenta implants in the lower uterine segment and partially or completely covers the cervical os, and placenta accreta is an abnormal attachment of the placenta to the uterine wall in which the villi adhere to or penetrate the myometrium.) Dilatation and curettage procedures predispose to later placenta accreta. The chance of having twins increases with maternal age up to 40 years of age and with parity up to seven. The risk of ectopic pregnancy is increased in women who use an intrauterine contraceptive device or have had pelvic inflammatory disease, previous abdominal-pelvic surgery, or repeated elective abortions.

The most likely diagnosis of the woman's second-trimester difficulties is hydatidiform mole. Missed abortion usually causes the uterus to be small, not large, for dates. Although the other conditions listed can cause an enlarged uterus, they are not associated with increased vomiting, signs of hyperthyroidism, or early pregnancy-induced hypertension. Hydatidiform mole is a developmental anomaly of the placenta in which chorionic villi are converted into vesicles. It may be benign or may become malignant.

Diagnosis of hydatidiform mole is best confirmed by ultrasound of the uterus. Sonograms of affected women may be similar to sonograms of a normal pregnancy, uterine myoma with an early pregnancy, or twins, but repeat scanning should eliminate the uncertainty. Women with molar disease are at greatest risk for persistent trophoblastic disease and choriocarcinoma. Elevated human chorionic gonadotropin (HCG) levels after pregnancy has been ended represent the continued presence of active trophoblastic tissue. HCG levels are useful in diagnosing molar pregnancies only if the levels are extremely high. Otherwise, they could reflect a normal singleton or multifetal pregnancy. If HCG is detectable after pregnancy, chemotherapy may be required. *(DeCherney, p 277; Gant, pp 246–250)*

395–397. (395-D, 396-E, 397-A) Vaginal adenosis can develop in women exposed in utero to diethylstilbestrol (DES). Cervical metaplasia associated with this disorder occurs at the squamocolumnar junction, usually at or near the external cervical os. Careful inspection, palpation, cytologic examination, and, if needed, colposcopy are necessary to search for the presence of clear cell adenocarcinoma of the vagina. This rare neoplasm can develop from vaginal adenosis in DES-exposed women. Regular visual, tactile, and cytologic examinations are important in the management of these women. The use of oral contraceptives is not contraindicated in DES-exposed women.

Monilial vaginitis causes a thick, white discharge and is associated with vulvitis; the treatment is clotrimazole (Lotrimin), miconazole (Monistat), or terconazole (Terazol). Genital herpes primary infection usually produces "cold sore" vesicular lesions externally or on the cervix and is associated with pain. Wolffian duct cysts occur on the lateral vaginal walls. *(Gant, p 52)*

398–400. (398-B, 399-C, 400-D) An android pelvis has prominent ischial spines, convergent sidewalls, a flat and forward-inclined sacrum, and a narrow, deep pubic arch. Although some of these characteristics can occur in other pelvic types (eg, ischial spines can be variable in size in anthropoid and platypelloid types), only the android pelvic type combines all these characteristics. During labor, the fetal head engages in the transverse or posterior diameter of the maternal android pelvis. Asynclitism (lack of parallelism between maternal pelvic planes and fetal presenting part), molding of the fetal head, and a prolonged second stage of labor are common with this pelvic type, as are transverse arrest and arrest in an occiput posterior position. Forceps deliveries commonly are required and are often difficult, leading to an increased incidence of perineal tears as well as increased fetal morbidity and mortality. *(Gant, pp 299–304)*

REFERENCES

Cunningham FG, MacDonald PC, Gant NF. *Williams Obstetrics.* 19th ed. East Norwalk, Conn: Appleton & Lange; 1993.

Gant NF, Cunningham FG. *Basic Gynecology and Obstetrics.* East Norwalk, Conn: Appleton & Lange; 1993.

DeCherney AM, Pernoll ML. Current Obstetric & Gynecologic Diagnosis & Treatment. 8th ed. East Norwalk, Conn: Appleton & Lange; 1994.

SUBSPECIALTY LIST: OBSTETRICS & GYNECOLOGY

Question Number and Subspecialty

331. Endocrinology of menstruation
332. Infections
333. Colposcopy
334. Breast pathology
335. Management of labor and delivery
336. Clinical gynecology

337. Clinical gynecology
338. Clinical obstetrics, abnormal
339. Clinical gynecology
340. Physiology of pregnancy
341. Newborn resuscitation
342. Clinical gynecology
343. Clinical obstetrics, normal
344. Prenatal diagnosis
345. Oncology, breast
346. Endocrinology, infertility
347. Clinical gynecology
348. Oncology
349. Obstetric anesthesia
350. Endocrinology, infertility
351. Pregnancy diagnosis
352. Management of abnormal labor
353. Clinical gynecology
354. Clinical gynecology
355. Physiology of labor
356. Oncology
357. Oncology
358. Oncology
359. Oncology
360. Teratology
361. Teratology
362. Genetics
363. Genetics
364. Clinical obstetrics, abnormal
365. Clinical gynecology
366. Clinical obstetrics, abnormal
367. Breast disease
368. Breast disease
369. Breast disease
370. Breast disease
371. Infectious disease
372. Infectious disease
373. Fetus, placenta, and newborn
374. Clinical obstetrics, abnormal
375. Precocious puberty
376. Physiology of pregnancy
377. Teratology
378. Newborn physiology
379. Clinical obstetrics, abnormal
380. Infertility
381. Endometriosis
382. Oncology
383. Oncology
384. Breast pathology
385. Obstetric complications of pregnancy
386. Abortion
387. Oncology
388. Reproductive endocrinology
389. Oncology
390. Oncology
391. Clinical obstetrics, abnormal
392. Clinical obstetrics, abnormal
393. Clinical obstetrics, abnormal
394. Clinical gynecology
395. Clinical gynecology
396. Clinical gynecology
397. Clinical gynecology
398. Clinical obstetrics, normal
399. Clinical obstetrics, normal
400. Clinical obstetrics, normal

Pediatrics

Stephan R. Glicken, MD

DIRECTIONS (Questions 401 through 426): Each of the numbered items or incomplete statements in this section is followed by answers or by completions of the statement. Select the ONE lettered answer or completion that is BEST in each case.

401. All the following statements about cystic fibrosis are true EXCEPT

    (A) the incidence in whites is about 1 in 2000

    (B) it may present in the newborn period with meconium ileus

    (C) it is an autosomal dominant disease

    (D) hepatic involvement is due to inspissated biliary secretions

    (E) chronic hypoxia, hypercapnia, and acidosis produce pulmonary hypertension

402. Which of the following statements in regard to fever in infants and children is NOT correct?

    (A) fever is generally of more concern in the very young infant than the older child

    (B) fever may be a manifestation of a noninfectious condition

    (C) the febrile response is initiated by release of interleukin-1 by macrophages and certain other cells

    (D) brain damage is likely when rectal temperature exceeds 40°C (104°F)

    (E) the central component of the febrile response is mediated by prostaglandins

403. A 14-month-old boy is taken to the emergency room with a fracture of the left femur sustained, according to his father, in a fall from his crib. Bruises are observed on both shoulders and on the back. The remainder of the examination is within normal limits. Which of the following evaluative procedures should be performed first?

    (A) skull CT scan

    (B) chest roentgenogram

    (C) lumbar puncture

    (D) retinoscopy

    (E) renal sonography

404. A 2-year-old girl feeds her 4-month-old brother 8 of her mother's prenatal iron pills (325 mg ferrous sulfate), 10 amoxicillin tablets (250 mg), and 9 fluoride tablets (1 mg). What is most likely to result if appropriate therapy is not undertaken?

    (A) hypercoagulable state caused by excessive vitamin K

    (B) tooth staining caused by exposure to amoxicillin

    (C) hepatic necrosis caused by iron toxicity

    (D) bowel necrosis caused by fluoride toxicity

    (E) hemolytic anemia caused by iron toxicity

405. A baby is born with ambiguous genitalia. Which of the following statements is correct?

    (A) the baby should undergo corrective surgery and should be reared as a female

    (B) adrenogenital syndrome must be ruled out

(C) the baby should be reared according to the appearance of its genitalia

(D) the baby's gender assignment should be determined by its chromosomal sex

(E) gender assignment must be made immediately to prevent parents and relatives from transmitting to the child their confusion about the sexual identity

406. Child abuse, including sexual abuse, is being recognized and reported with such increased frequency that it has reached epidemic proportions. Which of the following complaints is LEAST likely to be a clue to sexual abuse?

(A) encopresis

(B) secondary enuresis

(C) recurrent abdominal pain

(D) chronic cough

(E) school phobia

407. A specific pattern of abnormalities has been identified among infants born to mothers who consume moderate to large amounts of alcohol during their pregnancies. All of the following abnormalities are characteristic of these infants EXCEPT

(A) growth deficiency

(B) cardiac defects

(C) facial abnormalities

(D) major joint abnormalities

(E) mental retardation

408. The major clinical manifestations of rheumatic fever include all of the following EXCEPT

(A) carditis

(B) polyarthritis

(C) chorea

(D) erythema chronicum migrans

(E) subcutaneous nodules

409. An 8-month-old child presents with fever and respiratory distress. Auscultation of the chest reveals crackles and decreased breath sounds bilaterally. The child appears agitated and restless. The remainder of the physical examination is within normal limits. Chest roentgenogram reveals a normal heart size and bilateral pneumonia. Arterial oxygen tension is 50 mm Hg and carbon dioxide tension is 69 mm Hg. Which of the following is most appropriate in the management of this child at this time?

(A) endotracheal intubation and assisted ventilation

(B) oxygen and close observation

(C) oxygen and bronchial (postural) drainage

(D) administration of bronchodilators by aerosol

(E) insertion of a Swan–Ganz catheter

410. A 10-month-old girl is admitted to a hospital because of the insidious onset of fever, a brassy cough, inspiratory stridor, and mild respiratory distress—all symptoms of infectious croup. If this diagnosis is correct, the most likely causative agent is

(A) adenovirus

(B) respiratory syncytial virus

(C) parainfluenza virus

(D) *Haemophilus influenzae*

(E) *Corynebacterium diphtheriae*

411. A 2-year-old girl is admitted to the hospital with generalized tonic convulsions. Her history is unremarkable, and her physical examination is normal except for a slightly red throat and a slight fever. Her prolonged convulsions require intravenous administration of diazepam. White blood cell count is normal, and lumbar puncture only reveals elevated cerebrospinal fluid pressure. CT scan of her head shows cerebral edema but no signs of trauma. Which of the following should be the next diagnostic step?

    (A) free erythrocyte protoporphyrin level
    (B) viral cultures of cerebrospinal fluid
    (C) rapid slide (Monospot) test
    (D) antistreptolysin O titer
    (E) electroencephalography

412. A 4-year-old child manifests symptoms of fever, sore throat, and swollen lymph nodes. Spleen tip is palpable. Throat culture and rapid slide (Monospot) test results are negative. The next logical diagnostic procedure would involve

    (A) repeat throat culture
    (B) heterophil titer
    (C) Epstein–Barr virus titer
    (D) chest x-ray
    (E) bone marrow examination

413. Women with phenylketonuria (PKU) who are planning pregnancy should be advised that

    (A) a low phenylalanine diet should be initiated before conception
    (B) a low phenylalanine diet should be started as soon as pregnancy is confirmed
    (C) a low phenylalanine diet should be followed throughout the first trimester but can be stopped thereafter
    (D) a low phenylalanine diet has been shown to have little effect in preventing fetal damage
    (E) if phenylalanine levels are only mildly to moderately elevated, there is no need for dietary change

414. The major mode of transmission of HIV infection in young children today is

    (A) biting
    (B) transfusion
    (C) vertical transmission
    (D) horizontal transmission
    (E) sexual abuse

415. A 4-year-old child with moderate vesicoureteral reflux has had recurrent urinary tract infections despite adequate antibiotic prophylaxis. This child now should have

    (A) a 2-week course of intravenous antibiotics
    (B) repeat intravenous pyelography
    (C) renal arteriography
    (D) antireflux surgery
    (E) a course of vitamin C (ascorbic acid) in conjunction with antibiotic prophylaxis

416. All the following statements about nocturnal enuresis (bed-wetting) are true EXCEPT

    (A) the problem occurs in approximately one third of 4-year-old children
    (B) boys are affected more often than girls
    (C) there is often a familial predisposition to enuresis
    (D) small bladder capacity plays a causative role in many cases
    (E) significant emotional problems are found in most affected children

417. Which of the following malignant neoplastic processes has the highest rate of spontaneous regression?

    (A) neuroblastoma
    (B) Ewing's sarcoma
    (C) Wilms' tumor
    (D) acute myelogenous leukemia
    (E) Hodgkin's disease

418. Which of the following immunizations is currently recommended routinely for normal children in the United States?

    (A) smallpox vaccination
    (B) pneumococcal vaccine

(C) *Haemophilus influenzae* vaccine

(D) Salk inactivated polio vaccine

(E) Hepatitis A vaccine

419. Which of the following conditions is the leading cause of death in the United States of infants between the ages of 1 and 12 months?

(A) bacterial meningitis

(B) congenital heart disease

(C) congenital malformation syndromes

(D) accidental poisonings

(E) sudden infant death syndrome

420. Long-term therapy of sickle cell disease includes all of the following EXCEPT

(A) pneumococcal vaccine

(B) monthly benzathine penicillin injections

(C) iron supplementation

(D) folic acid

(E) acetaminophen for pain

421. A 9-year-old boy presents with a several-day history of progressive arm and leg weakness. He has been well except for an upper respiratory infection 2 weeks ago. The patient is alert and oriented. On repeated examination, the heart rate varies between 60 and 140 beats/min and the blood pressure varies between 90/60 and 140/90 mm Hg. Respirations are shallow with a rate of 50/min. There is symmetric weakness of the face and all four extremities. Deep tendon reflexes are absent. Sensation is intact. The most likely diagnosis is

(A) polymyositis

(B) myasthenia gravis

(C) transverse myelitis

(D) Guillain–Barré syndrome

(E) viral encephalitis

422. Which of the following statements concerning sensorineural hearing loss in children with bacterial meningitis is true?

(A) it occurs uncommonly (less than 5% of cases)

(B) it occurs more commonly when *Haemophilus influenzae* type b rather than

Streptococcus pneumoniae is the causative organism of the meningitis

(C) its onset often is late in the clinical course, after discontinuation of antimicrobial therapy

(D) prompt institution of antimicrobial therapy appears not to influence the incidence

(E) evoked-response audiometry is indicated only if there is clinically evident hearing loss

Questions 423 through 426

An 8-year-old girl is involved in a severe motor vehicle accident and sustains multiple injuries to her head, arms, and abdomen. She arrives at the local emergency room with profuse and pulsatile bleeding from her left upper arm; the blood is bright red. The left forearm is disfigured, and bone can be seen in the wound. Her respirations are periodic and her lips are cyanotic. Respiratory rate is 6/min, pulse is 160/min, and blood pressure is 80/40 mm Hg. Her abdomen is rigid, and hemorrhagic discoloration is present along the lateral flanks.

423. The first step in the management of the girl described above would be to

(A) stop the bleeding from her left arm

(B) insert an intravenous line and give a large volume of normal saline

(C) ensure airway patency

(D) give vasopressor agents intravenously

(E) splint her left arm

424. The next step in management would be to

(A) stop the bleeding from her left arm

(B) insert an intravenous line and give a large volume of normal saline

(C) ensure airway patency

(D) give vasopressor agents intravenously

(E) splint her left arm

425. The most important first step in evaluating the girl's rigid abdomen would be to

(A) obtain a flat-plate roentgenogram of her abdomen
(B) obtain an emergency liver–spleen scan
(C) obtain an emergency ultrasound of her abdomen
(D) obtain an emergency CT scan of her abdomen
(E) perform a paracentesis of her abdomen

426. In treating the girl's fracture in the emergency room, the girl's physician should

(A) splint the arm and cover the wound with sterile gauze
(B) splint the arm and debride the wound
(C) splint the arm and close the wound
(D) splint the arm and start intravenous antibiotics
(E) reduce and splint the fracture

DIRECTIONS (Questions 427 through 456): Each group of items in this section consists of lettered headings followed by a set of numbered words or phrases. For each numbered word or phrase, select the ONE lettered heading that is most closely associated with it. Each lettered heading may be selected once, more than once, or not at all.

Questions 427 through 429

For each description below, select the drug with which it is likely to be associated.

(A) acetylcysteine (Mucomyst)
(B) methylene blue
(C) deferoxamine
(D) amyl nitrite
(E) atropine

427. Useful in the treatment of acetaminophen poisoning

428. Useful in the treatment of organic phosphate (eg, Malathion) poisoning

429. Useful in the treatment of ferrous sulfate poisoning

Questions 430 through 432

For each congenital cardiac abnormality, select the most characteristic cardiac auscultatory finding.

(A) holosystolic murmur
(B) continuous "machinery" murmur
(C) wide, fixed splitting of the second heart sound
(D) systolic ejection murmur
(E) diastolic murmur

430. Ventricular septal defect

431. Pulmonary stenosis

432. Atrial septal defect

Questions 433 through 436

For each condition listed below, select the organism with which it is most closely associated.

(A) *Haemophilus influenzae* type b
(B) group A streptococcus
(C) *Mycoplasma pneumoniae*
(D) *Escherichia coli*
(E) *Pneumocystis carinii*

433. Neonatal sepsis

434. Epiglottitis

435. Cervical adenitis

436. Occult bacteremia

Questions 437 through 439

For each condition listed below, select the characteristic skin lesion with which it is most closely associated.

(A) vesicle
(B) pustule
(C) nodule
(D) macule
(E) bulla

E 437. Stevens–Johnson syndrome

A 438. Hand-foot-and-mouth syndrome

A 439. Chickenpox

Questions 440 through 443

For each condition listed below, select the peripheral blood smear finding with which it is most closely associated.

(A) target cells
(B) no abnormality
(C) hypersegmented polymorphonuclear leukocytes
(D) hypochromia
(E) red blood cell fragmentation

C 440. Folate deficiency

441. Hemolytic uremic syndrome

B 442. Anemia of chronic disease

D 443. Iron deficiency

Questions 444 through 447

For each clinical description listed below, select the microorganism with which it is most likely to be associated.

(A) *Mycoplasma pneumoniae*
(B) *Chlamydia trachomatis*
(C) *Pneumocystis carinii*
(D) *Neisseria meningitidis*
(E) *Bordatella pertussis*
(F) respiratory syncytial virus
(G) group B streptococcus
(H) *Haemophilus influenzae* type b

F 444. Bronchiolitis in an infant

A 445. Pneumonia in an otherwise healthy adolescent

C 446. Pneumonia in an infant born to a mother with HIV infection

G 447. Meningitis in a neonate

Questions 448 through 452

For each condition listed below, select the medication with which it is most likely to be associated in an infant or child.

(A) theophylline
(B) aspirin
(C) vancomycin
(D) phenytoin
(E) cefaclor
(F) loperamide
(G) diphenhydramine
(H) chloramphenicol
(I) tetracycline

D 448. Gingival hyperplasia

B 449. Reye syndrome

I 450. Dental staining

451. Red man syndrome

452. Gray baby syndrome

Questions 453 through 456

For each disorder listed below, select the measurable defect.

(A) factor IX deficiency
(B) abnormal white blood cell chemotaxis
(C) factor VIII deficiency
(D) hypoxanthine guanine phosphoribosyl-transferase deficiency
(E) abnormal hemoglobin synthesis
(F) defective NADPH oxidase system
(G) hexosaminidase A deficiency
(H) ornithine-transcarbamylase deficiency

453. Lesch–Nyhan syndrome

454. Chronic granulomatous disease

455. Hemophilia B

456. Tay–Sachs disease

ANSWERS AND EXPLANATIONS

401. **(C)** Cystic fibrosis is an autosomal recessive disorder common among whites. The incidence of the disorder is estimated to be about 1 in 2000. The disease is characterized by an unusual abnormality of the secretions of the exocrine glands. Meconium ileus is a common presenting feature in infants with cystic fibrosis. The disease has severe effects on the respiratory system, in which the viscid secretions obstruct the airways, predisposing to bacterial infections, bronchitis, chronic pneumonia, and bronchiectasis. The chronic changes in the lungs lead to hypoxia and hypercapnia, at times producing pulmonary hypertension and eventually cor pulmonale. Hepatic involvement is due to inspissated biliary secretions. Hepatic insufficiency results in hypoalbuminemia and edema. Portal hypertension with hypersplenism is com-

mon. Supplemental therapy with pancreatic enzymes is usually indicated. *(Rudolph et al, pp 1640–1650)*

402. **(D)** Fevers up to 40°C (104°F) rectally are common and fevers to 42.1°C (106°F) are not rare in young children. There is no evidence that these degrees of fever result in any permanent damage to the brain or other organs. This is in contrast to heat illnesses, such as heat stroke or malignant hyperthermia, where body temperatures may reach or exceed 42.2°C (108°F) and brain damage is common. Although most fevers are associated with infections, this is not invariably true. Intracranial hemorrhage, leukemia and other neoplasms, histiocytosis-X, and juvenile rheumatoid arthritis are just a few examples of noninfectious diseases in which fever is common. The mechanism of fever involves the release of interleukin-1 (previously referred to as endogenous pyrogen) by macrophages and certain other cells. This low-molecular-weight protein is carried by the blood to the brain, where it stimulates the release of prostaglandins in the temperature control center located in the anterior hypothalamic region. Antipyretic drugs, such as aspirin and acetaminophen, act by blocking the synthesis of prostaglandins in the hypothalamus. In young infants, fever is an especial source of concern because of the risk of serious infection. In this age group, localized infection often occurs in the absence of expected signs or symptoms. For example, nuchal rigidity is very infrequent in young infants with meningitis; the only finding may be fever and irritability. *(Dinarello et al)*

403. **(D)** When a child presents with atypical or multiple injuries, the possibility of child abuse must be a prime consideration. Because a significant percentage of pediatric emergency room visits are due to some kind of abuse or neglect, it is imperative that physicians have a high degree of suspicion in such cases as that described in the question. Injuries that result from being shaken by an adult and subtle head trauma are common findings in abused children. The retinas should always be examined for evidence of hemorrhage. Depending on symptoms and signs, bone roentgenograms, rib films, and CT scan of the head may be indicated in a total work-up of an abused child. Often, renal ultrasonography is advisable in the presence of flank mass or bloody urine. Caution must be observed if lumbar puncture is performed, because increased intracranial pressure may be present. Many hospitals have protocols for suspected child abuse cases, and trauma teams that include pediatricians, social workers, psychiatrists, nurses, and legal experts have aided in the treatment and rehabilitation of the victims and families of child abuse. *(Rudolph et al, pp 145–150,175–177)*

404. **(C)** Of the substances ingested, only iron and fluoride have any significant toxicity. The maximum amount of fluoride customarily contained in a tablet is 1 mg which is much less than a toxic dose for even a full bottle of 100 tablets. While amoxicillin may commonly cause lower gastrointestinal distress and diarrhea, it has no effect on developing teeth. Tetracycline is the antibiotic well known for this effect. Toxicologically, iron is very important. Its acute effects which may occur following an ingestion of 25 mg/kg of body weight, include acute corrosive necrosis of the stomach and bowel followed by acute hepatic necrosis. Management includes the induction of emesis followed by purging. Deferoxamine administration may reduce the serum iron concentration below toxic levels by chelation and consequent urinary excretion. *(Rudolph et al, pp 834–835)*

405. **(B)** Gender assignment of infants with ambiguous genitalia should be done urgently, but not at the expense of an accurate and thoughtful decision. Gender assignment should be based on the correct diagnosis and a reasonable prognosis for future functioning; these, more than chromosomal or gonadal sex characteristics, should be the overriding considerations. Therefore, as much information as can be gathered must be available before a decision is made. Particularly important points to consider include the fol-

lowing: (1) In a virilized chromosomal female, salt-losing adrenogenital syndrome must be ruled out by determination of 17-hydroxyprogesterone levels. Not only is this a life-threatening condition if left untreated, but if treated appropriately, fully normal sexual functioning, including fertility, can be restored. (2) In inadequately virilized males for whom male gender assignment is being contemplated, a consultation with a urologist is mandatory to determine whether correction is likely to produce a phallus capable of sexual functioning. One must also demonstrate that the baby is not relatively androgen-resistant and that there will be a response to testosterone with the onset of puberty. (3) In addition to careful examination of the external genitalia, one should examine the internal genitalia by means of vaginography, pelvic ultrasonography, laparoscopy, or even laparotomy, depending on the needs of the individual case. (4) Although it is desirable to retain as many of the patient's original characteristics as possible, one must keep in mind that a functional vagina can be constructed with much less difficulty than can a functional penis. (5) Certain individuals with dysplastic gonads and a Y chromosome are prone to tumor formation and may require gonadectomy. In summary, gender assignment is a complex problem with important consequences for the infant and the infant's family. It should be made urgently but not hastily after appropriate tests have been administered and specialists in the field of endocrinology, urology, pediatric gynecology, and child development have been consulted. *(Saenger, pp 1–17)*

406. **(D)** Children who are victims of sexual abuse often develop functional complaints, and it may be these complaints that first bring them to medical attention. School phobia, obviously, is functional in nature. Although most cases of school phobia represent a fear of separation from the parent rather than a fear of the school itself, in some cases it may result from someone in the school setting abusing the child. Encopresis, secondary enuresis (enuresis developing after bladder

control had been achieved and the child had been dry at night), and recurrent abdominal pain are common functional complaints that, occasionally, may be a clue to sexual abuse. Cough is the least likely of the symptoms listed to be functional in nature. *(Rudolph et al, pp 147–148)*

407. **(D)** The characteristics of fetal alcohol syndrome include (1) persistent growth deficiency that begins in utero and affects weight, height, and head circumference; (2) facial abnormalities such as micrognathia, short palpebral fissures, and a thin upper lip; (3) cardiac abnormalities, commonly septal defects; (4) minor limb abnormalities with some restriction of mobility and some alteration in palmar crease patterns; and (5) mental deficiency ranging from mild to severe. There is a decided relationship between the extent of abnormalities and the degree of mental retardation. Affected infants may present with hypoglycemia and alcohol withdrawal symptoms, which may last for 48 to 72 hours. The management of these infants consists of correction of the hypoglycemia. Otherwise, no specific therapy is indicated, but prevention by restriction of maternal alcohol consumption during pregnancy needs to be stressed. *(Rudolph et al, pp 193,419–420,2126)*

408. **(D)** Erythema marginatum, an evanescent, erythematous macular eruption with central clearing and a serpiginous border, is the characteristic skin lesion of rheumatic fever. Erythema chronicum migrans is the pathognomonic skin lesion of Lyme disease. *(Rudolph et al, pp 930,933,1518–1520)*

409. **(A)** This child has clear evidence of respiratory failure, which is a medical emergency. Administration of oxygen alone, although it might correct the hypoxemia, will not correct the hypercarbia and presumed respiratory acidosis. Immediate steps must be undertaken to restore effective alveolar ventilation so as to return arterial carbon dioxide levels to normal at the same time that oxygen is administered. The fact that this child appears restless is a clue to the severity of his respiratory insufficiency. In the absence of wheezing, it is unlikely that bronchodilators would be sufficiently effective to obviate the need for intubation. The fact that the roentgenogram reveals evidence of pneumonia rather than airway obstruction (no mention of hyperaeration), also makes it unlikely that bronchodilators would be effective. *(Newth)*

410. **(C)** Viruses are the causative agents in the vast majority of cases of infectious croup. The parainfluenza virus accounts for approximately 66% of the cases of infectious croup, with adenoviruses, respiratory syncytial, influenza, and measles viruses responsible for most of the remaining cases. The majority of cases of viral croup occur between the ages of 3 months and 5 years, whereas infectious croup caused by bacterial agents is more common between the ages of 3 and 7 years. *(Rudolph et al, pp 674–676)*

411. **(A)** In the differential diagnosis of acute cerebral edema with convulsions in a child, ingestion of toxic substances, including lead, must be considered early so that specific management can be initiated immediately. Although a diagnosis of acute lead encephalopathy can be suspected following (1) a history of pica, (2) the presence of basophilically stippled erythrocytes, (3) lead lines in the long bones, or (4) heavy metal densities visible on abdominal roentgenograms, none of these may be present. A direct measurement of serum lead levels is often difficult to obtain within a short time. In contrast, the free erythrocyte protoporphyrin level can be rapidly measured in many laboratories. A marked elevation in such a case is highly suggestive of lead poisoning. A rapid slide (Monospot) test is unlikely to be positive in the presence of a normal white blood cell count and normal differential blood count. An EEG is not likely to provide a diagnosis under the circumstances described in the question. *(Rudolph et al, pp 835–837,1890–1892)*

412. **(C)** Infectious mononucleosis may affect children of all ages. The rapid slide (Monospot) test response is positive in approximately 90% of infected persons; however,

younger children with mononucleosis may have a negative result. Moreover, many younger children have poor antibody response to the heterophil titer test. Specific serodiagnostic testing for the Epstein–Barr virus, the agent responsible for infectious mononucleosis, can confirm the diagnosis. A repeat throat culture, even if positive for β-hemolytic *Streptococcus,* may be of only partial value, because both infectious mononucleosis and streptococcal pharyngitis may be present simultaneously. Chest x-ray and bone marrow examinations would contribute little to the correct diagnosis. *(Ginsburg et al)*

413. **(A)** The effects of maternal phenylketonuria (PKU) on the fetus are still incompletely understood. Adverse effects correlate with the degree of hyperphenylalaninemia: women with mildly to moderately elevated levels have borne both developmentally normal and damaged children. It does appear that lowering the maternal phenylalanine level into the normal range by dietary means starting before conception affords optimal protection. However, this treatment must be supervised carefully by a physician who has special knowledge of amino acid metabolism, and it should be backed by a laboratory that can measure appropriate amino acid concentrations throughout pregnancy. *(Lipson et al)*

414. **(C)** Current screening practices have all but eliminated blood transfusion as a source of HIV infection. Today, most infections in young children are the result of vertical (perinatal) transmission of the virus from an infected mother. Sexual abuse certainly is a possible source of infection, but fortunately few such cases have been reported. Horizontal transmission of HIV (eg, in household or daycare settings) by biting or other behaviors, if it occurs at all, is extremely rare. *(Rogers)*

415. **(D)** Vesicoureteral reflux is the most common anatomic abnormality associated with recurrent urinary tract infection in children. Many cases of reflux are the result of an inadequate length of submucosal ureter immediately proximal to its opening into the bladder lumen, a condition that sometimes requires surgical correction. However, in other children reflux often appears to result from the direct effects of infection on ureteral tone and peristalsis. Thus, many children may outgrow mild degrees of reflux if they are maintained on prophylactic antibiotics until the condition resolves. Frequently, moderate to severe degrees of reflux require surgery. Failure of adequate antibiotic treatment to prevent infection is also a prime indication for surgery. Repeating intravenous pyelography or performing renal arteriography on an already diagnosed case is not useful, although a radionuclide scan may be very helpful to determine the present degree of reflux with a minimum of radiation exposure. Vitamin C, although reportedly useful in acidifying the urine to help prevent infection, does not enhance adequate antibiotic prophylaxis. Intravenous antibiotics would be necessary only if oral antibiotics were not successful in eradicating infection. *(Rudolph et al, pp 1388–1392)*

416. **(E)** Nocturnal enuresis (involuntary nighttime bed-wetting) is a common problem. There is often a family history (parent or sibling) of enuresis, and boys are affected more often than girls. Thirty percent of children still do not have nighttime bladder control by the age of 4 years. Even by the age of 12 years, fully 3% of children still have not developed complete nocturnal continence. Therefore, the age at which nocturnal enuresis is defined as a "problem" is somewhat arbitrary, but most authorities consider ages 5 to 6 years an appropriate time to consider intervention. Small bladder capacity is a common finding, but more significant urologic abnormalities are rare. Significant emotional problems are not found in most affected children. Evaluation of enuretic children involves a detailed history and physical examination, as well as urinalysis and urine culture. Contrast radiographic studies are indicated only if significant abnormalities are revealed by this initial evaluation. Treatment should be multifaceted and includes motivational counseling, bladder training exercises, enuresis alarms, and, under special cir-

cumstances, medication such as imipramine or anticholinergic drugs. *(Schmitt)*

417. **(A)** Neuroblastoma is a malignant neoplasm arising from sympathetic nervous tissue and may occur anywhere such tissue is found. It occurs almost exclusively in the first 6 years of life. The diagnosis is most often made during evaluation of an abdominal mass. Advanced stages of the disease are accompanied by systemic symptoms, such as fever, anemia, and weight loss. The diagnosis is almost always suggested by increased urinary excretion of vanillylmandelic acid or homovanillic acid or both. Treatments include surgery, radiation, and chemotherapy. Prognosis depends on the patient's age and the extent to which the disease has spread. Younger patients fare especially well. Of great interest is the fact that neuroblastoma has the highest rate of spontaneous regression of any of the malignancies that afflict humankind. However, the overall survival rate in most reported series approximates only 50%, and this figure has changed little during the past two decades. *(Rudolph et al, pp 1286–1289)*

418. **(C)** Of the vaccines listed in this question, only the *Haemophilus influenzae* vaccine currently is recommended in the United States for routine immunization of healthy children. Although both *Streptococcus pneumoniae* and *H. influenzae* type b are common pathogens in the pediatric patient, *H. influenzae* is the leading cause of bacterial meningitis in young children beyond the neonatal period. Pneumococcal vaccine currently is recommended only for certain high-risk children, for example those with sickle cell disease, nephrotic syndrome, or asplenia. Smallpox has been essentially eradicated from the world and routine vaccination no longer is recommended in any developed country. Hepatitis A vaccine is not routinely used. Immunization against polio is routinely accomplished with the live oral (Sabin) vaccine; the inactivated (Salk) vaccine is used only for patients who are immunocompromised, for example, those with leukemia or AIDS. *(Rudolph et al, pp 29–36)*

419. **(E)** Although meningitis, congenital heart disease, congenital malformations, accidents, and poisonings are major causes of childhood morbidity and mortality, sudden infant death syndrome (SIDS) heads the list of causes of death in infants between the ages of 1 and 12 months. SIDS is diagnosed when death in an infant occurs unexpectedly and without explanation; careful autopsy discloses no identifiable cause. SIDS occurs most commonly in infants between the ages of 2 and 5 months and affects boys more frequently than girls. Additional risk factors include low socioeconomic level, low birth weight, and a positive family history for SIDS. The incidence in the general population is approximately 2 cases per 1000 live births. No single cause explains all cases of SIDS; however, many cases are thought to result from abnormalities of respiratory control leading to cessation of breathing (apnea), especially during sleep. Methods of prevention currently being used include home monitoring of respiration and use of respiratory stimulants such as theophylline. *(Rudolph et al, pp 868–878)*

420. **(C)** Appropriate long-term therapy for sickle cell disease includes measures aimed at preventing bacteremia. Penicillin and pneumococcal vaccine are helpful. Because folic acid deficiency has been thought to be associated with sickle cell disease, folic acid should be administered daily. Acetaminophen is an appropriate analgesic. Iron deficiency does not usually occur in affected children, and supplementation is contraindicated. *(Rudolph et al, pp 1203–1207)*

421. **(D)** Progressive, symmetric motor weakness, areflexia, and autonomic instability, with mild or absent sensory signs, are typical features of Guillain-Barré syndrome. Frequently there is a history of infection (often respiratory) in the several weeks preceding clinical onset of the syndrome. Supportive evidence for the diagnosis includes elevation of cerebrospinal fluid protein concentration with a mild (10 or fewer cells/µL) mononuclear pleocytosis and slowing of nerve conduction velocities. *(Rudolph et al, pp 1668,1970–1972)*

422. (D) Sensorineural hearing loss is detected by evoked-response audiometry in between 5 and 10% of children with bacterial meningitis. Up to 30% of children with meningitis caused by *Streptococcus pneumoniae* will have hearing deficits. Hearing loss generally is noted early in the course of bacterial meningitis and occurs despite prompt initiation of appropriate antimicrobial therapy. All children with bacterial meningitis should have hearing assessment by evoked-response audiometry before or soon after hospital discharge. *(Rudolph et al, pp 544–548,575–576,162–165)*

423–426. (423-C, 424-A, 425-E, 426-A) Because the emergency treatment of multiple trauma patients mobilizes a large number of personnel and calls for a large number of interventions, management approach in the emergency room must be geared first to sequential evaluation of the patients' life support systems. This sequence constitutes the "ABC's" of emergency care: ensure or establish a patent airway; monitor and support breathing; and monitor and support circulatory status. In the evaluation of circulatory status, bleeding should be controlled and then volume losses replaced.

Probable intra-abdominal bleeding is an emergency situation requiring rapid assessment and treatment. Paracentesis is a quick and reliable way to check for intra-abdominal bleeding. Roentgenography and sonography are useful to perform after paracentesis, but only if time permits.

Emergency room treatment of an open fracture is best accomplished by splinting and covering the wound. Reducing an open fracture should be performed by an orthopedist. Debridement can be done and antibiotic therapy started when time permits. Whether and when to close the wound are decisions usually made after all the measures mentioned above have been taken. *(Fleischer et al, pp 1089–1101)*

427–429. (427-A, 428-E, 429-C) Acetylcysteine (Mucomyst) is quite effective in the treatment of acetaminophen overdose. If treatment is begun within 16 hours of ingestion, hepatotoxicity is significantly reduced. Organic phosphates (eg, Malathion, Parathion) are cholinesterase inhibitors used as insecticides. Atropine is the drug of choice in the treatment of poisonings with these agents. Deferoxamine chelates unabsorbed iron (ferrous sulfate) and facilitates the removal of this potentially toxic substance. Methylene blue is used in the treatment of nitrite or nitrate poisoning and amyl nitrate in cyanide poisoning. *(Rudolph et al, pp 817–818,829–830,834–835,842–843)*

430–432. (430-A, 431-D, 432-C) Ventricular septal defect characteristically produces a high-pitched harsh, holosystolic murmur well-localized to the left sternal border. Pulmonary stenosis produces a systolic ejection murmur maximal at the upper left sternal border, often with radiation to the back. Diastolic murmurs sometimes are audible in patients with either ventricular or atrial septal defects, but these diastolic sounds are not as characteristic as the findings described above. A continuous "machinery" murmur is characteristic of patent ductus arteriosus. *(Rudolph et al, pp 1466–1468,1468–1471,1485–1487, 1462–1464)*

433–436. (433-D, 434-A, 435-B, 436-A) With the exception of the group B streptococci, *Escherichia coli* is the most common cause of neonatal sepsis and meningitis in many medical centers. *Haemophilus influenzae* type b is a prominent cause of serious invasive bacterial disease in children between 1 month and 6 years of age. Conditions associated with the organism include meningitis, pneumonia, periorbital and facial cellulitis, and epiglottitis. Occult bacteremia is caused most commonly by *Streptococcus pneumoniae; H. influenzae* type b and *Neisseria meningitidis* are the other common causes of this condition. Cervical adenitis can be caused by a variety of microorganisms, including not only group A streptococcus but also *Staphylococcus aureus*, mycobacteria, and anaerobes. *(Rudolph et al, pp 536–544)*

437–439. (437-E, 438-A, 439-A) Stevens-Johnson syndrome (erythema multiforme major) is a hypersensitivity reaction that is believed to be immune-complex–mediated. Cutaneous lesions often are bullous, and mucous membrane involvement and systemic toxicity generally are present. Medications and/or infectious agents often are linked etiologically. Both hand-foot-and-mouth syndrome and chickenpox characteristically produce vesicular skin lesions. The former condition usually is a summertime illness caused by a variety of coxsackieviruses. The name of the condition derives from the fact that affected individuals often manifest vesicular lesions of the hands and feet as well as oral ulcers. *(Rudolph et al, pp 907,966,684–686,936–937,2082)*

440–443. (440-C, 441-E, 442-B, 443-D) Target cells can be observed in a variety of conditions, including thalassemia, thalassemia trait, and sickle hemoglobinopathies. Generally, there are no characteristic peripheral blood smear findings in the anemia of chronic disease although a low mean corpuscular volume (MCV) may be noted. Folate and vitamin B_{12} deficiency are associated with megaloblastic red blood cell changes (high MCV) and hypersegmentation of polymorphonuclear leukocytes. Iron deficiency anemia is characterized by hypochromia and microcytosis. The peripheral blood smear obtained from an individual with hemolytic uremic syndrome will demonstrate fragmentation of red blood cells and a reduced number of platelets. *(Rudolph et al, p 1174–1175)*

444–447. (444-F, 445-A, 446-C, 447-G) Bronchiolitis may be caused by a variety of viral pathogens, including parainfluenza, influenza, and adenovirus, but respiratory syncytial virus is by far the most common etiologic agent. *Mycoplasma pneumoniae* is the single most common agent of pneumonia among adolescents and young adults. As is the case for adults, *Pneumocystis carinii* pneumonia is the most common AIDS-defining illness among infants and children with HIV infection. Group B streptococcus, enteric gram-negative bacilli, and *Listeria monocytogenes* are the most frequent causes of bacterial meningitis during the newborn period. *(Rudolph et al, pp 536–544,672–675,686–688,1655)*

448–452. (448-D, 449-B, 450-I, 451-C, 452-H) Gingival hyperplasia occurs in about 40% of individuals receiving phenytoin therapy. It does not appear to be related to dosage. Epidemiologic studies suggest a strong statistical association between aspirin use during the prodromal illness and development of Reye's syndrome. As a consequence, aspirin use is discouraged for children with influenza, chickenpox, and other common viral infections. Teeth may be stained yellow, brown, or gray as a result of tetracycline use during tooth formation. The drug generally should not be administered to children less than about 8 years of age. Red man syndrome is characterized by the presence of flushing, fever, chills, and paresthesias. It occurs during or shortly following vancomycin infusion and is thought to be histamine-mediated. Gray baby syndrome is a form of circulatory collapse associated with excessive serum concentrations of unconjugated chloramphenicol. Neonates are particularly susceptible to this complication because of immaturity of their hepatic drug-metabolizing enzymes. *(Rudolph et al, pp 505,508,965,985,1154)*

453–456. (453-D, 454-F, 455-A, 456-G) Lesch–Nyhan syndrome is a disorder of purine metabolism characterized by severe mental retardation, cerebral palsy, choreoathetosis, and self-destructive biting. It has an X-linked mode of inheritance. Chronic granulomatous disease is inherited primarily in an X-linked manner. Defective phagocyte oxidative function leads to a propensity for certain serious bacterial and fungal infections. Hemophilia B is another X-linked disease, which accounts for about 12% of all individuals with hemophilia. The clinical manifestations are indistinguishable from classic hemophilia. Tay–Sachs disease is a genetic disorder predominantly affecting individuals of Ashkenazi–Jewish descent and characterized by progressive neurologic deterioration and seizures, usually beginning during the first year of life. *(Rudolph et al, pp 324,1230–1231, 1245,2025–2026)*

REFERENCES

Dinarello CA, Cannon JG, Wolff SM. New concepts on the pathogenesis of fever. *Rev Infect Dis.* 1988; 10:168.

Feigin RD, Cherry JD. *Textbook of Pediatric Infectious Diseases.* 3rd ed. Philadelphia, Pa: WB Saunders Co; 1992.

Fleischer GR, Ludwig S. *Textbook of Pediatric Emergency Medicine.* Baltimore, Md: Williams & Wilkins; 1993.

Ginsburg CM, Henle W, Henle G. Infectious mononucleosis in children: evaluation of Epstein-Barr virus-specific serologic data. *JAMA.* 1977;237:781.

Lipson A, Beuhler B, Bartley J, Walsh D, et al. Maternal hyperphenylalaninemia fetal effects. *J. Pediatr.* 1984; 104:216–220.

Newth CJL. Recognition and management of respiratory failure. *Pediatr Clin North Am.* 1979;26:617–618.

Rogers MF. AIDS in children: a review of the clinical, epidemiologic and public health aspects. *Pediatr Infect Dis.* 1985;4:230–236.

Rudolph AM, Hoffman JIE, Rudolph CD. *Pediatrics.* 20th ed. Stamford, Conn: Appleton & Lange; 1996.

Saenger P. Abnormal sex differentiation. *J Pediatr.* 1984; 104:1–17.

Schmitt BD. Nocturnal enuresis: an update on treatment. *Pediatr Clin North Am.* 1982;29:21–36.

SUBSPECIALTY LIST: PEDIATRICS

Question Number and Subspecialty

401. Genetics
402. Infection
403. Psychosocial examination
404. Toxicology
405. Structure, genetics
406. Psychosocial history taking
407. Toxicology, congenital defects
408. Cardiology
409. Respiratory system
410. Infection
411. Toxicology
      Metabolic problems
      Use of laboratory
412. Infection
413. Metabolic problems
      Definition of problems
      Management
414. Infection
415. Structure
      Infection
416. Growth and development
417. Neoplastic disease
418. Health maintenance, infection
419. Idiopathy
420. Hematology
421. Neurology
422. Neurology
423. Emergency medicine
424. Emergency medicine
425. Emergency medicine
426. Emergency medicine
427. Toxicology
428. Toxicology
429. Toxicology
430. Cardiology
431. Cardiology
432. Cardiology
433. Infection
434. Infection
435. Infection
436. Infection
437. Skin
438. Skin
439. Skin
440. Hematology
441. Hematology
442. Hematology
443. Hematology
444. Infection
445. Infection
446. Infection
447. Infection
448. Toxicology
449. Toxicology
450. Toxicology
451. Toxicology
452. Toxicology
453. Genetics
454. Genetics
455. Genetics
456. Genetics

C. Internal Medicine

Catherine E. DuBeau, MD

457. Galactorrhea, amenorrhea, and infertility all appear in association with which of the following disorders?

    (A) hyperthyroidism
    (B) hyperprolactinemia
    (C) hyperadrenocorticism
    (D) excessive growth hormone secretion
    (E) hypothyroidism

458. The drug of choice in preventing attacks of hereditary angioedema is

    (A) aminocaproic acid (Amicar)
    (B) tranexamic acid
    (C) danazol (Danocrine)
    (D) hydroxyzine (Atarax)
    (E) diphenhydramine (Benadryl)

459. Lyme disease can be described by which of the following statements?

    (A) it is due to a spirochetal infection
    (B) it is due to a deficiency of vitamin C
    (C) it is an autoimmune disease
    (D) it usually begins with a monoarticular arthritis
    (E) it is best treated with erythromycin

460. Each of the following can cause hypoglycemia EXCEPT

    (A) beta blockers
    (B) hepatoma
    (C) pituitary insufficiency
    (D) chronic renal failure
    (E) multiple endocrine neoplasia (MEN) syndrome, type II

461. Which of the following statements about Cushing's disease is true?

    (A) serum adrenocorticotropin (ACTH) levels usually are low
    (B) pituitary microadenoma usually is present
    (C) there is a high incidence of nonendocrine tumors
    (D) nonsuppression of cortisol production by the high-dose dexamethasone suppression test is a characteristic finding
    (E) treatment of choice is bilateral adrenalectomy

462. Hypercalcemia would NOT be expected to occur as a result of

    (A) lung carcinoma
    (B) sarcoidosis
    (C) hypothyroidism
    (D) administration of thiazide drugs
    (E) administration of lithium

463. The most common cause of bacterial meningitis in adults is

   (A) *Streptococcus pneumoniae*
   (B) *Neisseria meningitidis*
   (C) *Hemophilus influenzae*
   (D) *Staphylococcus aureus*
   (E) *Staphylococcus epidermidis*

464. Zollinger–Ellison syndrome is associated with all of the following conditions or laboratory findings EXCEPT

   (A) severe peptic ulcer disease
   (B) diarrhea
   (C) basal gastric acid hypersecretion
   (D) hypergastrinemia
   (E) lack of response to secretin stimulation tests

465. The predominant immunoglobulin deposited in the glomeruli and skin of persons with Henoch–Schönlein purpura is

   (A) immunoglobulin A
   (B) immunoglobulin D
   (C) immunoglobulin E
   (D) immunoglobulin G
   (E) immunoglobulin M

466. The best test to determine the earliest signs of depletion of body iron stores is

   (A) plasma ferritin
   (B) plasma iron
   (C) plasma transferrin
   (D) red cell free protoporphyrin
   (E) bone marrow iron stain

467. The roentgenograms shown on page 130 are from a patient who has had a sudden onset of back pain. The vertebra most commonly affected by the disease process shown is

   (A) C-7
   (B) T-4
   (C) T-12
   (D) L-4
   (E) S-1

468. Primary biliary cirrhosis can be described by all of the following statements EXCEPT

   (A) 90% of affected individuals are men
   (B) pruritus, fatigue, and jaundice are common
   (C) serum transaminase levels are normal or slightly elevated
   (D) serum cholesterol level is elevated
   (E) the most common causes of death are hepatic failure and bleeding esophageal varices

469. Antimitochondrial antibodies are found in 90% of patients with

   (A) primary biliary cirrhosis
   (B) chronic active hepatitis
   (C) seminoma
   (D) choriocarcinoma
   (E) systemic lupus erythematosus

470. Common findings in hemochromatosis include all of the following EXCEPT

   (A) diabetes mellitus
   (B) diabetes insipidus
   (C) impotence
   (D) hepatocellular carcinoma
   (E) pseudogout

471. Mitral valve prolapse can be described by which of the following statements?

   (A) most affected individuals are asymptomatic
   (B) men are affected more often than women
   (C) ventricular arrhythmias are common
   (D) mitral regurgitation frequently develops
   (E) congestive heart failure frequently develops

Figures for use with question 467.

472. A 61-year-old man complains of weakness and loss of weight. His voice is hoarse. Examination reveals tongue enlargement, hepatomegaly, pedal edema, and a purpuric rash on the face and neck. Urinalysis shows a protein/creatinine ratio >4.0. Diagnosis may be made by

(A) liver-spleen scan
(B) 24-hour urine determination of protein
(C) subcutaneous fat biopsy
(D) urine protein electrophoresis
(E) urine protein immunophoresis

473. Acanthocytosis nigricans is NOT associated with

(A) Stein–Leventhal syndrome
(B) type II diabetes mellitus
(C) acromegaly
(D) adenocarcinoma of the colon
(E) starvation

474. A 65-year-old man presents with worsening shortness of breath, orthopnea, and paroxysmal nocturnal dyspnea. Examination reveals jugular venous distention, bibasilar rales, S₃ gallop, and pedal edema. His chest roentgenogram is shown on page 131. The physiologic abnormality NOT associated with this condition is

(A) increased sympathetic nervous system activity
(B) venous and arteriolar vasoconstriction
(C) increased myocardial contractility
(D) increased plasma renin activity
(E) decreased sodium and water excretion

Figure for use with question 474.

475. A 67-year-old executive who has coronary artery disease is to undergo elective cholecystectomy. Perioperative cardiac risk would be increased if

(A) jugular venous distention is present
(B) five premature ventricular contractions per minute are noted on ECG
(C) an S_4 gallop is heard
(D) he had coronary artery bypass grafting in the past
(E) general endotracheal anesthesia is used

476. A 48-year-old chef is admitted to the coronary care unit with chest pain and diaphoresis. During the next 24 hours he develops ECG changes and enzyme elevations typical of an acute myocardial infarction. On the second day he is found to have a new harsh systolic murmur. The most likely diagnosis is

(A) papillary muscle rupture
(B) left ventricular thrombus
(C) extension of the area of infarction
(D) coronary artery dissection
(E) aortic valve vegetation

Questions 477 through 479

A 25-year-old woman has intermittent diplopia. She says she chokes on her food and regurgitates it, sometimes through her nose. Physical examination reveals drooping eyelids and bilateral facial muscle weakness without atrophy; deep tendon reflexes are normal.

477. The most likely diagnosis for the woman described is

(A) familial periodic paralysis
(B) muscular dystrophy
(C) polymyositis
(D) myasthenia gravis
(E) multiple sclerosis

478. The pathogenesis of this woman's disorder involves

(A) an inflammatory process in the muscles
(B) antibodies directed against acetylcholine receptors
(C) slow-growing virus infection
(D) periodically depressed potassium levels
(E) a congenital inherited disorder

479. The best way to confirm this woman's diagnosis would be by

(A) observing long-term change in symptoms after injection of edrophonium
(B) observing long-term change in symptoms after administration of potassium
(C) demonstrating a decrease in muscle response to repetitive nerve stimulation
(D) demonstrating an increase in muscle response to repetitive nerve stimulation
(E) performing nerve conduction studies

Questions 480 and 481

A 35-year-old woman has systemic lupus erythematosus manifested only by polyarthritis, which is successfully treated with ibuprofen. Now, however, she presents with headache, stiff neck, and fever; examination of cerebrospinal fluid shows pleocytosis.

480. The first step in the management of this woman's disease would be to

   (A) start treatment with penicillin
   (B) start treatment with cortisone
   (C) start treatment with a third-generation cephalosporin and an aminoglycoside
   (D) increase ibuprofen dosage
   (E) stop ibuprofen

481. With the proper treatment, the woman's symptoms abate. Symptoms would likely return, however, if

   (A) antibiotics were stopped too soon
   (B) cortisone was stopped too abruptly
   (C) ibuprofen was restarted
   (D) immunosuppressive drug therapy was omitted
   (E) antibiotic coverage for anaerobic organisms was omitted

Questions 482 through 484

A 50-year-old woman suddenly develops extreme weakness in the proximal muscles of her hips and thighs and then the shoulder girdle. The ocular muscles are unaffected and the distal muscles are spared. There is mild atrophy of the affected muscles, and deep tendon reflexes are only slightly reduced. She does not complain of muscle pain.

482. The most likely diagnosis for the woman described is

   (A) polymyalgia rheumatica
   (B) muscular dystrophy
   (C) myasthenia gravis
   (D) polymyositis
   (E) thyrotoxicosis

483. The woman's diagnosis is best confirmed by which of the following tests?

   (A) sedimentation rate
   (B) serum creatine phosphokinase concentration
   (C) thyroid function tests
   (D) tensilon test
   (E) muscle biopsy

484. The treatment of choice for the woman's disease is

   (A) an anticholinesterase drug
   (B) an immunosuppressive drug
   (C) cortisone
   (D) thyroidectomy
   (E) thymectomy

DIRECTIONS (Questions 485 through 506): Each group of items in this section consists of lettered headings followed by a set of numbered words or phrases. For each numbered word or phrase, select the ONE lettered heading that is most closely associated with it. Each lettered heading may be selected once, more than once, or not at all.

Questions 485 through 488

For each deficiency of a component of complement listed below, select the disease state with which it is most likely to be associated.

   (A) recurrent *Neisseria* infection
   (B) recurrent pyogenic infection
   (C) recurrent urticaria
   (D) hereditary angioedema
   (E) systemic lupus erythematosus

485. CH_{50}

486. C3 deficiency

487. C8 deficiency

488. $C\overline{1}MINH$ deficiency

Questions 489 through 492

All the following drugs are used in treating ulcer disease. Match each drug with its mechanism of action.

(A) inhibits acid secretion by blocking the action of histamine on H_2 receptors

(B) inhibits *Helicobacter pylori*

(C) neutralizes gastric acid

(D) forms a protective coat over the ulcer crater by binding to necrotic ulcer tissue

(E) reduces serum gastrin concentration

A **489.** Cimetidine

C **490.** Antacids

B **491.** Antibiotics

D **492.** Sucralfate

Questions 493 through 496

For each set of clinical findings below, select the brain lesion most likely to be the cause.

(A) hemispheric lesion

(B) thalamic lesion

(C) midbrain lesion

(D) pontomedullary lesion

(E) none of the above

A **493.** Pupils reactive and 3 mm in diameter; intact ocular movements; localized response to painful stimuli

B **494.** Pupils reactive and 3 mm in diameter; intact ocular movements; decorticate posturing

C **495.** Pupils unreactive and 5 mm in diameter; unpaired ocular movements; decorticate posturing

D **496.** Pupils unreactive and 5 mm in diameter; ocular movements cannot be elicited; no motor response to pain

Questions 497 through 500

For each disease listed below, select the associated physical finding.

(A) decreased fremitus, trachea shifted toward affected side

(B) increased fremitus

(C) absent fremitus

(D) hyperresonance, low diaphragms

(E) decreased fremitus, trachea shifted away from affected side

C **497.** Pneumothorax

D **498.** Bronchial asthma

A **499.** Lobar obstruction

B **500.** Pneumonia

Questions 500 through 504

For each statement listed below, select the associated abnormality.

(A) aortic stenosis

(B) mitral stenosis

(C) aortic regurgitation

(D) tricuspid regurgitation

(E) idiopathic hypertrophic subaortic stenosis

D **501.** May be a complication of an inferior wall infarction

C **502.** Associated with largest degree of left ventricular thickening

B **503.** Atrial arrythmias and recurrent pulmonary embolism feared complications

A **504.** Loudness of murmur can be misleading in severe cases

Questions 505 and 506

For the nutrients listed below, select the appropriate statement.

    (A) body stores are limited

    (B) must be replaced parenterally in deficiency states

    (C) neurological abnormalities may occur in the absence of anemia

    (D) small intestinal bacteria an important source

    (E) agonist drug interactions important cause of anemia

505. Folate

506. Cobalamin (Vitamin B_{12})

DIRECTIONS (Questions 507 through 519): Each of the numbered items or incomplete statements in this section is followed by answers or by completions of the statement. Select the ONE lettered answer or completion that is BEST in each case.

507. *Staphylococcus aureus* endocarditis in intravenous drug abusers

    (A) is less common than *Staphylococcus epidermitis* endocarditis

    (B) preferentially involves the tricuspid valve

    (C) should not be treated with valve replacement surgery

    (D) is commonly associated with murmurs and peripheral stigmata

    (E) rarely results in septic pulmonary emboli

508. Diagnostic features of allergic bronchopulmonary aspergillosis include all of the following EXCEPT

    (A) eosinophilia

    (B) positive skin test for *Aspergillus fumigatus*

    (C) precipitans to *Aspergillus*

    (D) peripheral bronchiectasis on chest roentgenogram

    (E) sputum cultures positive for *Aspergillus*

509. The factor that signifies a good prognosis in rheumatoid arthritis is

    (A) eosinophilia

    (B) female sex

    (C) thrombocytosis

    (D) low rheumatoid factor titers

    (E) age over 65 years

510. A routine lipid screen in a 32-year-old woman reveals hypertriglyceridemia. Secondary causes to be ruled out exclude

    (A) hyperthyroidism

    (B) loop diuretics

    (C) inhaled beta agonists

    (D) use of progestins

    (E) excessive alcohol consumption

511. A 60-year-old man with malignant lymphoma presents with the findings seen in the picture on page 135. These findings last for 2 to 4 days and recur periodically. This condition differs from its related hereditary form by low levels of

    (A) $\overline{C1}INH$

    (B) C1

    (C) C4

    (D) C5

    (E) C2

512. Propylthiouracil is useful in the treatment of hyperthyroidism. Its action does NOT include

    (A) blocking the organification and coupling process

    (B) inhibiting iodine trapping and organification

    (C) blocking proteolysis of hormone from thyroglobulin

    (D) blocking hormone release

    (E) inhibiting peripheral conversion of T4 to T3

Figure for use with question 511.

513. A late complication of the acquired immuno-deficiency syndrome is

(A) progressive weight loss
(B) *Pneumocystis carinii* pneumonia
(C) cognitive impairment
(D) Kaposi's sarcoma
(E) Candida esophagitis

514. An immunologic abnormality usually associated with the acquired immunodeficiency syndrome is

(A) decreased levels of IgG
(B) decreased levels of IgA
(C) decreased number of B lymphocytes
(D) decreased number of T8 lymphocytes
(E) anergy in delayed hypersensitivity tests

515. Evidence of infection with hepatitis B virus is seen in association with which of the following disease states?

(A) Henoch–Schönlein purpura
(B) mixed cryoglobulinemia
(C) Wegener's granulomatosis
(D) Sjögren's syndrome
(E) proliferative glomerulonephritis

516. A 63-year-old man complains of worsening headache and right-sided weakness. CT of the head is shown below. The most likely diagnosis is

(A) aneurysmal bleed
(B) brain tumor
(C) lacunar infarct
(D) vasculitis
(E) toxoplasmosis infection

517. Bacteremia resulting from contaminated intravenous fluids is most likely to be caused by

(A) *Staphylococcus aureus*

(B) *Staphylococcus epidermidis*

(C) *Escherichia coli*

(D) *Enterobacter agglomerans*

(E) *Candida albicans*

518. A 43-year-old man complains of fatigue, headache, anorexia, and a dull ache in the left upper quadrant of his abdomen. Examination reveals a mass extending just below the left costal margin; the mass is presumed to be an enlarged spleen. Which of the following would NOT be a possible cause of this man's illness?

(A) Polycythemia vera

(B) idiopathic thrombocytopenic purpura

(C) folate deficiency

(D) brucellosis

(E) immune hemolytic anemia

519. A 26-year-old man is found to have acute leukemia. Three weeks after initiation of chemotherapy he has a body temperature spike to 38.9°C (102°F), with a white blood cell count of 500/mm. Which of the following is true regarding this clinical situation?

(A) antibiotics should be given if a source of infection can be identified

(B) normal chest roentgenographic findings would eliminate pneumonia as the cause of the fever

(C) bacteremia, if present, would most likely be caused by *Pseudomonas* and other gram-negative bacilli

(D) chemotherapy and tumor lysis are the most likely cause of fever

(E) empiric antifungal therapy should be initiated immediately

ANSWERS AND EXPLANATIONS

457. **(B)** Galactorrhea, amenorrhea, and infertility together are suggestive of excessive secretion of prolactin by the pituitary gland. Hyperprolactinemia is the most common pituitary hypersecretory disorder and occurs in almost 20% of women with secondary amenorrhea. Women who have prolactin levels less than 25 ng/ml and galactorrhea resulting from an increased sensitivity of their mammary glands to prolactin usually do not have amenorrhea. Amenorrhea may be associated with hyperadrenocorticism and hypothyroidism but usually not with galactorrhea. *(Isselbacher, pp 2025–2029)*

458. **(C)** The drugs of choice in preventing attacks of hereditary angioedema are the anabolic steroids with diminished androgenic effects, such as danazol and stanozolol. These drugs not only decrease the number of recurrent attacks but also stimulate the synthesis of normal $\overline{C1}$MINH in affected persons. ε-Aminocaproic acid and tranexamic acid, which inhibit the conversion of plasminogen to plasmin, previously were used to prevent attacks. Antihistamines, such as hydroxyzine and diphenhydramine, should not be used in the treatment or prevention of hereditary angioedema. *(Isselbacher, pp 1634–1638)*

459. **(A)** Lyme disease is due to the spirochete *Borrelia burgdorferi* transmitted by the tick *Ixodes dammini*. The initial sign usually is a characteristic skin lesion, erythema chronicum migrans, that typically develops on the trunk or lower body. Later on, affected persons experience recurrent attacks of arthritis. The disease resolves faster in patients treated with either penicillin or tetracycline; erythromycin is not an effective treatment of Lyme disease. *(Isselbacher, pp 745–747)*

460. **(E)** Hypoglycemia can occur in MEN I (Wermer's syndrome), which includes islet cell tumors as well as hyperparathyroidism and pituitary adenomas. Hypoglycemia is not a complication of MEN II (Sipple's syndrome), characterized by hyperparathroidism, medullary carcinoma of the thyroid, and pheochromocytoma. Beta blockers, sulfonylureas, insulin, salicylates, and alcohol can cause hypoglycemia. Hepatomas and other extrapancreatic tumors may provoke hypoglycemia through unknown mechanisms. Hypoglycemia may occur in pituitary insufficiency as a result of the absent or reduced secretion of growth hormone and ACTH. In many adults, however, hypoglycemia can be prevented by glucocorticoid replacement alone. Hypoglycemia occurs in some patients with chronic renal failure. One suggested cause is that marked muscle wasting reduces the availability of alanine from muscle for use by the liver and kidney in gluconeogenesis. *(Isselbacher, pp 2000–2006)*

461. **(B)** Cushing's *syndrome* is due to increased adrenal cortisol production, regardless of etiology. Cushing's *disease* usually is caused by a pituitary microadenoma producing high adrenocorticotropin (ACTH) levels. In most patients, cortisol levels would be suppressed as a result of the high-dose dexamethasone suppression test. Transsphenoidal microsurgical removal of the microadenoma is the treatment of choice in most centers. *(Isselbacher, pp 1960–1965)*

462. **(C)** Hypercalcemia often is associated with malignancies and is due either to skeletal metastasis or to a humoral substance secreted by the tumor. Hypercalcemia accompanying sarcoidosis appears to be due to enhanced synthesis of vitamin D. Thiazide diuretics cause hypercalcemia by decreasing the urinary clearance of calcium. Lithium may cause a mild hypercalcemia by elevating plasma parathormone levels. Calcium levels in persons with hypothyroidism are either normal or low as a result of decreased bone turnover. *(Isselbacher, pp 2151–2165)*

463. **(A)** *Streptococcus pneumoniae* is responsible for between 30 and 50% of cases of bacterial meningitis in adults, and *Neisseria meningi-*

tidis between 10 and 35% of cases. *Hemophilus influenzae* meningitis occurs primarily in children, and group B *Streptococcus* meningitis usually affects infants. *Staphylococcus* is the most common cause of bacterial meningitis associated with shunting procedures. Acute otitis media and mastoiditis, recent head injury, sickle cell anemia, chronic alcoholism, immunoglobulin deficiency, and splenectomy all predispose to infection with *S. pneumoniae*. *(Isselbacher, pp 2296–2302)*

464. **(E)** The Zollinger–Ellison syndrome is characterized by severe peptic ulcer disease and, in many patients, diarrhea. Basal gastric acid hypersecretion and hypergastrinemia are due to the presence of pancreatic gastrinomas, which are nonbeta islet-cell tumors. Serum gastrin levels increase markedly following the injection of secretin or gastrointestinal hormone (GIH). In normal subjects and in persons with duodenal ulcer, serum gastrin levels either do not increase or increase slightly after secretin stimulation. Most affected individuals can be successfully treated with H_2-receptor antagonists, such as cimetidine, at higher dosages than are used to treat common duodenal ulcers. An attempt also should be made to remove the gastrinoma. *(Isselbacher, pp 1375–1377)*

465. **(A)** Henoch–Schönlein purpura is one of the few diseases in which immunoglobulin A (IgA) is the predominant immunoglobulin deposited in the glomeruli and skin. In many other glomerulopathies, IgG and IgM are the predominant immunoglobulins deposited in glomeruli. Henoch-Schönlein purpura generally has a benign course characterized by arthralgias, abdominal pain, and nonthrombocytopenic purpura in addition to glomerulonephritis. However, progressive renal failure may occur in a small percentage of patients. Treatment is usually symptomatic. *(Isselbacher, pp 1674)*

466. **(E)** A stain of the bone marrow with Prussian blue stain detects depletion of marrow iron stores, the earliest sign of iron deficiency. As the extent of iron deficiency increases, plasma ferritin levels fall and subsequently there is a rise in plasma transferrin. Plasma iron and transferrin saturation fall and free erythrocyte protoporphyrin increases when the amount of available iron declines below the minimal amount required for erythropoiesis. *(Isselbacher, pp 1723–1725)*

467. **(C)** The most common site of vertebral fracture in persons with idiopathic osteoporosis is middle and lower thoracic and upper lumbar vertebral bodies. More caudal or distal fractures are less likely to be due to idiopathic osteoporosis. Osteoporosis occurs most frequently in postmenopausal women but also occurs in younger women and in men. It is important to rule out secondary and potentially reversible forms of osteoporosis, such as glucocorticoid excess, hyperparathyroidism, thyrotoxicosis, multiple myeloma, and immobilization. Both estrogen supplementation and calcium supplementation have been shown to retard postmenopausal bone loss, but the increased risk of endometrial carcinoma with estrogen replacement may make this a less acceptable treatment. *(Isselbacher, pp 2172–2177)*

468. **(A)** Primary biliary cirrhosis, an uncommon type of cirrhosis, is associated with the presence of antimitochondrial antibodies. Ninety percent of patients with primary biliary cirrhosis are women. The disease has an insidious onset: fatigue and pruritus are early symptoms. Hyperlipidemia, especially elevation of unesterified cholesterol, is common in affected individuals. Serum alkaline phosphatase levels are very high but transaminase levels are normal or only slightly elevated. The most common causes of death are hepatic failure and bleeding from esophageal varices. *(Isselbacher, pp 1487–1488)*

469. **(A)** The most characteristic immunologic abnormality associated with primary biliary cirrhosis is the presence of antimitochondrial antibodies, which are found in 90% of affected individuals. This antibody is predominantly IgG. Antimitochondrial antibodies also can be detected in persons with other liver diseases but with a much lower frequency (less than 10%) and usually in low titer. *(Isselbacher, pp 1487–1488)*

470. **(B)** In hemochromatosis the principal organs involved with excessive iron storage, leading to parenchymal damage and fibrosis, are the liver, pancreas, heart, and gonads. Diabetes occurs in the majority of patients and more than 80% demonstrate abnormalities of glucose tolerance. Testicular atrophy and fibrosis cause impotence. Diabetes insipidus does not occur because the pituitary and hypothalamus are not involved. Cirrhosis is usually present when the diagnosis is established, and hepatocellular carcinoma develops in 25 to 40% of patients. Chondrocalcinosis (pseudogout) is found in 25 to 50% of patients. Other common manifestations include cardiac involvement with congestive heart failure and arrhythmias. Melanin deposition causes increased skin pigmentation with a characteristic slate gray color. *(Isselbacher, pp 2069–2073)*

471. **(A)** Most patients with mitral valve prolapse are asymptomatic. Ventricular arrhythmias are uncommon, and mitral valve regurgitation and congestive heart failure develop infrequently. Women are affected more commonly than men. *(Isselbacher, pp 1058–1059)*

472. **(C)** The clinical features of the patient described in the question suggest amyloidosis, a disorder characterized by extracellular deposition of fibrous protein in various tissues and organs. Amyloidosis may be primary or may be associated with an underlying disease such as myeloma or rheumatoid arthritis. It may present with skin lesions, macroglossia, hepatomegaly, malabsorption, proteinuria, congestive cardiomyopathy, or orthostatic hypotension. Diagnosis is based on the typical findings and demonstration of amyloid fibrils by Congo red staining under polarized light. Abdominal subcutaneous fat pad aspirate or rectal submucosal biopsy are often performed. Bone marrow, kidney, liver, skin, and endomyocardial biopsy specimens may also show positive findings. Liver scan

findings are nonspecific for amyloidosis, as is the amount of protein in a 24-hour urine specimen. Urine protein electrophoresis and immunophoresis testing can help establish whether amyloidosis is immunoglobulin-related, but they are not diagnostic of amyloidosis. *(Isselbacher, pp 1625–1630)*

473. **(E)**   Acanthosis nigricans is a velvety hyperpigmentation, typically found on the neck, axillae, and groin. It is most commonly associated with obesity but also is associated with gastrointestinal malignancies and endocrinopathies, including insulin-resistant diabetes mellitus, the Stein–Leventhal syndrome, acromegaly, Cushing's disease and Addison's disease. *(Isselbacher, pp 297–298)*

474. **(C)**   The chest roentgenogram that accompanies the question displays cardiomegaly and bilateral pulmonary vascular congestion with cephalad redistribution of the vessels. Together with the history and examination, these findings are consistent with a diagnosis of congestive heart failure. Several adaptive mechanisms allow the normal heart to continue to function in the face of changing loads: the Frank–Starling principle (increased resting muscle length allows increased muscle tension), increased adrenergic tone (which increases heart rate and contractility), and myocardial hypertrophy and dilation. When these mechanisms fail, CHF occurs. Physiologic abnormalities that may accompany CHF include arteriolar and venous constriction (as a result of increased sympathetic tone), increased renin activity (a result of renal vasoconstriction), increased aldosterone levels, and increased proximal tubular reabsorption of sodium and water. *(Isselbacher, pp 998–1009)*

475. **(A)**   Physicians are often confronted with the difficult task of evaluating for noncardiac surgery those patients with known cardiac disease. The best-studied group of such patients are those with coronary artery disease, for whom several risk factors have been identified. Previous myocardial infarction (especially within the last 6 months), age beyond

70 years, jugular venous distention, and S$_3$ gallop, aortic stenosis, rhythm other than sinus, more than five premature ventricular contractions per minute, emergency procedures, and thoracic, aortic, or upper abdominal surgery all increase the risk of surgery. Conversely, the patient's sex, location of the previous MI, method of anesthesia, stable angina pectoris, and previous coronary artery bypass grafting have not been associated with increased risk. *(Goldman)*

476. **(A)**   A new systolic murmur appearing after an acute infarct requires immediate evaluation because it may indicate a lesion requiring surgical correction. Mitral regurgitation resulting from papillary muscle rupture occurs in almost 1% of all affected persons and may progress quickly to severe congestive failure. Papillary muscle dysfunction without actual rupture may also result in a new murmur. Interventricular septal rupture may occur; it progresses to cardiogenic shock in almost 50% of cases. Ventricular aneurysm formation is another cause of a new murmur following an infarction. Left ventricular thrombus formation is an associated complication but is clinically silent and usually is detected by echocardiography. Coronary artery dissection is a cause, not a consequence of a heart and does not usually cause a murmur. Extension of the area of infarction would not in itself cause a new murmur. Murmurs resulting from valvular vegetations occur in endocarditis, which would be unlikely in this setting. *(Isselbacher, pp 1066–1077)*

477. **(D)**   The woman described has typical signs and symptoms of myasthenia gravis. Women in the third decade of life are most commonly affected. Ocular weakness is a very common presenting sign and is usually transitory. Facial and pharyngeal muscle weakness also are common. *(Isselbacher, pp 2393–2396)*

478. **(B)**   It is now believed that myasthenia gravis is an autoimmune disease. Most patients (85%) produce antibodies that bind to acetylcholine receptors. (Complement is also found on the receptors.) Affected skele-

tal muscle is unable to synthesize acetylcholine receptors at a rate sufficient to enable the muscle to function properly. *(Isselbacher, pp 2393–2396)*

479. **(C)** Demonstrating a characteristic decreased response of affected muscle to repetitive nerve stimulation is important in the diagnosis of myasthenia gravis. Injection of neostigmine may be used for diagnosis if the edrophonium test is equivocal. *(Isselbacher, pp 2393–2396)*

480–481. **(480-E, 481-C)** Systemic lupus erythematosus can cause a number of unusual drug side effects. For example, administration of ibuprofen for arthritis can lead to aseptic meningitis, which subsides when the drug is withdrawn but returns if the drug is reintroduced. Salicylate hepatitis is more common in persons with systemic lupus erythematosus. These persons also seem to develop decreased renal blood flow at a greater rate than in unaffected persons when given any nonsteroidal antiinflammatory drug. *(Isselbacher, pp 1643–1648)*

482–484. **(482-D, 483-E, 484-C)** Polymyositis is an inflammatory disease that usually involves the proximal muscles of the upper and lower extremities. Ocular muscles are unaffected, unlike myasthenia gravis, and there is minimal atrophy. This syndrome may occur as an isolated illness or in association with a characteristic skin rash (dermatomyositis). Polymyositis may also be associated with such malignancies as lung, breast, colon, and prostate cancer. The diagnosis of polymyositis is confirmed by muscle biopsy showing an inflammatory reaction and widespread destruction of muscle fibers. Ancillary findings include elevated serum levels of creatine phosphokinase, aldolase, glutamicoxaloacetic transaminase, and lactic dehydrogenase. Sedimentation rate also is elevated, and electromyograms are abnormal. Cortisone is the drug of choice for the treatment of polymyositis. If this treatment fails, immunosuppressive drugs can be tried. The end point of initial therapy is restoration of strength and normalization of muscle enzymes. Although drug therapy may sometimes be discontinued, most patients require long-term treatment. *(Isselbacher, pp 2379–2383)*

485–488. **(485-E, 486-B, 487-A, 488-D)** Deficiencies in complement components are associated with rheumatic disorders, especially systemic lupus erythematosus; total functional hemolytic complement (CH_{50}) may be low. Also, complement deficiencies have been associated with Henoch-Schönlein purpura. C3 has a central role in both the classical and alternate pathways of complement activation. Deficiency of C3 is associated with recurrent pyogenic infections, which are often severe and life-threatening. Deficiencies of C6, C7, and C8 are associated with recurrent meningococcal meningitis or gonacoccal arthritis.

A deficiency of $\overline{C1}$MINH as well as the presence of nonfunctioning $\overline{C1}$MINH is associated with hereditary recurrent and sometimes life-threatening angioedema. Increased vascular permeability in this syndrome is mediated by a kininlike substance liberated from C2 by the unopposed action of C1 esterase and plasmin. Prophylactic use of anabolic steroids with attenuated androgenic effects raises the levels of $\overline{C1}$MINH and prevents attacks of angioedema. *(Isselbacher, pp 1554–1555,1558–1559)*

489–492. **(489-A, 490-C, 491-B, 492-D)** A variety of agents are available to treat ulcer disease. Cimetidine inhibits gastric acid secretion by blocking the action of histamine on H_2 receptors. Patients with duodenal ulcer are treated for 4 to 6 weeks, whereas patients with gastric ulcer are treated until the ulcer heals, as demonstrated either by roentgenography or endoscopy. It has also been shown that a bedtime dose of cimetidine prevents recurrent duodenal ulceration in most patients. Antacids neutralize gastric acid and when given 1 and 3 hours after meals and at bedtime are effective in promoting the healing of duodenal ulcers. It is not known if prophylactic therapy with antacids prevents recurrent duodenal ulcers. Antibiotic regimens can eradicate *Helicobacter pylori* infection, which may be an important etiologic agent in some duodenal ulcers. Sucralfate heals ulcers by forming a protective coat over the ulcer crater by binding to necrotic ulcer tissue; in addition, it absorbs bile acids. It may be used as the primary treatment of duodenal ulcer disease. *(Isselbacher, pp 1363–1382)*

493–496.   (493-A, 494-B, 495-C, 496-D)   In evaluating a comatose patient, a physician must determine the level of the lesion and thus the severity of the coma. The site of supratentorial structural lesions of the central nervous system can be localized according to the pattern of clinical findings. Individuals with hemispheric lesions have reactive pupils 3 mm in diameter, intact ocular movements, and a localized motor response to painful stimuli. As the lesion progresses to the thalamic level, decorticate posturing develops. When the defect involves the midbrain, the pupils enlarge (5 mm) and become unreactive, and ocular movements are impaired. When the process affects the pontomedullary portion of the brain, ocular movements cannot be elicited, and there is no motor response to painful stimuli. It is very important to differentiate between supratentorial lesions and a metabolic encephalopathy in a comatose patient in order to know whether surgical intervention or medical therapy is needed. In patients with metabolic coma, anatomic localization is not possible: scattered, anatomically inconsistent central nervous system findings are found on examination. For example, findings of a pontomedullary lesion may be associated with hemispheric signs in the same patient. *(Isselbacher, pp 146–153)*

497–500.   (497-C, 498-D, 499-A, 500-B)   Careful physical examination is often very helpful in the diagnosis of common pulmonary diseases. Pneumothorax is characterized by absent fremitus, hyperresonant or tympanic percussion, and absent breath sounds on auscultation; the diaphragm would be in the normal position. Hyperresonance also is found in bronchial asthma, associated also

with low diaphragm (from hyperinflation), prolonged expiration, and inspiratory and expiratory wheezes. Lobar obstruction or atelectasis is associated with decreased fremitus with a tracheal shift toward the affected side, dullness on percussion, and absent breath sounds. On the other hand, a consolidation from pneumonia would have increased fremitus, percussive dullness, and bronchial breath sounds. Large pleural effusions are associated with decreased fremitus and tracheal deviation away from the affected side. *(Isselbacher, pp 1145–1146)*

501–504.   (501-D, 502-C, 503-B, 504-A)   Tricuspid regurgitation is often functional and can occur when right ventricular papillary muscles are damaged by an inferior infarction. Both chronic aortic stenosis and aortic regurgitation often result in left ventricular dilation and hypertrophy; however, the increase in left ventricular end-diastolic volume that occurs with aortic regurgitation can result in tremendous left ventricular thickening, with hearts at autopsy weighing up to 1000 g. Atrial arrhythmias occur with increasing frequency as the course of moderately severe mitral stenosis progresses; recurrent pulmonary emboli are an important cause of morbidity late in the course. While the murmur of aortic stenosis is generally grade 3/4 in patients with moderately severe obstruction, when severe stenosis is accompanied by heart failure the murmur may be soft and brief. *(Isselbacher, pp 939–940)*

505–506.   (505-A, 506-C)   Since folate stores in the body are limited, deficiency occurs within several months if dietary intake or intestinal absorption decreases. Drugs that antagonize folate metabolism, usually by inhibiting dihydrofolate reductase, are a very common cause of megaloblastic anemia. Because the dietary intake of cobalamin, or vitamin B_{12}, is usually greater than daily requirements, body stores are usually built up and sustained. Overgrowth of small intestinal bacteria may divert cobalamin from the host, resulting in anemia; treatment with antibiotics may eliminate the problem. Neurological abnormalities in cobalamin deficiency are caused by demyelination in the peripheral nerves, spinal cord, and cerebrum; these may be evident even when the hematocrit and red blood cell indices are normal. (Isselbacher, pp 1728–1730)

507. **(B)** Over half the cases of endocarditis in intravenous drug abusers are caused by *Staphylococcus aureus*. The tricuspid valve is preferentially involved (50% of cases), followed by the aortic (25%) and mitral (20%) valves. Cardiac murmurs and peripheral stigmata are rare with endocarditis in intravenous drug abusers, especially when the tricuspid valve is involved. Septic and aseptic pulmonary emboli are common. If positive blood cultures persist on antibiotic therapy for the treatment of endocarditis, surgical valve replacement is necessary in all cases. (Isselbacher, pp 565–566)

508. **(D)** Bronchopulmonary aspergillosis occurs in individuals with extrinsic asthma whose airways become a culture medium for *Aspergillus fumigatus*. Clinical criteria used to establish a diagnosis of bronchopulmonary aspergillosis include a history of pulmonary infiltrates, the presence of asthmatic symptoms, and a positive immediate skin test to *A. fumigatus*. Precipitins to *Aspergillus*, sputum cultures growing *Aspergillus*, and eosinophilia are important laboratory findings. Chest roentgenograms typically show central bronchiectasis. (Isselbacher, pp 861–862)

509. **(D)** Rheumatoid arthritis tends to be less severe in males than in females. Also, the disease generally is less severe if associated with an acute onset rather than an insidious onset, which is more common. Eosinophilia and thrombocytosis are associated with a poorer prognosis. (Isselbacher, pp 1648–1655)

510. **(E)** The many causes of secondary hypertriglyceridemia include hypothyroidism, chronic renal failure, nephrotic syndrome, diabetes mellitus, glycogen storage disease, acute stress states, and rarely the dysgammaglobulinemias (multiple myeloma, macro-globulinemia, and systemic lupus erythematosus). Drugs that may raise triglyceride levels are thiazide diuretics, beta blockers, estrogens, corticosteroids, and retinoids. Women who start with modest triglyceride elevations can have enormous increases in their triglyceride levels and face the risk of attacks of acute pancreatitis when placed on oral contraceptives. Corticosteroids often raise triglyceride levels, sometimes in association with the development of glucose intolerance. Hypertriglyceridemia, at times severe, is a common side effect of the use of retinoids. (Wyngaarden et al, p 1087)

511. **(A)** The picture shows an angioedematous eruption on the right hand, which is associated with the absence of C1MINH. Lymphoproliferative disorders such as malignant lymphoma are associated with an acquired form of C1MINH deficiency that differs from hereditary angioedema (familial C1MINH deficiency) in its lack of a familial element and reduction in C1/C1. C2 and C4 are reduced in both disorders. C5a is an anaphylatoxin. (Isselbacher, pp 1554–1556)

512. **(B)** Steps involved in the synthesis of thyroid hormone include (1) trapping of iodine by follicular cells; (2) organification of the iodine by linking it to tyrosines on thyroglobulin; (3) coupling two of these tyrosines to form iodothyronines; and (4) proteolysis and release of thyroid hormones from thyroglobulin stored as colloid in the follicular lumen. Tetraiodothyronine (T_4) is converted in peripheral tissues to triiodothyronine (T_3). Propylthiouracil blocks organification and coupling within the thyroid and also reduces the conversion of T_4 to T_3. (Wyngaarden, pp 1248–1271)

513. **(C)** Persons with acquired immunodeficiency syndrome (AIDS) frequently present with opportunistic infections, especially *Pneumocystis carinii* pneumonia. Also common in these persons is the otherwise rare dermal malignancy, Kaposi's sarcoma. One of the most striking early clinical features is progressive weight loss out of proportion

to any reduction in food intake. *Candida* esophagitis usually occurs at the onset of the disease or in the course of therapy for opportunistic infections. Cognitive impairment from AIDS-related dementia, however, usually occurs later in the course of the disease. *(Isselbacher, pp 1566–1618)*

514. **(E)** Patients with acquired immunodeficiency syndrome have a profound immunologic deficit similar to that associated with DiGeorge syndrome. Lymphopenia is usually present along with skin-test anergy because the immunodeficiency is largely within the T lymphocyte population. Numbers of B lymphocytes usually are normal. Levels of IgG and IgA usually are elevated in response to opportunistic infections. *(Isselbacher, pp 1566–1618)*

515. **(B)** Two thirds of patients with mixed cryoglobulinemia have evidence of infection with hepatitis B virus. This virus also has been found in the serum of 30 to 40% of patients with polyarteritis nodosa. Because hepatitis B virus has been found in vascular lesions along with immunoglobulin and complement, vasculitis in these individuals might be due to immune complexes containing the hepatitis antigen. *(Isselbacher, pp 1458–1480)*

516. **(B)** The CT scan that accompanies the question reveals near the left cortex a solitary, rounded, discrete lesion that enhances with contrast and has mild surrounding edema. The history, examination, and CT scan suggest a brain tumor, either primary or metastatic. Further work-up should be aimed at uncovering an occult primary tumor, if any. Common sources occur at the lungs, kidneys, colon, and breasts. Chest roentgenogram, intravenous pyelography, gastrointestinal series, or mammography might therefore be indicated. A myelogram or lymphangiogram would not be helpful for most patients. If an occult primary tumor cannot be found, biopsy of the brain lesion may be indicated. *(Stein, pp 2220–2222)*

517. **(D)** Infections with contaminated intravenous infusions involve organisms that are potentially pathogenic and survive well in water. These include *Enterobacter agglomerans, Pseudomonas cepacia, Citrobacter freundii, Klebsiella,* and *Serratia*. A large-scale national epidemic involved *Enterobacter agglomerans,* which became suspect when a large number of patients receiving IV fluids from one supplier developed bacteremia with this relatively uncommon blood culture isolate. *(Isselbacher, pp 583–586)*

518. **(C)** The mass extending below the left costal margin is likely an enlarged spleen. Splenomegaly has an extensive differential diagnosis that falls into several general categories: infections (eg, acute bacterial infections), diseases of disordered immunoregulation (eg, Felty's syndrome), conditions with disordered splenic blood flow (eg, cirrhosis and idiopathic thrombocytopenic purpura), diseases with abnormal erythrocytes (eg, spherocytosis), infiltration by abnormal material (eg, amyloidosis), extramedullary hematopoiesis (polycythemia vera), and malignant tumors (eg, lymphoma). Folate deficiency causes anemia but not splenomegaly. *(Wyngaarden, pp 982–983)*

519. **(C)** The leading cause of death in cancer patients is infection. Fever developing during the course of treatment for cancer demands careful investigation for infection by all classes of pathogens: bacteria, viruses, yeasts, and protozoans. Pneumonia is common but difficult to diagnose. There is scant sputum production, and often the chest roentgenographic findings are misleadingly normal. Gram-negative bacilli are responsible for most pneumonias and bacteremias. The skin, mucous membranes, and catheter sites are common portals of entry. In the absence of an obvious source of infection, it is essential to begin empirical antibiotic therapy aimed at the most common organisms. An antipseudomonal penicillin plus an aminoglycoside is a commonly used regimen. Both chemotherapy and the tumor lysis syndrome can cause fever, but infection is much more likely to be the cause. *(Wyngaarden, pp 1067–1072)*

REFERENCES

Isselbacher KJ, Braunwald E, Wilson JD, et al, eds. *Harrison's Principles of Internal Medicine.* 13th ed. New York, NY: McGraw-Hill Book Co; 1994.

Goldman L, Caldera DL, Nussbaum SR, et al. Multifactorial index of cardiac risk in noncardiac surgical patients. *N Engl J Med.* 1977;297:845.

Stein JH, ed. *Internal Medicine.* Boston, Mass: Little, Brown & Co; 1987.

Wyngaarden JB, Smith LH Jr, Bennett JC, eds. *Cecil's Textbook of Medicine.* 19th ed. Philadelphia, Pa: WB Saunders Co; 1992.

SUBSPECIALTY LIST: INTERNAL MEDICINE

Question Number and Subspecialty

457. Endocrinology
458. Allergy and immunology
459. Infectious disease
460. Endocrinology
461. Endocrinology
462. Endocrinology
463. Infectious disease
464. Gastroenterology
465. Nephrology
466. Blood diseases
467. Rheumatology
468. Gastroenterology
469. Gastroenterology
470. Gastroenterology
471. Cardiology
472. Rheumatology
473. Blood disorders
474. Cardiovascular system diseases
475. Cardiovascular system diseases
476. Cardiovascular system diseases
477. Neurology
478. Neurology
479. Neurology
480. Rheumatology
481. Rheumatology
482. Rheumatology
483. Rheumatology
484. Rheumatology
485. Allergy and immunology
486. Allergy and immunology
487. Allergy and immunology
488. Allergy and immunology
489. Gastroenterology
490. Gastroenterology
491. Gastroenterology
492. Gastroenterology
493. Neurology
494. Neurology
495. Neurology
496. Neurology
497. Pulmonary medicine
498. Pulmonary medicine
499. Pulmonary medicine
500. Pulmonary medicine
501. Cardiology
502. Cardiology
503. Cardiology
504. Cardiology
505. Internal medicine
506. Internal medicine
507. Infectious disease
508. Allergy and immunology
509. Rheumatology
510. Endocrinology
511. Allergy and immunology
512. Endocrinology
513. Allergy and immunology
514. Allergy and immunology
515. Rheumatology
516. Neurology
517. Infectious diseases
518. Gastroenterology
519. Oncology

Surgery

Morris D. Kerstein, MD and David Coll, MD

DIRECTIONS (Questions 520 through 557): Each of the numbered items or incomplete statements in this section is followed by answers or by completions of the statement. Select the ONE lettered answer or completion that is BEST in each case.

520. The most specific test for diagnosing and localizing pheochromocytoma is

   (A) CT scan
   (B) sonography
   (C) nephrotomography
   (D) ^{131}I-metaiodobenzylguanidine scan
   (E) abdominal aortic angiography

521. Relative contraindications for single-digit reimplantation include all of the following EXCEPT

   (A) old age and associated medical problems
   (B) amputation of the thumb
   (C) amputation of the index finger
   (D) crush injuries
   (E) associated life-threatening injuries

522. A severely traumatized patient who has been receiving prolonged parenteral alimentation develops diarrhea, mental status depression, alopecia, and perioral and periorbital dermatitis. Administration of which of the following trace elements is most likely to reverse these complications?

   (A) iodine
   (B) zinc
   (C) selenium
   (D) silicon
   (E) tin

523. All the following statements concerning tracheoesophageal fistula developing after tracheal intubation with a cuffed tracheostomy tube are true EXCEPT

   (A) an indwelling nasogastric tube is a predisposing factor
   (B) the incidence increases with the duration of tracheal intubation
   (C) positive-pressure ventilation contributes to its development
   (D) violent coughing following the ingestion of food is a common symptom
   (E) it is best managed by nonsurgical measures

524. A 55-year-old man seeks medical attention for a painless, slow-growing mass that has persisted for 15 years and is located below and in front of his right ear. This growth is most likely

   (A) a parotid adenocarcinoma
   (B) a mucoepidermoid carcinoma
   (C) a mixed tumor
   (D) an undifferentiated carcinoma
   (E) a sarcoma

525. Increased intracranial pressure is correctly described by all of the following statements EXCEPT

   (A) it can result from head injury
   (B) it can result from an intracranial tumor
   (C) it can be relieved by solute diuresis
   (D) it is an indication to perform a spinal tap
   (E) it can be treated with ventriculostomy

526. All of the following statements correctly describe wound contraction EXCEPT

(A) onset is concurrent with the appearance of granulation tissue
(B) myofibroblasts are believed to be the responsible agent
(C) it is slowed by radiation
(D) it is inhibited by partial or full-thickness skin grafts
(E) it is inhibited by epidermal grafts

527. Acute compartment syndrome typically is characterized by all of the following EXCEPT

(A) pain on stretching the muscles
(B) absent arterial pulsations
(C) the presence of paresthesia or anesthesia
(D) the presence of paresis or paralysis
(E) increased intracompartment pressure

528. All the following statements concerning venous thromboembolism in patients undergoing total hip replacement are true EXCEPT

(A) clinical diagnosis is unreliable
(B) the incidence of pulmonary embolism is underestimated
(C) emboli commonly originate from thigh veins
(D) emboli commonly originate from calf veins
(E) labeled-fibrinogen scanning is not helpful in the diagnosis

529. All the following drugs are beneficial in decreasing the incidence of deep vein thrombosis in patients with hip fracture EXCEPT

(A) warfarin
(B) dextran
(C) heparin
(D) aspirin
(E) dipyridamole

530. Retroperitoneal hematoma should be routinely explored EXCEPT if it is

(A) expanding
(B) associated with pelvic fracture

(C) posterior to the lesser sac
(D) related to hepatic flexure laceration
(E) related to splenic flexure laceration

531. All the following statements concerning basal cell carcinoma are correct EXCEPT

(A) its incidence increases with age
(B) it is more common in exposed than unexposed parts of the skin
(C) it occurs commonly among persons with light-colored skin
(D) it arises from the basal layer of epidermis
(E) metastatic spread to lymph nodes is common

532. Clark's classification of melanoma is based on the

(A) level of tissue invasion
(B) depth of tissue invasion
(C) width of the lesion
(D) presence or absence of nodal metastasis
(E) none of the above

533. The radiographic abnormality seen on the roentgenogram on page 147 may result from all the following conditions EXCEPT

(A) perforation of a duodenal ulcer
(B) perforation of a sigmoid diverticulum
(C) peritoneal dialysis
(D) rupture of the gallbladder
(E) laparotomy

534. A man who underwent total thyroidectomy 24 hours ago now complains of a generalized "tingling" sensation and muscle cramps. Appropriate treatment would include

(A) intravenous infusion of calcium gluconate
(B) administration of oxygen by mask
(C) administration of an anticonvulsant
(D) administration of a tranquilizer
(E) neurologic consultation

Figure for use with question 533.

535. Vital capacity is best described as the volume of air

(A) inhaled during normal respiration

(B) expelled during passive expiration

(C) remaining in the lungs after passive expiration

(D) actively exchanging with pulmonary venous blood

(E) able to be expelled following maximal inspiration

536. Prolonged exposure to para-aminobiphenyl is associated with the development of

(A) basal cell carcinoma

(B) urinary bladder carcinoma

(C) lung carcinoma

(D) large-bowel carcinoma

(E) pancreatic carcinoma

537. All the following statements concerning adenocarcinoma of the small intestine are true EXCEPT

    (A) it is the most frequent primary malignant small-bowel tumor
    (B) presenting features are those of intestinal obstruction
    (C) its incidence is higher in persons with immunoglobulin deficiency
    (D) its incidence is higher in persons with Crohn's disease
    (E) the prognosis is worse, stage for stage, than with colonic carcinoma

538. Somatic (muscle) protein malnourishment can be identified by all of the following indices EXCEPT

    (A) body weight
    (B) creatinine-height index
    (C) triceps skin-fold measurement
    (D) mid-arm muscle circumference
    (E) serum transferrin level

539. The most common site of aortic transection in deceleration injuries is

    (A) the root of the aorta
    (B) at the level of the right innominate artery
    (C) at the level of the left innominate artery
    (D) near the origin of the left subclavian artery
    (E) in the middle portion of the descending thoracic aorta

540. The most common site of gastrinoma is the

    (A) gastric antrum
    (B) duodenum
    (C) pancreas
    (D) spleen
    (E) gallbladder

541. Avascular necrosis is most likely to occur in fracture dislocations involving the

    (A) femoral head
    (B) shaft of the femur

    (C) shaft of the humerus
    (D) scapula
    (E) clavicle

542. Flexible esophagogastroduodenoscopy is indicated for all of the following EXCEPT

    (A) the acute phase after corrosive ingestion
    (B) gastric ulcer
    (C) upper GI bleeding
    (D) dysphagia
    (E) epigastric pain with normal roentgenogram findings

543. All of the following statements concerning Hirschsprung's disease are correct EXCEPT that

    (A) constipation is the most frequent presenting feature
    (B) enterocolitis is the major cause of death
    (C) severity of the symptoms corresponds with the extent of bowel involvement
    (D) acetylcholinesterase activity is increased in the aganglionic segment of the bowel
    (E) serum and erythrocyte acetylcholinesterase activity is increased

544. Serum gastrin level is elevated in all of the following EXCEPT

    (A) Zollinger–Ellison syndrome
    (B) gastric outlet obstruction
    (C) retained antrum after Billroth II gastrectomy
    (D) pernicious anemia
    (E) uncomplicated duodenal ulcer

545. A 38-year-old man, previously in good health, suddenly develops severe abdominal pain radiating from the left loin to groin and associated with nausea, perspiration, and the need for frequent urination. He is restless, tossing in bed, but has no abnormal findings. The most likely diagnosis is

    (A) herpes zoster
    (B) left ureteral calculus
    (C) sigmoid diverticulitis

(D) torsion of the left testicle

(E) retroperitoneal hemorrhage

546. A kidney from one identical twin is transplanted in the iliac fossa of the other. This type of transplantation is described as

(A) an orthotopic autograft

(B) a heterotopic isograft

(C) an orthotopic isograft

(D) an orthotopic allograft

(E) a heterotopic xenograft

547. Loss of limb is most likely to occur in injuries involving the

(A) external iliac artery

(B) internal iliac artery

(C) superficial femoral artery

(D) deep femoral artery

(E) popliteal artery

548. Persons with burns over large areas of their bodies may have daily calorie requirements as great as

(A) 1000 kcal

(B) 1500 kcal

(C) 2000 kcal

(D) 2500 kcal

(E) 3000 kcal

549. In a patient with a stab injury to the femoral artery, the treatment of choice is

(A) ligation of both transected ends

(B) end-to-end anastomosis

(C) interposition of autogenous vein graft

(D) interposition of homologous arterial graft

(E) interposition of Dacron graft

Questions 550 through 552

A 56-year-old man comes to the hospital. For the past 5 days he has had colicky abdominal pain, vomiting, abdominal distention, and constipation.

550. All the following measures are appropriate in the management of the man described EXCEPT

(A) rehydration

(B) nasogastric decompression

(C) supine and erect x-rays of the abdomen

(D) abdominal sonography

(E) serum electrolyte determination

551. The man described undergoes barium enema examination. The findings on barium enema, shown on page 150, are most compatible with a diagnosis of

(A) mechanical small-bowel obstruction

(B) intussusception

(C) volvulus

(D) carcinoma of the colon

(E) diverticulitis

552. During definitive surgical treatment of the lesion shown on the barium enema, the left ureter is accidentally transected at the level of the pelvic brim. The most appropriate management of this complication would include

(A) ureteroneocystostomy

(B) ureteroureterostomy

(C) anastomosis of the two cut ends over a "double J" stent

(D) nephrectomy

(E) ligation of the transected ends

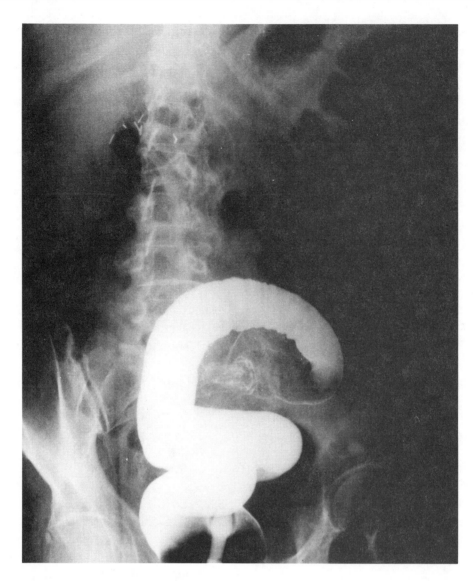

Figure for use with questions 551 and 552.

Questions 553 through 557

A 19-year-old woman is now arriving in the emergency room after an automobile accident that caused injury to several of her organ systems.

553. The first priority in the management of this woman would be to

(A) insert an intravenous line

(B) insert a Foley catheter

(C) perform a thorough neurologic examination

(D) examine her airway

(E) check her blood pressure

554. The woman described, while still in the emergency room, becomes progressively less responsive, but there are no focal neurologic signs. Increased intracranial pressure is suspected. Appropriate treatment measures include all of the following EXCEPT

(A) head elevation

(B) hypoventilation

(C) administration of mannitol

(D) administration of furosemide

(E) ventriculostomy

555. The woman described undergoes exploratory laparotomy for a suspected intra-abdominal injury. Complete transection of the body of the pancreas is found. The treatment of choice is

(A) distal pancreatectomy

(B) repair of the pancreatic duct over a stent

(C) anastomosis of both transected ends to a defunctionalized loop of bowel

(D) ligation of both transected ends

(E) ligation of the proximal transection and anastomosis of the distal end to a loop of bowel

556. During the second week after surgery, the woman becomes tachypneic and hypoxic. Pulmonary wedge pressure remains normal. Adult respiratory distress syndrome (ARDS) is suspected. All of the following statements concerning ARDS are true EXCEPT

(A) it is associated with sepsis

(B) chest roentgenogram typically shows a fluffy infiltrate

(C) functional residual capacity is increased

(D) lung compliance is decreased

(E) right-to-left shunting occurs

557. To improve her respiratory status, the woman is placed on a respirator. With the addition of positive end-expiratory pressure (PEEP), she suddenly develops restlessness, hypotension, and more profound hypoxemia. The most likely diagnosis is

(A) pulmonary embolism

(B) myocardial infarction

(C) decreased venous return

(D) tension pneumothorax

(E) cerebrovascular accident

DIRECTIONS (Questions 558 through 561): Each group of items in this section consists of lettered headings followed by a set of numbered words or phrases. For each numbered word or phrase, select the ONE lettered heading that is most closely associated with it. Each lettered heading may be selected once, more than once, or not at all.

Questions 558 through 561

For each of the following clinical situations, select the type of transplantation being described.

(A) heterotopic isograft

(B) heterotopic xenograft

(C) orthotopic autograft

(D) orthotopic isograft

(E) orthotopic allograft

558. Transplantation between genetically dissimilar individuals of the same species, and the transplanted part is placed at its normal anatomic location

559. Transplantation between genetically identical individuals, and the transplanted part is placed at an extra-anatomic location

560. Transplantation between genetically identical individuals, and the transplanted part is placed at its normal anatomic location

561. Transplantation between two different species, and the transplanted organ is placed at an extra-anatomic location

DIRECTIONS (Questions 562 through 585): Each of the numbered items or incomplete statements in this section is followed by answers or completions of the statement. Select the ONE lettered answer or completion that is BEST in each case.

562. The most likely cause of sudden cardiopulmonary collapse in a patient with blunt thoracic injury is

(A) rib fracture
(B) hemothorax
(C) pneumothorax
(D) pulmonary contusion
(E) chylothorax

563. The most frequent cause of spontaneous pneumothorax is

(A) carcinoma of the lung
(B) tuberculosis
(C) pyogenic abscess of the lung
(D) emphysema
(E) rupture of small blebs

564. The absolute contraindication for lung resection in a patient with lung cancer is

(A) involvement of more than one ipsilateral lobe
(B) ipsilateral mediastinal node involvement
(C) chest wall invasion
(D) liver metastases
(E) pleural effusion

565. The overall 5-year survival rate of patients with carcinoma of the lung is

(A) 5%
(B) 10%
(C) 20%
(D) 40%
(E) 80%

566. A 50-year-old man comes to the emergency room with a history of vomiting of 3 days' duration. His past history reveals that for approximately 20 years, he has been getting epigastric pain, lasting for 2 to 3 weeks, during early spring and autumn. He remembers getting relief from pain by taking milk and antacids. Physical examination showed a fullness in the epigastric area with visible peristalsis, absence of tenderness, and normal active bowel sounds. The most likely diagnosis is

(A) gastric outlet obstruction
(B) small bowel obstruction
(C) volvulus of the colon
(D) incarcerated umbilical hernia
(E) cholecystitis

567. In the above patient, the most likely metabolic consequences include all of the following EXCEPT

(A) systemic alkalosis
(B) hypercalcemia
(C) hypokalemia
(D) hypovolemia
(E) hypochloremia

568. All the following statements concerning hematemesis are true EXCEPT

(A) it refers to vomiting of blood from a source proximal to the ligament of Treitz
(B) hematocrit level is not an accurate indicator of blood loss
(C) melena does not occur unless there is bleeding of at least 500 mL of blood
(D) stools may remain positive for occult blood up to 3 weeks following bleeding
(E) factors influencing the degree of azotemia include status of bacterial flora of the gut, site of bleeding, and liver function tests

569. Gastrin secretion is enhanced by

(A) antral distention
(B) antral acidification
(C) presence of fat in the antrum

(D) sympathetic nerve stimulation

(E) duodenal acidification

570. A 45-year-old woman, mother of four children, comes to the emergency room complaining of the sudden onset of epigastric and right upper quadrant pain, radiating to the back, associated with vomiting. On examination, tenderness is elicited in the right upper quadrant, bowel sounds are decreased, and laboratory data shows leukocytosis, normal serum levels of amylase, lipase, and bilirubin. The most likely diagnosis is

(A) acute cholecystitis

(B) perforated peptic ulcer disease

(C) myocardial infarction

(D) acute pancreatitis

(E) sigmoid diverticulitis

571. The most useful diagnostic test to confirm the diagnosis is

(A) a two-way roentgenogram of the abdomen

(B) ultrasonography of the upper abdomen

(C) barium swallow

(D) HIDA scan

(E) peritoneal lavage

572. A patient is operated on with the presumptive diagnosis of acute appendicitis. However, at operation, the appendix and cecum are found to be normal. Terminal ileum for a distance of approximately 30 cm is red, edematous, and thickened with creeping of the mesenteric fat onto the ileum. There is no dilation of the bowel proximal to the area of involvement. The remainder of the small bowel is normal. The appropriate operative procedure is

(A) closure of the abdomen

(B) appendectomy

(C) ileostomy proximal to the area of involvement

(D) side-to-side ileo-transverse colostomy

(E) right hemicolectomy

573. Biopsy of a 4-cm rectal tumor shows it to be a villous adenoma with atypia. The most appropriate management of this tumor includes

(A) photocoagulation of the tumor

(B) electrocoagulation of the tumor

(C) transanal excision of the tumor

(D) abdominoperineal resection

(E) external beam radiation

574. All the following statements concerning cyclosporine are true, EXCEPT

(A) it is a fungal cyclic peptide

(B) it inhibits formation of cytotoxic T cells

(C) its use leads to permanent tolerance

(D) it interferes with production of lymphokine interleukin-2

(E) it is nephrotoxic

575. All the following statements concerning left ventricular aneurysm are true EXCEPT

(A) it results from transmural infarction of the myocardium

(B) progressive enlargement and rupture are common

(C) the majority are located in the antrolateral portion of the left ventricle

(D) aneurysms less than 5 cm in diameter have a negligible hemodynamic effect

(E) operation is indicated for symptomatic aneurysms

576. All the following statements concerning splenic injury are true EXCEPT

(A) nonoperative management in children is more likely to be successful than in adults

(B) CT scan is the diagnostic modality of choice

(C) splenic salvage is contraindicated in the presence of concomitant major abdominal injuries

(D) the risk of postsplenectomy sepsis is highest during the first 2 years after splenectomy

(E) *Pseudomonas aeroginosa* is the most frequent organism responsible for postsplenectomy sepsis

577. The most frequent benign tumor of the lung is

(A) hamartoma
(B) lipoma
(C) carcinoid
(D) fibroma
(E) rhabdomyoma

578. All the following statements concerning mixed venous hemoglobin saturation (SvO_2) are true EXCEPT

(A) normal SvO_2 is 50%
(B) normal mixed venous oxygen tension (PvO_2) is 40 mm Hg
(C) SvO_2 is the best single predictor of cardiac output
(D) SvO_2 is a sensitive means to track the accuracy of the peripheral oxygen delivery
(E) a persistent PvO_2 less than 28 mm Hg is associated with hyperlactemia and death

579. The antibiotic of choice for treating patients with *Clostridium difficile* enterocolitis is

(A) penicillin
(B) gentamicin
(C) streptomycin
(D) metronidazole
(E) tetracycline

580. The most likely testicular tumor in a 25-year-old man is

(A) Leydig's cell tumor
(B) choriocarcinoma
(C) seminoma
(D) teratocarcinoma
(E) androblastoma

581. A neonate has persistent vomiting of bile-stained material. A two-way abdominal roentgenogram shows "double bubble" sign. The most likely diagnosis is

(A) annular pancreas
(B) duodenal atresia
(C) congenital hypertrophic pyloric stenosis
(D) Meckel's diverticulum
(E) none of the above

582. Maternal polyhydramnios is associated with

(A) esophageal atresia
(B) duodenal atresia
(C) jejunal atresia
(D) all of the above
(E) none of the above

583. All the following statements concerning sacrococcygeal teratoma are true except that

(A) it is more common in males
(B) it may present as a postsacral mass
(C) it may present as a retrorectal mass
(D) it is prone to malignant degeneration
(E) it should be excised promptly

584. Following bilateral femoral embolectomy, a patient with atrial fibrillation becomes oliguric and passes red-colored urine. All the following measures may be appropriate in this patient's management EXCEPT

(A) administration of sodium bicarbonate
(B) administration of mannitol
(C) aggressive hydration
(D) determination of serum potassium
(E) cessation of heparin

585. Anal incontinence in a patient with rectal prolapse is primarily due to

(A) loss of anal rectal angle
(B) weakness of endopelvic fascia
(C) stretching of pudendal nerves
(D) all of the above
(E) none of the above

ANSWERS AND EXPLANATIONS

520. **(D)** Although CT scan, MRI, sonography, nephrotomography, and angiography may demonstrate a mass, these techniques by themselves cannot confirm the diagnosis of

pheochromocytoma. In ^{131}I-metaiodobenzyl-guanidine scanning, the agent is selectively taken up by adrenal tumors and is helpful in the diagnosis of pheochromocytoma in both adrenal and extra-adrenal locations. This scan is also helpful in the diagnosis of medullary hyperplasia. (*Thompson and Vinik, pp 139–148; Schwartz, pp 1286–1292*)

521. **(B)** Advances in microsurgery techniques have enabled successful reimplantation of digits. Whether or not the digit should be reimplanted is sometimes an issue. In the consideration of reimplantation, the chances for return of function should be evaluated. There are no absolute indications or contraindications for reimplantation of a digit. In general, digital reimplantation is contraindicated in elderly patients with concomitant medical disorders, in patients with associated life-threatening injuries, and in cases of amputation of a single digit—with the exception of the thumb. The type of injury is another factor influencing the decision. A severe crush injury with extensive damage to the parts is a relative contraindication. (*Schwartz and Shires, pp 73–97; Schwartz and Ellis, p 2009*)

522. **(B)** Symptoms of zinc deficiency include diarrhea, mental changes, alopecia, and periorbital, perinasal, and perioral dermatitis. Persons who have cirrhosis, who are receiving steroids, who have excessive loss of gastrointestinal secretions, or who are severely traumatized are at risk for zinc deficiency. Deficiency states resulting from inadequate ingestion of selenium, silicon, and tin have not been described. Deficiency of iodine produces hypothyroidism. (*Grant, pp 155–170; Sabiston, p 142*)

523. **(E)** Tracheoesophageal fistula is a serious complication of tracheostomy and tracheal intubation. The presence of a nasogastric tube, positive-pressure ventilation, and prolonged periods of intubation are predisposing factors. The complication should be suspected when an intubated patient develops violent coughing after swallowing food or saliva. The recommended treatment is primary closure of the fistulous opening in the trachea and the esophagus with a transposed regional muscle flap interposed between the trachea and esophagus. Nonsurgical corrective measures are associated with a higher rate of mortality. (*Conley, pp 288–289*)

524. **(C)** Mixed tumor of the salivary gland (pleomorphic adenoma) is the most frequently occurring tumor of the parotid gland (70%). It is slow growing, with a tendency for recurrence after removal. Mucoepidermoid carcinomas vary in the degree of their malignancy and are classified as either low-grade or high-grade tumors. Adenocarcinoma and undifferentiated carcinoma are fast-growing tumors that carry a poor prognosis. Sarcomas of the parotid gland are rare. (*Cummings, pp 1029–1078*)

525. **(D)** The skull is a rigid cavity, so expansion of its contents leads to increased intracranial pressure. Both brain edema resulting from trauma and space-occupying lesions within the skull increase intracranial pressure. Solute diuresis, corticosteroids, elevation of the head of the bed, and ventriculostomy are helpful in reducing the pressure. Spinal tap is contraindicated because of the danger of herniation of the brain. (*Schwartz et al, p 1832*)

526. **(E)** Wound contraction, an important aspect of wound healing, can result in deformity. Dependent on myofibroblasts present in granulation tissue, wound contraction is slowed by radiation, administration of steroids, and splinting. The most effective measure for preventing wound contraction is partial or full-thickness skin grafts. Epidermal grafts do not prevent wound contraction. The reason for the differences observed between epidermal grafts and partial or full-thickness grafts is not well understood. (*Greenfield et al, pp 1960–1961*)

527. **(B)** Differentiation among acute compartment syndrome, arterial occlusion, and neuropraxia is not always easy (in fact, these conditions may coexist). However, accurate diagnosis is essential for proper management.

Typical acute compartment syndrome is characterized by the following findings: pain on stretching the muscles; the presence of paresthesia or anesthesia; the presence of paralysis or paresis; and increased intracompartment pressure. Arterial pulsation is present but may require detection by Doppler technique. In a typical case of arterial occlusion, pulsations are absent and intracompartment pressure is normal. In neuropraxia, arterial pulsations and intracompartment pressure remain normal. In addition, pain on stretching the muscles will be absent. Difficult diagnostic situations may require the use of Doppler technique, arteriography, and intracompartment pressure measurements. *(Greenfield et al, pp 1998–1999)*

528. **(D)** ^{125}I-fibrinogen scanning and venography are positive in less than half the patients who have clinical evidence of venous thrombosis. Pulmonary emboli have been shown to arise from thigh veins. Detection of thrombi in thigh veins with labeled-fibrinogen scan is difficult for two reasons: (1) the scan is not sensitive in the thigh, and (2) interpretation is rendered difficult by accumulation of fibrinogen in the operated site. *(Greenfield, pp 1766–1768)*

529. **(C)** Warfarin, dextran, and aspirin have been found to be efficacious in preventing deep venous thrombosis. Hemorrhagic complications are fewer with aspirin compared with warfarin. One disadvantage of dextran is that because it must be administered parenterally it may cause allergic reactions. Dipyridamole is less effective than warfarin, dextran, and aspirin. Though effective in medical and general surgical patients, low-dose heparin, has, for unexplained reasons, been found to be ineffective in preventing deep vein thrombosis. Low molecular weight heparin is also efficacious in preventing DVT in this patient group. *(Sabiston, p 311)*

530. **(B)** Retroperitoneal hematoma may be a manifestation of serious retroperitoneal injury, such as laceration of hepatic and splenic flexure or injury to the pancreas, blood vessels, and renal parenchyma. Serious complications such as continued hemorrhage, abscess formation, and arteriovenous fistula may develop. The best method of avoiding these complications is by exploration. Combined pelvic hematoma, which is not associated with bladder injury but is associated with pelvic fracture, is not routinely explored. This type of hematoma resolves spontaneously, and exploration may result in uncontrollable bleeding. *(Feliciano, pp 615–650)*

531. **(E)** Basal cell carcinoma arises from the basal layer of epidermis. It is a slow-growing tumor, and distant spread is infrequent. Exposure to ultraviolet radiation (bright sunlight) is a predisposing factor to the development of basal cell carcinoma. The longer the duration of exposure, the greater the likelihood of disease. Not surprisingly, then, exposed parts of the skin are more vulnerable than unexposed regions; moreover, the cancer is more common among persons with light-colored skin, because they lack the pigment melanin, which protects against ultraviolet ray penetration into the skin. *(Browse, pp 54–56)*

532. **(A)** Clark's classification of melanoma is based on the level of invasion and not on the actual depth of the tumor. In level I, the lesion has not penetrated the basement membrane. In level II, the lesion extends to the papillary dermis, and in level III, the lesion has penetrated the papillary and reticular dermis junction. In level IV, the reticular dermis is invaded. The subcutaneous tissue is invaded in level V. This classification provides prognostic information concerning the probability of lymph node metastasis and survival. In general, the higher the level, the higher the incidence of metastasis to lymph nodes and, consequently, the poorer the survival. *(Sabiston, pp 605–608)*

533. **(D)** The radiographic abnormality seen on the roentgenogram presented in the question (and again on page 157) is pneumoperitoneum, which occurs following perforation of hollow viscera containing air. Air can gain

Figure for use with answer 533.

entry into the peritoneal cavity during laparotomy and air insufflation of fallopian tubes, as well as from penetrating injuries of the abdominal wall. In the roentgenogram, pneumoperitoneum can be recognized by the presence of air both inside and outside the bowel lumen (the arrows point to the wall of the intestine). *(Greenfield, pp 1137)*

534. (A) During total thyroidectomy, parathyroid glands may inadvertently be removed or their vascular supply interrupted. Hypoparathyroidism may then develop, the manifestations of which include tingling, muscle cramps, convulsions, and a positive Chvostek's sign. These symptoms are dramatically relieved by intravenous administration of calcium. Oral calcium and vitamin D are administered for long-term correction of hypocalcemia. *(Hardy, p 402)*

535. (E) Vital capacity is an important measure of respiratory function. It is defined as the maximum volume of air a person can expel following a maximum inspiratory effort. When vital capacity is normal, significant restrictive pulmonary disease is not present. Acutely decreased vital capacity indicates decreased ventilatory reserve. *(Marini, p 114)*

536. **(B)** Carcinoma of the urinary bladder has been linked to several predisposing factors. The development of bladder carcinoma is associated with the ingestion of chemicals that are excreted in urine as conjugated ortho-aminophenols; among these chemicals are beta-naphthylamine and para-aminobiphenyl. Chronic schistosome infection and vesicle calculus also have been identified as predisposing factors. *(Schwartz et al, p 1761)*

537. **(E)** Despite the large surface area of the small-bowel mucosa, the incidence of adenocarcinoma of the small bowel, the most frequent neoplasm of the small bowel, is rare. However, the incidence is higher in persons with immunoglobulin A deficiency or Crohn's disease. Presenting features are signs and symptoms of small-bowel obstruction. Prognosis is poor, because the disease is usually difficult to identify. Stage for stage, the survival rates of colonic carcinoma and small-bowel carcinoma are no different. *(Greenfield, pp 756–757)*

538. **(E)** Body protein is distributed in two compartments: somatic (muscle) and visceral (all other protein). Loss of weight and decreases in the creatinine-height index, triceps skinfold measurement, and mid-arm muscle circumference all indicate somatic protein malnourishment. Visceral protein depletion causes decreased serum albumin and transferrin levels. Visceral protein depletion also results in decreased total lymphocyte count. *(Bartlett et al, pp 128–130)*

539. **(D)** In deceleration injuries, laceration involving the aorta most frequently occurs just distal to the left subclavian artery. The tear may be complete or partial. Diagnosis is difficult; aortography is helpful in establishing the diagnosis. *(Feliciano, pp 423–430)*

540. **(C)** Gastrinoma produces Zollinger-Ellison syndrome, which is associated with markedly elevated gastric acid secretion and ulcer disease of the upper gastrointestinal tract. The most common site of occurrence is the pancreas. However, gastrinoma has been known to occur in the gastric antrum, duodenum, spleen, and ovary. Removal of the gastrinoma can result in a cure. A thorough search must be made at surgical exploration to locate the tumor, which in early stages will be small. The gastrinoma triangle is defined as the junction of the cystic and common bile ducts, second and third portion of the duodenum, and the division of the pancreatic neck and body. 90% of gastrinomas are located here. *(Greenfield, pp 838–841)*

541. **(A)** Avascular necrosis results when, following a fracture, the blood supply to a bone fragment is disrupted. The femoral head, humeral head, scaphoid, and talus, because of their precarious blood supply, are particularly vulnerable to this complication. A dense appearance of the bone on x-ray is a diagnostic clue. Radioisotope scanning can detect avascular necrosis at an earlier stage than is possible with roentgenography. *(Hardy [1988], p 1211)*

542. **(A)** Upper GI fiberendoscopy is a safe and useful procedure for diagnosing GI disorders. It is indicated for treating symptomatic patients with upper abdominal pain, nausea, and weight loss, even though abnormalities are absent on roentgenography. Endoscopy can reveal lesions overlooked on roentgenograms. Contraindications to this procedure include an uncooperative patient, recent ingestion of corrosives, and recent peptic ulcer perforation. *(Greenfield, p 676)*

543. **(C)** Although constipation is the most common presenting feature of Hirschsprung's disease, some patients suffer from diarrhea. The severity of symptoms does not correlate well with the extent of bowel involvement. Enterocolitis, a major cause of death, requires vigorous treatment. This complication can occur even after removal of the aganglionic segment of the bowel. Increased acetylcholinesterase activity has been noted in the serum, affected aganglionic bowel, and erythrocytes of afflicted persons. *(Lavery, pp 151–175; Schwartz, pp 1702–1703)*

544. (E) Elevated serum gastrin is found in patients with and without peptic ulcer disease. Hypergastrinemia affects patients with gastrinoma, G-cell hyperplasia, gastric stasis, retained antrum, renal failure, and massive small-bowel resection. Most studies have shown no difference in gastrin level between uncomplicated duodenal ulcer patients and those persons in a control group. Pernicious anemia commonly is associated with loss of intrinsic factor secondary to atrophic gastritis. The atrophic gastritis and loss of acid secretion is what stimulates the hypergastrinemic state. (*Greenfield, pp 666–667*)

545. (B) Contraction of hollow organs against obstruction or excessive contraction causes colic. Typical ureteral colic is severe, sudden in onset, radiates from loin to groin, and is associated with an urge to urinate. Blood clots and calculi in the ureter can cause colic, the latter being more frequent. Urine examination demonstrates macroscopic or microscopic hematuria. (*Tanagho, pp 272–275*)

546. (B) Based on the genetic relationship between the donor and the recipient, transplants are classified as either (1) autografts, in which the same individual acts as both donor and recipient; (2) isografts, in which the donor and recipient are genetically identical; (3) allografts, in which the donor and recipient are genetically dissimilar but belong to the same species; or (4) xenografts, in which the donor and recipient belong to different species. In orthotopic transplants, the transplanted part is placed in its normal anatomic location. In heterotopic transplants, the transplanted part is placed in a different anatomic location. (*Sabiston, p 340*)

547. (E) Arterial injuries below the level of the adductor hiatus result in more amputations than in other sites. Early diagnosis and prompt revascularization improve the chance for limb preservation. Blunt injury is associated with a higher incidence of limb loss, probably because of compression of collateral vessels from the tissue swelling. (*Feliciano, pp 819–847*)

548. (E) Major trauma, surgical complications, and infection are characterized by hypermetabolism. Calorie requirements are highest among burn victims. The daily energy requirement has been found to be 25 kcal/kg of body weight plus 40 kcal/% of body surface burned. (*Sabiston, pp 197–198*)

549. (B) The best results are obtained by repair of an injured vessel by direct anastomosis. This may not be feasible when a segment of the vessel is lost, and repair cannot be performed without tension. In these situations, an interposition graft may be required. Ligation of the transected ends may lead to ischemic necrosis. (*Feliciano, pp 819–847*)

550. (D) Abdominal ultrasonography has no role in the diagnosis or management of intestinal obstruction. Serum electrolyte determination helps in identifying the electrolyte disturbances that have taken place. Fluid loss needs to be corrected with rehydration. Nasogastric suction helps in decreasing abdominal distention. (*Greenfield, pp 733–740*)

551. (D) An annular constricting lesion with overhanging edges is typical of annular carcinoma of the colon. Mechanical small-bowel obstruction results in multiple air-fluid levels in distended small-bowel loops. Intussusception produces a "corkscrew" appearance on barium enema, and sigmoid volvulus produces a "bird's beak" appearance. In diverticulitis, extravasation of barium outside the lumen of the colon typically is seen. (*Greenfield, pp 1014–1031*)

552. (C) The ureters may be injured during pelvic operations. It is important to recognize the injury, because early diagnosis and prompt treatment produce good results. Factors to be considered following the injury are whether the ureter needs to be repaired, the method of repair (if repair is necessary), and the measures required for minimizing the consequences of the injury. End-to-end anastomosis is a simple, feasible procedure when there is no loss of a segment of the transected ureter. When injury is close to the bladder, ureteroneocystostomy is the procedure of choice. When there is loss of ureteral substance, ureteroureterostomy (anastomosis to the opposite ureter) should be considered. Nephrectomy may be a reasonable choice if there is loss of renal function and ureteral injury is at a higher level. Ligating the transected ends should not be done. *(Tanagho, p 317, Schwartz, p 1768)*

553. **(D)** In a patient with multiple injuries, the first treatment priority is airway maintenance. Once the patency and adequacy of the airway are established, the other emergency procedures, such as control of external bleeding, can begin. Although detailed physical examination is needed in establishing a definitive diagnosis, the condition of an injured patient may not permit a detailed examination, and, in any event, emergency treatment must be instituted immediately. *(Feliciano, pp 123–138)*

554. **(B)** Increased intracranial pressure from any cause results in decreased cerebral perfusion. To minimize further brain damage, it is essential to decrease intracranial pressure, which can be effected by a combination of measures: elevation of the head of the patient; administration of a hyperosmotic agent (mannitol) to shift fluid from the intercellular compartment to the vascular compartment; and institution of diuretic therapy. Removal of mass lesions, such as a hematoma or necrotic brain tissue, should be performed if necessary. Hyperventilation should be instituted (hypoventilation is contraindicated). Hypocapnia resulting from hyperventilation causes vasoconstriction, decreasing intracranial pressure. *(Schwartz, pp 1833–1835; Feliciano, pp 267–278)*

555. **(A)** The treatment of choice for complete transection of the body of the pancreas is distal pancreatectomy. This is a relatively simple and safe procedure and does not produce pancreatic insufficiency. Although the other procedures listed in the question may be feasible, in multitrauma patients the simplest and fastest procedure should be selected. *(Schwartz and Ellis, pp 495–496)*

556. **(C)** In a patient with multiple trauma who becomes tachypneic and hypoxemic despite adequate oxygen delivery, adult respiratory distress syndrome (ARDS) should be suspected. The clinical syndrome is characterized by noncardiac pulmonary edema, decreased lung compliance, decreased functional residual capacity, and a right-to-left shunt. Because ARDS is often associated with sepsis, a search should be made to identify a source of infection. *(Schwartz, pp 123–130)*

557. **(D)** Positive end-expiratory pressure (PEEP) is associated with two significant complications: pneumothorax and decreased venous return resulting from increased intrathoracic pressure. Pneumothorax causes a sudden worsening of a patient's condition, with increasing restlessness and progressive hypoxemia. Treatment consists of insertion of a chest tube. *(Schwartz, pp 128–129)*

558–561. **(558-E, 559-A, 560-D, 561-B)** Transplants are grouped into four classes based on the genetic relationship between the donor and recipient. In an autograft, the same individual acts as both donor and recipient. In isograft transplants, the donor and recipient are genetically identical, and in allograft transplants, donor and recipient are genetically dissimilar but belong to the same species. In xenograft transplants, donor and recipient belong to different species. The terms orthotopic and heterotopic refer to the anatomic location of the transplanted part. When the transplanted part is placed in its normal anatomic location, it is an orthotopic transplantation. In heterotopic transplantation, the part is transplanted to an extra-anatomic location. *(Sabiston, p 340)*

562. **(C)** The most frequent injury following blunt chest trauma is rib fracture. Unless associated with flail chest, rib fractures do not cause cardiopulmonary problems. Hemothorax can cause cardiopulmonary collapse if it is due to bleeding from intercostal vessels (high-pressure system). Hemothorax resulting from bleeding from lung parenchyma (low-pressure system) spontaneously stops.

Chylothorax, secondary to blunt trauma, is very rare. Pulmonary contusion can cause cardiopulmonary collapse but is of gradual onset and unlikely to present as an acute episode. Pneumothorax, especially tension pneumothorax, acutely can cause cardiorespiratory collapse and may prove fatal unless promptly treated. (*Schwartz et al, pp 672–684*)

563. **(E)** Rupture of small blebs located in the apex of the lung is the most frequent cause of spontaneous pneumothorax. The condition is more frequent in men between the ages of 20 and 40 years. Prior to recognition of this entity, tuberculosis was considered to be the frequent cause of spontaneous pneumothorax. Chronic bronchitis and emphysema account for 10% of the cases of pneumothorax. (*Schwartz et al, pp 704–707*)

564. **(D)** Vocal cord paralysis indicates involvement of recurrent laryngeal nerve. Tumor invasion of the left recurrent laryngeal nerve in the aortopulmonary window is generally considered an indication of nonresectability. However, recurrent laryngeal nerve may be involved above the level of the aortic arch by direct tumor extension, in which case resection is not contraindicated. Some patients with chest wall invasion are cured following enbloc resection, and it therefore is not an absolute contraindication for resection. Tumors with ipsilateral mediastinal node involvement could be resected with a reasonable chance for cure. Malignant cells in pleural effusion indicate noncurability, but before a patient is denied a chance for cure, the presence of malignant cells in the effusion has to be proved beyond doubt. Involvement of more than one lobe has no bearing on prognosis as long as the patient's preoperative ventilation parameters will allow for safe resection. Metastasis to the liver is an absolute contraindication for resection, since lung cancer in this circumstance is not curable. (*Schwartz et al, pp 741–745; Sabiston, p 751*)

565. **(B)** The overall survival rate is approximately 10%. Five-year survival rate following surgical resection is 20 to 35%. In patients with T1 lesions, with no nodal or distant metastases, the survival rate is approximately 80%. (*Sabiston, p 1755*)

566. **(A)** In a patient who is known to have had symptoms of peptic ulcer disease for many years and presents with nausea and vomiting, one should consider gastric outlet obstruction, which can be due to exacerbation of the ulcer and edema or to scar tissue formation. Usually in these patients, epigastric fullness, with visible peristalsis going from the left side to the right, will be seen. A succussion splash may be audible. The history of periodicity and pain relief by taking antacids also favors a diagnosis of previous peptic ulcer disease. Patients with umbilical hernia will have a mass in the region of the umbilicus. Patients with acute cholecystitis usually present with the sudden onset of pain, radiating to the back, with fever and chills. Volvulus of the sigmoid colon presents with constipation and abdominal distention. Vomiting is a late feature. Small-bowel obstruction would be associated with a history of colicky abdominal pain, nausea, and vomiting. Patients will usually have hyperactive high-pitched bowel sounds. (*Greenfield, pp 674–688*)

567. **(B)** With persistent vomiting, the patient loses fluid, resulting in dehydration (hypovolemia). Loss of hydrogen ions and loss of potassium and chloride in the vomited gastric contents leads to alkalosis, hypokalemia, and hypochloremia. Because of hypovolemia, adrenocortical and renal mechanisms are stimulated to conserve sodium at the expense of potassium and hydrogen ions. Excretion of potassium in the urine further aggravates hypokalemia. The kidneys then compensate for the loss of potassium by conserving potassium and excreting more hydrogen ions which results in a paradoxical aciduria and self perpetuating metabolic alkalosis. (*Schwartz et al, p 71*)

568. **(C)** The term hematemesis refers to vomiting of blood from a source extending from the pharynx to ligament of Treitz. The most frequent causes are peptic ulcer disease, esophageal varices, and Mallory–Weiss syndrome. Melena refers to passage of black-colored stools. Melena can occur with as little as 50 mL of blood loss. Melena may persist for 5 days after bleeding; stools for occult blood may remain positive for up to 3 weeks. Hematocrit is not an accurate measure of blood loss, as it takes time for hemodilution to occur. The blood in the gastrointestinal tract is acted upon by bacterial flora, resulting in the production of ammonia, which in the liver is converted to urea. Alteration of bacterial flora, as well as the status of the liver function, can influence the degree of azotemia. *(Schwartz et al, pp 1032–1033)*

569. **(A)** Gastrin secretion is stimulated by vagal stimulation, antral distention, and by the presence of protein in the antrum. Antral acidification decreases gastric secretion by a feedback mechanism. Acid secretion fortunately ceases when antral pH reaches 1.5. The same is true with duodenal acidification. *(Schwartz et al, pp 1127–1128)*

570–571. **(570-A, 571-D)** Women are more often affected by gallstones than men. Pregnancy predisposes for the occurrence of gallstones. Gallstones may remain asymptomatic or may cause symptoms when they cause obstruction to the cystic duct. The usual presenting symptom is biliary colic, which is experienced as epigastric pain, radiating to the back and associated with nausea and vomiting. The presence of tenderness in the right upper quadrant and leukocytosis under these circumstances are very indicative of acute cholecystitis. The diagnosis of gallstones is best confirmed by ultrasonography. Ultrasonography also provides details about the presence of gallstones, the wall of the gallbladder, and also the presence or absence of tenderness over the gallbladder during the examination. In only 20% of the cases, gallstones are seen on a two-way roentgenogram of the abdomen. Barium swallow in this instance is of no help. Failure to visualize the gallbladder with HIDA scan indicates cystic duct obstruction. In a majority of the patients acute cholecystitis is secondary to cystic duct obstruction. Lack of visualization may also oc-

cur in patients who have had a previous cholecystectomy (history is helpful) or agenesis of the gallbladder (rare). Peritoneal lavage in this instance will be of no help, except in detecting fluid, which may contain leukocytes. *(Sreenivas, pp 69–77; Schwartz, pp 1378–1379)*

572. **(B)** From the description, the diagnosis in this patient is acute regional enteritis. Incidental finding of regional enteritis in patients operated upon for presumed diagnosis of acute appendicitis is medically treated, unless there is proximal obstruction. The risk of operating on patients with regional enteritis is formation of fistula and abscess, especially if the area to be resected is involved with the disease process. However, if the cecum and the appendix are not involved, it is advisable to perform appendectomy. In this instance, it would be safe and, if the patient were to have a recurrence in the future, at least acute appendicitis would no longer be a possible diagnosis and the patient could be treated for an exacerbation of regional enteritis. *(Schwartz et al, pp 1310–1311)*

573. **(C)** Villous adenoma is a premalignant condition. The incidence of carcinoma increases as the tumor increases in size, and the finding of a 4-cm lesion with induration has an almost 90% risk for carcinoma. The specimen that is being submitted for biopsy examination may not be truly representative of the entire lesion. Carcinoma may be present deep within the tumor. Therefore, to exclude malignancy, the tumor should be excised in its entirety and submitted for histologic examination. If an infiltrating tumor is seen, further treatment will be required. Photocoagulation and electrocoagulation of the tumor will destroy the tumor and may not provide the information as to its nature. Abdominal perineal resection should not be performed unless there is histologic proof of the presence of carcinoma. External beam radiation is not indicated in this situation. *(Schwartz et al, pp 1270–1271)*

574. **(C)** Cyclosporine, a fungal-cyclic peptide, has revolutionized clinical transplantation. Its one disadvantage is that it is nephrotoxic. Cy-

closporine does not appear to affect precursor hemopoietic cells. It acts by interfering with the production of lymphokine interleukin-2, which is needed for lymphocyte proliferation. Expansion antigen-responsive clones of T lymphocyte are thereby suppressed. Once cyclosporine is discontinued, rejection can resume. Other adverse effects include neurotoxicity, hirsutism, hypercalemia, and hepatotoxicity. *(Schwartz et al, p 398)*

575. (B) Ventricular aneurysm occurs as a result of transmural myocardial infarction, primarily affecting the anterior aspect of the ventricle. Most of the aneurysms are therefore present on the antromedial portion of the left ventricle. Their natural history is to develop 4–8 weeks after a transmural MI, and to remain stable in size. Aneurysms less than 5 cm in diameter have negligible hemodynamic affect and require no operative intervention. Operation is indicated for symptomatic aneurysms. However, the symptoms the patient experiences could be secondary to ischemic disease of the heart. Progressive enlargement and rupture is uncommon. Prognosis depends on the residual ventricular function. *(Schwartz et al, pp 864–867)*

576. (E) Because of the risk of postsplenectomy sepsis, attempts should be made for splenic salvage when possible. Attempts at splenic salvage is contraindicated in patients with multiple concomitant injuries, as it prolongs the operation and increases blood loss. Among children, approximately two thirds respond favorably to nonoperative management. Nonoperative management is contraindicated in the presence of hypotension, which persists when more than 50% of the child's circulating volume is transfused within 24 hours, in the presence of concomitant major injuries, and in the presence of a shattered spleen, which is not amenable to repair. The risk of postsplenectomy sepsis persists throughout life, the highest incidence being in the first 2 years following splenectomy. The most frequent organisms responsible for postsplenectomy sepsis include *Pneumococcus*, *Meningococcus*, and *Haemophylus in-*

fluenzae. The mortality rate is approximately 50% when sepsis occurs. *(Sabiston, pp 1111–1113, 1131–1132)*

577. (A) Hamartoma is the most frequent benign tumor of the lung. It presents as a density on chest roentgenogram, and it occurs usually during the fifth and sixth decades of life. Operation is often required to differentiate it from lung carcinoma. *(Schwartz et al, p 751–752)*

578. (A) The average mixed venous oxygen tension is 40 mm Hg. The PvO_2 of 40 mm Hg corresponds to mixed venous oxygen saturation of 75%. Since SvO_2 of 75% corresponds to the steep portion of the oxyhemoglobin dissociation curve, small changes in peripheral oxygenation result in significant changes in SvO_2. Therefore, SvO_2 is sensitive in tracking adequacy of oxygen delivery to tissues. A normal SvO_2 ensures physiologic balance between oxygen delivery and oxygen consumption. A sudden fall in SvO_2 could result from decreased cardiac output, arterial oxygen desaturation, dropping hemoglobin, or increased oxygen consumption. Persistent PvO_2 less than 28 mm Hg has been reported with hyperlactemia and death. *(Greenfield, p 171)*

579. (D) *Clostridium difficile* enterocolitis occurs as a complication of broad-spectrum antibiotic treatment. Symptoms may appear as late as 6 weeks following antibiotic treatment. The organism, which is resistant to broad-spectrum antibiotics, produces toxin that causes necrosis of the colonic mucous membrane. Orally administered metronidazole is the drug of choice. Vancomycin is also effective against *Clostridium difficile*, but due to its expense is often reserved for refractory cases. *(Schwartz et al, pp 1226–1228)*

580. (C) The majority of testicular tumors occurring in young adults are malignant tumors. The tumors may originate from germinal or nongerminal cells. Those that arise from germinal cells include seminoma (the most common), embryonal cell carcinoma, choriocarcinoma, teratocarcinoma. Leydig cell tumors and androblastoma originate from nongerminal cells and may produce excess testosterone. Benign tumors such as fibroma can occur but are rare. *(Schwartz et al, pp 1764–1765)*

581. **(B)** Persistent bilious vomiting is a sign of intestinal obstruction, distal to the ampulla of Vater. Double bubble on a two-way abdominal roentgenogram is caused by air in the distended stomach and duodenum. The picture is most compatible with duodenal atresia, which typically presents in the neonate. *(Schwartz et al, p 1696)*

582. **(D)** Under normal circumstances, the fetus swallows amniotic fluid and the fluid is absorbed by the gastrointestinal tract. The absorbed fluid is then excreted through the kidneys. Any obstruction to the gastrointestinal tract interferes with this process and the mother runs the risk of developing polyhydramnios. Infants born to mothers with polyhydramnios should have the gastrointestinal tract investigated to rule out obstruction. Polyhydramnios is defined as greater than 2 liters of amniotic fluid. *(Sabiston, pp 1151–1152)*

583. **(A)** Sacrococcygeal teratoma frequently occurs in females (80%). The tumor usually presents as a mass posterior to the sacrum. It may also present as a retrorectal tumor between the rectum and the sacrum and may not be obvious externally. At birth, most of sacrococcygeal tumors are benign and subsequently undergo malignant degeneration. Prognosis is worse when excision is delayed beyond 2 months of birth. Therefore the tumor should be excised promptly. *(Sabiston, p 1183)*

584. **(E)** Reperfusion of an ischemic extremity can result in metabolic acidosis hyperkalemia from necrotic muscle. Rhabdomyolysis releases myoglobin, which can precipitate in acid urine, causing obstruction to renal tubules and subsequent renal failure. Serum potassium has to be monitored for hyperkalemia. If present, glucose and insulin are administered to drive the potassium into the cell, thus decreasing its level in the serum. Sodium bicarbonate is given to alkalinize urine and prevent precipitation of myoglobin. Mannitol or other osmotic diuretics are given to flush the kidney of any precipitates. Aggressive and adequate hydration is required to assure brisk diuresis and euvolemia. Heparin should be continued, since the risk of further embolization from the underlying cardiac condition persists. *(Sabiston, pp 320–324)*

585. **(C)** Anal and urinary incontinence in patients with rectal prolapse is due to stretching of pudendal nerves, resulting in neuromuscular dysfunction. Loss of anal rectal angle, loose endopelvic fascia, and stretching of the anal sphincter are associated with rectal prolapse but do not cause incontinence. Rectal prolapse should be repaired to prevent stretching of pudendal nerve and resulting incontinence. *(Sabiston, p 962)*

REFERENCES

Bartlett RH, Whitehouse WH, Turcotte JS. *Life Support Systems in Intensive Care.* Chicago, Ill: Year Book Medical Publishers Inc; 1984.

Bravermann LE, Utinger RD, eds., *Werner & Ingbar's The Thyroid: A Fundamental Clinical Text.* 6th ed. Philadelphia, Pa: Lippincott; 1991.

Browse NL. *An Introduction to the Symptoms and Signs of Surgical Disease.* Chicago, Ill: Year Book Medical Publishers Inc; 1978.

Conley JJ, ed. *Complications of Head and Neck Surgery.* Philadelphia, Pa: WB Saunders Co; 1979.

Cummings CW, et al, ed. *Otolaryngology—Head and Neck Surgery.* 2nd ed. St. Louis, Mo: Mosby Year Book; 1993.

David JA. *Wound Management.* Springhouse, Pa: Springhouse Corp; 1986.

Feliciano DV, Moore EE, Mattox KL, eds. *Trauma.* 3rd ed. Stamford, Conn: Appleton & Lange; 1996.

Grant JP. *Handbook of Total Parenteral Nutrition.* Philadelphia, Pa: WB Saunders Co; 1980.

Greenfield LJ, et al. *Surgery: Scientific Principles and Practice.* Philadelphia, Pa: JB Lippincott Co; 1993.

Hardy JD, ed. *Hardy's Textbook of Surgery.* Philadelphia, Pa: JB Lippincott Co; 1988.

Juhl JH. *Paul and Juhl's Essentials of Roentgen Interpretation.* New York, NY: Harper & Row Publishers Inc; 1993.

Lavery IC. The surgery of Hirschsprung's disease. *Surg. Clin North Am.* 1983;63:161–175.

Marini JJ. *Respiratory Medicine and Intensive Care for the House Officer.* Baltimore, Md: Williams & Wilkins; 1987.

Sabiston DC, ed. *Textbook of Surgery.* 14th ed. Philadelphia, Pa: WB Saunders Co; 1991.

Santiani B. False aneurysms following arterial reconstruction. *Surg Gynecol Obstet.* 1981;152:357–363.

Schwartz SI, Ellis H, eds. *Maingot's abdominal operations,* 9th ed. Norwalk, Conn: Appleton & Lange; 1990.

Schwartz SI, Shires GT, Spencer FC, eds. *Principles of Surgery.* 6th ed. New York, NY: McGraw-Hill Book Co; 1994.

Sreenivas VI. *Acute Disorders of the Abdomen: Diagnosis and Treatment.* New York, NY: Springer-Verlag New York, Inc; 1980.

Tanagho EA, McAninch JW. *Smith's General Urology.* 13th ed. Norwalk, Conn: Appleton & Lange; 1992.

Thompson NW, Cheung SY. Diagnosis and treatment of functioning and nonfunctioning adrenocortical neoplasms including incidentalomas. *Surg Clin North Am.* 1987;67(2):423–436.

Thompson NW, Vinik AI, eds. *Endocrine Surgery Update.* New York, NY: Grune and Stratton, Inc; 1983.

Vander AJ. *Renal Physiology.* 5th ed. New York, NY: McGraw-Hill Book Co; 1995.

SUBSPECIALTY LIST: SURGERY

Question Number and Subspecialty

520. Endocrinology
521. Trauma
522. Nutrition
523. Thoracic surgery
524. Head and neck
525. Neurosurgery
526. Wound healing
527. Orthopedics
528. Vascular surgery, orthopedics
529. Orthopedics
530. Trauma
531. Neoplasms
532. Neoplasms
533. Abdominal surgery
534. Endocrinology
535. Physiology
536. Urology
537. Gastrointestinal tract
538. Nutrition
539. Vascular surgery, trauma
540. Gastrointestinal tract
541. Orthopedics
542. Gastrointestinal tract
543. Gastrointestinal tract
544. Gastrointestinal tract
545. Genitourinary system
546. Immunology, transplantation
547. Trauma
548. Nutrition
549. Trauma
550. Gastrointestinal tract
551. Gastrointestinal tract
552. Urology
553. Trauma
554. Neurology, trauma
555. Pancreas, trauma
556. Physiology
557. Pulmonary surgery
558. Transplantation
559. Transplantation
560. Transplantation
561. Transplantation
562. Critical care, trauma
563. Pulmonary surgery
564. Pulmonary surgery, neoplasm
565. Pulmonary surgery
566. Gastrointestinal tract, surgical physiology
567. Gastrointestinal tract, surgical physiology
568. Gastrointestinal tract
569. Gastrointestinal tract, endocrine system
570. Gastrointestinal tract
571. Gastrointestinal tract
572. Gastrointestinal tract
573. Gastrointestinal tract
574. Transplantation
575. Cardiovascular surgery
576. Trauma
577. Neoplasm
578. Surgical physiology
579. Surgical infection
580. Urology, neoplasm
581. Gastrointestinal tract
582. Gastrointestinal tract
583. Neoplasm
584. Critical care
585. Gastrointestinal tract

Psychiatry

Mark Schultz, MD

DIRECTIONS (Questions 586 through 628): Each of the numbered items or incomplete statements in this section is followed by answers or by completions of the statement. Select the ONE lettered answer or completion that is BEST in each case.

586. All the following statements regarding the use of placebos in treating patients with non-specific physical complaints or puzzling pain syndromes are true EXCEPT

    (A) when emotional stress accompanies physical discomfort there is a higher probability for positive response to placebo

    (B) patients who respond to placebo complain of fewer somatic symptoms than do placebo nonresponders

    (C) positive placebo response is evidence that the pain had no physiologic basis

    (D) placebos are most often administered to disliked patients

    (E) positive placebo response should not cause the physician to curtail the usual diagnostic efforts

587. All the following statements concerning temporal lobe epilepsy are true EXCEPT

    (A) ictal phenomena may include episodes of intense rage

    (B) auditory hallucinations may occur during seizures

    (C) personality changes are apparent only during seizure activity

    (D) abnormal sexual behavior may be a presenting complaint

    (E) affected persons often have no memory of behavioral changes

588. Catatonic behavior can be best defined as a state of

    (A) extreme motor activity that is often violent and apparently pointless

    (B) generalized muscular rigidity

    (C) "waxy flexibility" in which subjects maintain any posture in which an examiner positions them

    (D) stupor or mutism not attributable to organic cause

    (E) profound psychomotor disturbance not attributable to organic causes

589. All the following statements regarding bulimia are true EXCEPT

    (A) binge eating is usually followed by a sense of euphoric well-being

    (B) bulimic episodes may occur in persons suffering from anorexia nervosa

    (C) bulimic persons are well aware of their disordered eating patterns

    (D) it most often affects young women

    (E) it tends to persist for several years

590. Which of the following statements concerning the kinetics and clinical effects of benzodiazepines is true?

    (A) short-half-life benzodiazepines are associated with a later onset of withdrawal signs than long-half-life benzodiazepines

    (B) long-half-life benzodiazepines may be associated with residual sedation even weeks after the medication is discontinued

(C) the metabolism of short-half-life agents is more influenced by old age than is that of long-half-life agents

(D) long-half-life agents are more efficacious in the treatment of anxiety symptoms

(E) lorazepam has a longer half-life than chlordiazepoxide

591. Compared with low-potency antipsychotic medications, high-potency antipsychotic medications tend to be associated with

(A) less anticholinergic activity and lower incidence of extrapyramidal side effects

(B) less anticholinergic activity and higher incidence of extrapyramidal side effects

(C) greater anticholinergic activity and lower incidence of extrapyramidal side effects

(D) greater anticholinergic activity and higher incidence of extrapyramidal side effects

(E) greater anticholinergic activity and greater α-adrenergic blockade

592. The clinical efficacy of antipsychotic medications is generally proportionate to the in vitro ability of the drug to

(A) decrease presynaptic reuptake of norepinephrine

(B) block postsynaptic dopamine receptors

(C) produce adrenergic blockade

(D) exert an atropinelike effect at the synapse

(E) increase general cerebral activation as measured by electroencephalography

593. A 22-year-old man is brought to the emergency room after sustaining an abdominal injury in a motor vehicle accident. Laparotomy and subsequent splenectomy are performed. Postoperative course is unremarkable until the third hospital day, when he exhibits apprehension, generalized twitching, tremors, and nausea. On the fourth hospital day he suffers a single generalized tonic–clonic seizure. After recovering, he admits that for the past 8 months he has been "popping yellow jackets" at a rate equivalent to roughly 1000 mg of pentobarbital per day. The most appropriate first step in this man's management would be to

(A) give a loading dose of intravenous phenytoin followed by a daily phenytoin regimen

(B) perform a sleep-deprived electroencephalogram to assess the risk of continued seizure activity

(C) begin a regimen of pentobarbital, 1000 mg daily

(D) administer intramuscular phenobarbital, 200 mg, followed by oral phenobarbital, 30 mg every 8 hours

(E) give 200 mg of oral pentobarbital and observe for sedation, slurred speech, or nystagmus

594. When compared to school-age children with conduct disorder, children who develop conduct disorder as adolescents

(A) are more likely to display persistent psychopathology

(B) are more likely to engage in aggressive behaviors

(C) are more likely to be diagnosed with antisocial personality disorder as adults

(D) are less likely to have relatively normal peer relationships

(E) show a lower male-to-female ratio among affected individuals

595. The maxim guiding the court in child custody disputes is "serve the best interest of the child." In cases involving custody of school-age children, this maxim has been interpreted to support all the following statements EXCEPT

(A) natural parents retain an inherent right to custody

(B) the mental health of the contending parents should be considered

(C) the physical health of the contending parents should be considered

(D) the willingness of each contending parent to encourage the child to maintain a close relationship with the other parent should be considered

(E) the child's preference should be considered

596. The cognitive deterioration that accompanies Alzheimer's disease may be associated with a deficiency of the neurotransmitter

(A) norepinephrine

(B) γ-aminobutyric acid

(C) serotonin

(D) acetylcholine

(E) dopamine

597. A 25-year-old woman is brought to the emergency room. She presents with confusion, bizarre and contorted posturing, marked diaphoresis, and abdominal distress. She is found to be tachycardic and has a rectal temperature of 39.4°C (103°F). Complete blood cell count and lumbar puncture results are normal. Review of outpatient records reveals that the woman has been receiving chlorpromazine for the treatment of schizophrenia. A potentially life-threatening medication side effect that must be considered in this case is

(A) acute dystonic reaction

(B) akathisia

(C) tardive dyskinesia

(D) neuroleptic malignant syndrome

(E) chlorpromazine allergic reaction

598. A severely emotionally ill woman, diagnosed as having schizoaffective illness, takes the following psychotropic medications: nortriptyline, fluphenazine, benztropine, lorazepam, and triazolam. She consults her gynecologist because of a variety of complaints, and hyperprolactinemia is discovered. Of the woman's medications, the one most likely to be causing her hyperprolactinemia is

(A) nortriptyline

(B) fluphenazine

(C) benztropine

(D) lorazepam

(E) triazolam

599. All the following are currently used as psychologic tests of personality functioning EXCEPT the

(A) Rorschach Test

(B) Thematic Apperception Test

(C) Word Association Test

(D) Bender Gestalt Test

(E) Sentence Completion Test

600. The M'Naghten rule is associated in American jurisprudence with

(A) protocols for civil commitment

(B) the insanity defense

(C) the right to psychiatric treatment

(D) maintaining confidentiality

(E) guidelines for expert testimony

601. Which of the following statements concerning suicide is true?

(A) persons who repeatedly attempt suicide are at low risk for eventually killing themselves

(B) discussing suicide with persons suspected of feeling suicidal increases their risk of suicide

(C) depressed persons who commit suicide usually do so after their depression has begun to abate

(D) persons with schizophrenia are at low risk for suicide

(E) persons who commit suicide usually leave few clues of their intentions

602. According to the theories of Erik Erikson, the developmental task of school-age children (6 to 11 years) is to resolve the psychosocial crisis of

(A) trust versus mistrust

(B) autonomy versus shame and doubt

(C) intimacy versus isolation

(D) ego integrity versus despair

(E) industry versus inferiority

603. Jean Piaget is best known for his theories on the

(A) development of intelligence

(B) roots of human aggression

(C) types of intrapsychic defense mechanisms

(D) meaning of symbols

(E) importance of infant-mother bonding

604. According to classical psychoanalytic theory, obsessive-compulsive personality in an adult is linked to which of the following stages of psychosexual development?

(A) oral stage

(B) anal stage

(C) phallic stage

(D) latency stage

(E) genital stage

605. All the following statements concerning the stress of life events are true EXCEPT

(A) divorce generally is considered a severe stress

(B) the birth of a child generally is considered a severe stress

(C) such events as vacations and recognition of job or school accomplishments reduce overall life stress

(D) the intensity of stress associated with a particular event may be magnified if the event occurs during a time of year in which stressful events have occurred in the past

(E) listing relevant life stresses is part of a complete diagnosis by criteria established in the *Diagnostic and Statistical Manual of Mental Disorders*

606. Which of the following statements concerning the risk of development of schizophrenia is true?

(A) children born to a schizophrenic mother but adopted by nonschizophrenic parents develop schizophrenia at a rate equal to that of the general population

(B) one third of persons with schizophrenia have a schizophrenic first-degree relative

(C) young adults with schizoid personality disorder nearly always develop schizophrenia

(D) boys are three times as likely as girls to develop schizophrenia during young adulthood

(E) disordered patterns of family communication are thought to be a predisposing factor in the development of schizophrenia

607. The epidemiology of major affective disorders can be described by all of the following statements EXCEPT

(A) women are more likely than men to develop bipolar I disorder (manic–depressive disorder)

(B) women are more likely than men to develop major depressive disorder

(C) bipolar I disorder tends to appear before the age of 30 years

(D) the frequency of major depressive disorder remains steady throughout adulthood

(E) as many as one-fourth of all Americans with recurrent major depressive disorder never fully recover between depressive episodes

608. The unconscious feelings that arise within a psychotherapist during psychotherapy are described by the term

(A) projection
(B) countertransference
(C) acting out
(D) identification
(E) introjection

609. Anorexia nervosa can be described by all the following statements EXCEPT

(A) prognosis is more favorable in younger adolescents than in older adolescents
(B) boys develop anorexia nervosa much less often than do girls
(C) affected persons typically believe they remain overweight despite marked weight loss
(D) affected persons typically are rebellious and delinquent
(E) mortality rate is said to be from 5% to 20%

610. The 1976 court case *Tarasoff v The Regents of the University of California* produced a landmark decision concerning the obligation of psychiatrists to

(A) maintain confidentiality in record keeping
(B) administer treatment in emergency situations
(C) assist in court-mandated competency hearings
(D) search for the "least restrictive" treatment setting for persons facing commitment
(E) warn persons threatened by their patients

611. Defining the usefulness of psychotherapy has been a difficult area of research and debate. Which of the following statements regarding psychotherapy is true?

(A) most types of outpatient psychotherapy subscribe to long-term, exploratory models
(B) continuous psychotherapy, ie, with no planned end, is contrary to a medical model of treatment
(C) a recommendation that no treatment is necessary can be appropriate for a variety of conditions
(D) consultation over one or two appointments should not be expected to provide therapeutic relief
(E) psychodynamic interventions should not be employed during consultation

612. Individuals who have bulimia nervosa and individuals who have anorexia nervosa would be LEAST likely to share which of the following clinical features?

(A) life-threatening change in body weight
(B) vomiting to limit caloric intake
(C) severe disturbance in body image
(D) dysphoria after consuming food
(E) response to antidepressant drugs

613. The *Diagnostic and Statistical Manual of Mental Disorders* (DSM) uses a multiaxial system for patient evaluation. Each axis provides a different set of descriptors and method of classification. One *DSM* axis has been devoted (for adult patients) exclusively to

(A) family history
(B) psychodynamic formulation
(C) estimated intelligence
(D) physical problems
(E) substance abuse disorders

614. Factors likely to interfere with the accuracy of the dexamethasone suppression test include

(A) advanced age

(B) obesity

(C) concurrent administration of tricyclic drugs

(D) recently concluded administration of tricyclic drugs

(E) none of the above

615. Antisocial personality disorder is considered to be

(A) synonymous with criminal behavior

(B) the male counterpart of histrionic personality disorder

(C) amenable to pharmacologic treatment with antiandrogenic agents

(D) correlated with electroencephalographic studies suggesting cortical immaturity

(E) a variant of malingering

616. Women suffering from postpartum psychiatric disorders would be most likely to demonstrate

(A) onset of symptoms within 12 hours of childbirth

(B) marked lability of mood

(C) visual hallucinations

(D) pseudoseizures

(E) grandiose delusions involving the baby

617. Social phobia can be described by which of the following statements?

(A) it is the diagnostic term for excessive shyness

(B) its lifetime prevalence is nearly that of alcohol dependence

(C) despite outward appearances of depressed mood, persons with social phobia in fact rarely develop major depression

(D) drug treatments are typically unsuccessful

(E) attempts at social skills training tend to worsen the condition by increasing feelings of being different and bizarre

618. Methadone maintenance therapy often is recommended for treating persons addicted to heroin. Methadone is considered useful because it

(A) does not cause euphoria

(B) is not associated with tolerance

(C) does not produce depressive side effects

(D) is not an opioid

(E) none of the above

619. True statements regarding disulfiram therapy include which of the following?

(A) tolerance to its effects develops rapidly and doses require frequent adjustment

(B) users may develop severe reactions to topical agents, like cosmetics, that contain alcohol

(C) it is the treatment of choice for persons who otherwise refuse to involve themselves in alcohol rehabilitation programs

(D) it is indicated in the treatment of persons with a history of psychotic disorders exacerbated by alcohol

(E) it is useful in treating pregnant alcoholic women, to lessen the risk of fetal alcohol syndrome

620. Which of the following statements about the extrapyramidal side effects of antipsychotic drugs is true?

(A) many extrapyramidal side effects mimic signs of worsening psychosis

(B) the frequency of acute dyskinetic reactions is directly proportional to dosage of antipsychotic medication

(C) tardive dyskinesia is an idiosyncratic complication of first-time use of antipsychotic drugs

(D) haloperidol produces few extrapyramidal side effects compared to most other antipsychotic drugs

(E) none of the above

621. Tricyclic antidepressant drugs have which of the following pharmacologic properties?

(A) potentiation of the reuptake of norepinephrine

(B) inhibition of noradrenergic function

(C) enhancement of activity of guanethidine and related drugs

(D) cholinergic activation

(E) atropinelike activity

622. Which of the following statements concerning sociologic factors in suicide risk is true?

(A) women are at higher risk than men

(B) persons older than 65 years of age are at higher risk than persons between 25 and 35 years of age

(C) blue-collar workers are at higher risk than persons in professional occupations

(D) wartime is associated with a higher suicide risk than peacetime

(E) a history of alcohol abuse is a risk factor for accidental death but not for suicide

623. The limbic system of the brain is presumed to be the region most concerned with the operation and expression of emotions. Components of the limbic system include the

(A) hypothalamus

(B) nucleus accumbens

(C) nucleus of Meynert

(D) hippocampus

(E) reticular formation

624. The so-called first-rank, or schneiderian, symptoms of schizophrenia include all the following EXCEPT

(A) auditory hallucinations

(B) somatic delusions

(C) thought broadcasting

(D) thought insertion

(E) catatonia

625. Paranoid schizophrenia can be described by which of the following statements?

(A) affected persons quickly lose the ability to function appropriately in social encounters

(B) age of onset generally is earlier than in other types of schizophrenia

(C) cognitive impairment tends to progress more rapidly than in other types of schizophrenia

(D) hallucinations and delusions often are grandiose in nature

(E) it is associated with paranoid personality disorder

626. Electroconvulsive therapy (ECT) can be described by which of the following statements?

(A) ECT is contraindicated in the treatment of psychotic depression

(B) ECT can cause depressed persons to exhibit manic symptoms

(C) transient memory loss occurs rarely after each ECT treatment

(D) morbidity and mortality are greater than with antidepressant drug therapy

(E) unilateral ECT is no longer recognized as a valid treatment

627. Amphetamine abuse can be described by which of the following statements?

(A) tolerance to amphetamines develops slowly

(B) recommended treatment of chronic abuse is with behavioral therapy

(C) amphetamine psychosis is easily distinguishable from paranoid schizophrenia

(D) withdrawal after chronic abuse can lead to a severe manic episode

(E) acute overdose can cause convulsions and coma

628. Moderate mental retardation can be described by which of the following statements?

   (A) it is the most common category of retardation in the United States

   (B) affected persons are considered trainable but not educable

   (C) affected persons usually are unable to perform routine self-care

   (D) the IQ range is 50 to 70

   (E) none of the above

DIRECTIONS (Questions 629 through 647): Each group of items in this section consists of a list of lettered headings followed by a set of numbered words or phrases. For each numbered word or phrase, select the ONE lettered heading that is most closely associated with it. Each lettered heading may be selected once, more than once, or not at all.

Questions 629 through 632

For each psychiatric disorder listed below, select the diagnostic class of which it is a member.

   (A) dissociative disorder
   (B) somatoform disorder
   (C) mood disorder
   (D) anxiety disorder
   (E) psychotic disorder
   (F) organic mental disorder
   (G) sexual disorder
   (H) impulse control disorder

629. Conversion disorder

630. Cyclothymic disorder

631. Social phobia

632. Multiple personality disorder

Questions 633 through 640

Below are several quotes from persons being evaluated for a possible psychiatric disorder. For each of the quotes that follow, select the psychologic process that would most closely apply.

   (A) illusion
   (B) delusion
   (C) hallucination
   (D) phobia
   (E) neurosis
   (F) fugue
   (G) obsession
   (H) compulsion

633. "I directed Hurricane Andrew to destroy Florida!"

634. "Every night before I go to sleep I need to check the door nine times to make sure it's locked"

635. "I don't care what the tests show, I know I'm pregnant"

636. "Look at the silver angel on the ceiling" (an alcoholic person is looking at a metal sprinkler on the ceiling)

637. "Look at the silver angel on the ceiling" (the person, not an alcoholic, is looking at a plain white ceiling)

638. "My father was cold and cruel. No wonder I hate men!"

639. "I'm deathly afraid of spiders"

640. "Elvis speaks to me and tells me how to lead my life"

Questions 641 through 647

For each psychiatric disorder below, select the medication most likely to be effective.

(A) fluoxetine

(B) clozapine

(C) alprazolam

(D) triazolam

(E) benztropine

(F) lithium carbonate

(G) haloperidol

641. Stress-related insomnia

642. Major depressive episode (new onset)

643. Major depressive episode (partially treated with an adequate dosage of antidepressant medication)

644. Obsessive–compulsive disorder

645. Schizophrenia intractable to common antipsychotic drugs

646. Adjustment disorder with anxiety

647. Extrapyramidal reaction to antipsychotic medication

ANSWERS AND EXPLANATIONS

586. **(C)** Research has shown that a high percentage of physicians have actually prescribed placebos, although infrequently. House staff surveyed were found to use placebo for at least one patient yearly. At the same time, little formal training for placebo use is provided. Data show that physicians perceive placebo users and responders as "problem" patients. However, the placebo response is a real phenomenon, the physiologic mechanism of which is poorly understood. What is clear is that patients who are under stress are more likely to obtain relief from placebos. It should be noted that placebo use can be a responsible tool for pain control re-gardless of the cause of the pain. Therefore, a positive response is not a diagnostic indicator; it simply represents a successful intervention in relieving a patient's discomfort or pain. Obviously, diagnostic efforts should not be affected by placebo response, and a careful evaluation should proceed without compromise. (*Goodwin et al*)

587. **(C)** Although temporal lobe epilepsy may present as dramatic bursts of unusual behaviors or feelings (ictal episodes), there may also be complex interictal changes. These may include pervasive changes in sexual interest (predominantly hyposexuality), increased social aggressiveness, hyperreligiosity, and paranoia. Patients with temporal lobe epilepsy also have an increased incidence of symptoms of schizophreniform psychosis (eg, auditory hallucinations and delusions). The presence of these psychotic symptoms may correlate chronologically with electroencephalgram-recorded spike activity in the temporal lobe. Similarly, behavioral idiosyncrasies may occur unpredictably, and affected individuals may be observed carrying out complex but automatic behaviors when temporal discharges are occurring. Thorough neurologic work-up including electroencephalographic studies is necessary to differentiate temporal lobe epilepsy from functional psychiatric illness. (*Kaplan and Sadock, vol 1, pp 721–722*)

588. **(E)** The term "catatonic behavior" refers to a variety of psychomotor disturbances that are not attributable to an organic cause. Catatonic excitement is a state of extreme motor activity that appears pointless and disorganized and may become violent and aggressive. Catatonic rigidity can involve all muscle groups and render a person completely stiff. Catatonic negativism is defined by persons resisting any outside force or doing the opposite of anything asked of them. Patients with catatonic waxy flexibility will maintain any position in which they are placed, as would a wax figure or a doll. Catatonic posturing refers to a voluntary posing in bizarre positions or maintenance of strange facial contor-

tions over a long time period. Catatonic stupor is a generalized and profound decrease in psychomotor activity; affected persons may be virtually oblivious to their surroundings. Individuals may suddenly shift among the various catatonic states: quiet and treatable patients may rapidly become active and aggressive. Catatonic patients are at increased risk for malnutrition, exhaustion, dehydration, and self-inflicted injury. It is important to rule out organic brain disorders, such as meningitis and exposure to toxic substances, before diagnosing catatonic schizophrenia. (*Kaplan and Sadock, vol 1, pp 538–539,751*)

589. **(A)** Bulimia is an eating disorder in which copious amounts of food are ingested rapidly over a brief time period (usually less than 2 hours). Affected persons are painfully aware that such binge eating is unhealthy but feel that the impulsive eating is beyond control. Binges are characteristically followed by a profound sense of failure and depression. This condition tends to persist for several years, with occasional remissions. It most commonly affects adolescent or young adult women. First symptoms may be associated with a major life change, such as leaving home or starting work. Bulimia may also occur as one aspect of the related eating disorder anorexia nervosa. (*Kaplan and Sadock, vol 2, pp 1362–1367*)

590. **(B)** One way to begin to differentiate clinically among the many benzodiazepines currently marketed for the treatment of anxiety is to divide them according to half-life. The long-acting agents include diazepam and chlordiazepoxide. They are metabolized in several steps, by hepatic oxidation, and therefore have biologically active metabolites. The short-acting agents include oxazepam and lorazepam. They are metabolized by glucuronide conjugation to inactive metabolites. Both groups are equally efficacious in the treatment of anxiety, in either single-dose or multiple-dose regimens. However, when multiple-dose treatment is indicated, it is important to be aware of the pharmacokinetic difference between these agents.

The time lag before onset of medication effect will depend on the absorption rate. Diazepam has been found to act more rapidly and more profoundly than the less well absorbed oxazepam. However, because of longer half-life, diazepam accumulates extensively in the body during multiple-dose regimens, with corresponding clinical side effects such as excessive sedation. Because of their slow elimination rate, long-acting agents may produce sedation 2 weeks or more after the agent is discontinued. There may also be increased risk of dangerous interaction with other substances, including alcohol. On the other hand, short-acting agents accumulate less and are more rapidly eliminated. Abrupt discontinuation of these agents may precipitate sudden onset of withdrawal symptoms, including increased anxiety, insomnia, and autonomic nervous system disturbance. One distinction between these agents that must be emphasized is that hepatic oxidation tends to be much more influenced by the aging process than does the glucuronidation process by which the short-acting agents are metabolized. Thus, elderly individuals may be much more prone to the dangers of drug accumulation when receiving long-half-life benzodiazepines. This is the basis for the opinion that short-half-life benzodiazepines are the drugs of choice in treating anxiety in the geriatric population. (*Salzmann et al*)

591. **(B)** High-potency antipsychotic medications include the piperazine-substituted phenothiazines, such as trifluoperazine, and members of the butyrophenone class, such as haloperidol. These medications are effective antipsychotics at relatively low dosages and generally produce less sedation, less anticholinergic activity, and less α-adrenergic blockade than do the low-potency antipsychotics, such as chlorpromazine, thioridazine, and perphenazine. High-potency antipsychotics do produce a higher incidence of extrapyramidal side effects, including acute dystonic reactions. This phenomenon may reflect the fact that these agents have less intrinsic anticholinergic activity. Awareness of the side effects of the various antipsychotics

is often the key determinant in choosing the best agent for each patient. Certain patients will have difficulty with the sedating effects of medication. A dehydrated patient may be prone to hypotension secondary to α-adrenergic blockade. Other patients may be extremely susceptible to acute dystonic reactions. A patient's entire health profile should be considered when choosing an antipsychotic medication. *(Kaplan and Sadock, vol 2, pp 2003–2011)*

592. **(B)** The clinical efficacy of an antipsychotic medication is generally proportional to its in vitro ability to block dopamine receptors. This finding is one of the major supports of the so-called dopamine hypothesis of schizophrenia, which holds that schizophrenic symptoms stem from an imbalance of dopaminergic systems in the brain. It remains to be seen if all antipsychotic medications are active in direct proportion to their ability to produce dopamine blockade. Antipsychotic medications tend to vary in the extent to which they affect multiple neurotransmitter systems in different parts of the brain. The dopamine hypothesis has yet to be fully validated. *(Kaplan and Sadock, vol 2, pp 1994–1995)*

593. **(E)** Physical dependence develops when significant amounts of barbiturates are ingested chronically over a course of weeks or months. Abstinence symptoms usually develop within 72 hours after the last drug ingestion. Early withdrawal signs include anxiety, insomnia, orthostatic hypotension, and mixed gastrointestinal complaints. Grand mal seizures may occur; they generally begin between the third and seventh day of withdrawal and may present as single episodes or as status epilepticus. Onset of seizures often heralds deterioration into frank delirium. The management of barbiturate withdrawal requires the accurate assessment of the patient's level of dependence (drug abusers are notoriously inaccurate in reporting their usual intake). In the "test dose" method to establish drug requirement during detoxification from barbiturates, a patient is given 200 mg of pentobarbital orally and assessed over the next hour. Patients who become very drowsy or exhibit coarse nystagmus may require no more than 600 mg daily. Patients who become only mildly drowsy with fine nystagmus may require 800 mg daily in divided doses. Patients with no response whatsoever probably will require more than 1200 mg daily. Once the maintenance dose is established and the patient is stabilized, the dose can be slowly tapered, by 10% daily. *(Tupin et al, pp 141–143)*

594. **(E)** Conduct disorder causes affected children to display persistent, disruptive, often violent behaviors toward other people and toward elements in their social systems. Behaviors can be aggressive, destructive, deceitful, manipulative, intimidating, cruel, truant and rebellious. In general, conduct disorder is more severe and intractable if it develops in younger children (childhood-onset type) than in older children (adolescent-onset type). Childhood-onset conduct disorder is more likely to be associated with later diagnosis of antisocial personality disorder. Male-to-female ratio of affected individuals is higher in childhood-onset conduct disorder than in the adolescent-onset type. *(APA, pp 85–91)*

595. **(A)** In recent years, the concept of what is in "the best interests of the child" in custody disputes has become more sophisticated. Many factors must be considered in evaluating the claims of the contending parents, including their physical and mental fitness, their ability to provide affection and protection, and their willingness to allow the child to maintain a close relationship with the non-custodial parent. It is no longer a given that natural parents have an indisputable right to custody, if other caregivers are deemed more appropriate. *(Kaplan and Sadock, vol 2, p 2765)*

596. **(D)** Major deficiencies in acetylcholine content in the brain are linked with the cognitive losses associated with Alzheimer's disease. The nucleus of Meynert is the richest site of acetylcholine in the brain. Recent studies of brain tissues of affected persons have demon-

strated that the amount of acetylcholine localized in these neurons is depleted and that the efferent pathways from the nucleus show signs of degeneration. *(Cummings and Benson, pp 64–71)*

597. **(D)** Neuroleptic malignant syndrome (NMS) is an uncommon but important side effect of psychotropic medication use. It is characterized by severe extrapyramidal reactions, autonomic disturbances, and hyperthermia. This syndrome is associated with a mortality rate of 20%. Anticholinergic treatment, generally helpful in common acute dystonic reactions, seems of only limited usefulness in NMS. NMS is believed to result from extensive dopamine blockade; bromocriptine, a dopamine agonist, has been of value in the treatment of NMS. *(Mueller et al)*

598. **(B)** Among psychotropic drugs, antipsychotic preparations are most likely to cause hyperprolactinemia. Release of prolactin is inhibited by dopamine. Therefore, the central dopamine receptor blockade produced by antipsychotic drugs leads to elevated prolactin production. *(Hales and Frances, pp 195–197)*

599. **(D)** When properly administered and interpreted by an experienced clinician, psychologic tests offer a significant contribution to understanding psychiatric illness. These tests can be powerful tools in clarifying issues of psychiatric diagnosis, psychodynamics, and patient management. Standardized psychologic tests provide a fairly objective means for comparing behavior with available normative data representative of a larger reference group. Psychologic tests of personality functioning include the Thematic Apperception Test, Word Association Test, Sentence Completion Test, and Rorschach Test. The Bender Gestalt Test is a test of visuomotor coordination. *(Kaplan and Sadock, vol 1, pp 544–557)*

600. **(B)** In 1843, Daniel M'Naghten, a disturbed Scottish woodcutter, attempted to kill the British Prime Minister. He mistook the Prime Minister's secretary for the Prime Minister

and shot and killed him. In the subsequent trial, M'Naghten's counsel argued that his client suffered from a mental illness and therefore did not know the difference between right and wrong and could not comprehend the nature or consequences of his actions. Although modified over time, these criteria for an insanity defense have become widely adopted in the United States. The current American Law Institute standard states that a person is not responsible for criminal conduct if, at the time of such conduct and as a result of mental disease or defect, a person lacked substantial capacity either to appreciate the wrongfulness of the actions (intent) or to conform conduct to the requirements of the law (voluntary conduct). *(Kaplan and Sadock, vol 2, pp 2763–2764)*

601. **(C)** Successful clinical intervention with persons known or suspected to be suicidal can be hampered by several popular myths regarding suicide. Fallacious notions are many, including "persons who have attempted suicide and failed are not serious about killing themselves" and "persons who talk about killing themselves don't do it" and "mentioning suicide to depressed persons can put the idea in their head." In persons with schizophrenia, suicide risk is especially high early in the course of their illness as well as during times of transition in their lives. The most dangerous phase of depression in relation to suicide is during successful convalescence; possible reasons for this phenomenon include abatement of psychomotor retardation, fear of relapse, and guilt over the effect the depression had on others. *(Kaplan and Sadock, vol 2, pp 1739–1752)*

602. **(E)** The psychoanalyst Erik Erikson has theorized that ego development proceeds from birth through eight identifiable stages marked by specific psychosocial crises. Infants are faced with the task of developing basic trust in the world and in themselves. As they grow older, children sequentially develop a sense of autonomy (ages 1 to 2 years), initiative (3 to 5 years), and industry (6 to 11 years) as they successfully meet developmental challenges. The psychosocial crises of adolescents and young adults are identity versus role confusion, and intimacy versus isolation, respectively. People successfully meet the challenges of adulthood by providing a suitable nurturing environment for themselves and the generation that follows ("generativity"); once past the generative stage, older adults can reflect back on their lives with either satisfaction ("ego integrity") or despair. *(Kaplan and Sadock, vol 1, pp 481–484)*

603. **(A)** Jean Piaget, a Swiss psychologist, has been described as the leading pioneer in researching the development and refinement of human intelligence. According to Piaget, human intelligence passes through four major stages of development: the sensorimotor stage (up to 2 years of age), during which individuals acquire the skills of self-regulation and the notion of object permanence; the preoperational stage (roughly 2 to 5 years), during which language skills are refined, the concept of "me" and "mine" is developed, and the functional significance of objects is appreciated; the concrete operational stage (5 to 11 years), during which children learn to quantify and categorize; and formal operational period, characterized by the ability to engage in abstract thought. Piaget's work has led to the understanding of how children's abilities to adapt and learn are dependent on the current stage of development of intelligence. *(Kaplan and Sadock, vol 1, pp 292–296)*

604. **(B)** The second stage of psychosexual development, the anal stage occurs in children from 1 to 3 years of age, a period in which they gain control over elimination of wastes by mastering sphincter function. The interactions between parents and children around toilet training impart an aggressive nature to the mastery—or lack of mastery—of sphincter control; conflicts regarding separation and independence also arise. Thus, in the anal stage are the roots of an individual's sense of independence, initiative, and cooperation; unsuccessful or impaired resolution of anal-stage conflicts can lead to such personality traits as stubbornness, orderliness,

and frugality, which are common manifestations of the obsessive-compulsive personality. Modern theoriticians also identify early struggles with self-esteem and intimacy as possible causative factors. *(Kaplan and Sadock, vol 1, pp 442–447,468)*

605. **(C)** Among the most severe life stresses are death of a spouse or other close family member, divorce or marital separation, and pregnancy and birth of a child. The intensity of stress can be heightened if it is associated with other stresses or occurs during a time of year marked by past stressful events (anniversary reaction). In general, any change—positive or negative—in a person's life represents a source of stress. Listing relevant life stresses comprises Axis IV of a complete DSM diagnostic formulation. *(APA, pp 29–30)*

606. **(E)** Determination of risk for the development of schizophrenia has been approached from a variety of directions. Genetic factors, for example, appear to be important, as evidenced by a high concordance rate for schizophrenia in monozygotic twins and an increased risk in adopted children whose biologic mothers were schizophrenic; on the other hand, fewer than 15% of schizophrenic individuals have schizophrenic first-degree relatives. Although persons who develop schizophrenia may have been previously diagnosed as having other psychiatric disorders, there appears to be no disorder that clearly predisposes to schizophrenia. Males and females develop the illness with approximately the same frequency. *(APA, pp 274–278; Kaplan and Sadock, vol 1, pp 907–909)*

607. **(A)** The two most common forms of major affective disorder are major depressive disorder (so-called unipolar disease) and bipolar I disorder (manic–depressive illness). It has been estimated that as many as 25% of American women and 12% of American men have experienced a major depressive episode. As many as one-fourth of individuals with recurrent major depressive disorder do not recover fully between bouts of illness. Although major depressive episodes can arise

any time during adulthood, bipolar I disorder tends to appear in young adulthood. Depression is diagnosed more often in women than in men; bipolar I disorder is diagnosed about equally in both sexes. *(Kaplan and Sadock, vol 1, pp 1080–1083)*

608. **(B)** During the course of psychotherapy, patients develop feelings toward the therapist that recreate feelings they have had toward significant persons in their life, a phenomenon called transference. Identification of these feelings and the behaviors they provoke is crucial, especially in insight-oriented psychotherapy. However, during the course of conducting psychotherapy, therapists, too, develop feelings and reactions as memories of situations from their past are evoked. These countertransference feelings provide the therapist with valuable clues regarding how people in the patient's life may have reacted to the patient. Countertransference may also serve to pinpoint areas within the therapist's own unconscious that may prejudice the ability to offer nondirective, unbiased treatment. *(Kaplan and Sadock, vol 1, pp 470–471)*

609. **(D)** Anorexia nervosa, a disorder predominantly but not exclusively affecting females, is characterized by obsessional weight loss and disordered body image. Other behavioral features include food binges, self-induced vomiting, and abuse of laxatives. Affected persons typically are described as pleasant, polite overachievers. Mortality rate is as high as 20%, with death caused by dehydration, electrolyte imbalances, and other manifestations of starvation. The prognosis is better if affected persons are younger and if intervention is begun before weight loss has become marked. *(Herskowitz and Rosman, pp 228–239)*

610. **(E)** Psychiatrists often come into contact with persons who, by virtue of emotional illness or personality, are potentially dangerous. Despite the fact that most studies refute the notion that psychiatrists are better able than other practitioners to predict danger-

ousness, several court decisions in recent years have made psychiatrists responsible to some degree for protecting persons endangered by their patients. In the landmark *Tarasoff* case in 1976, the California Supreme Court ruled that "when a therapist determines or . . . should determine that his patient presents a serious danger of violence to another, he incurs an obligation to use reasonable care to protect the intended victim against such danger." More recent court decisions have extended the scope of this obligation still further. *(Halleck, pp 77–82)*

611. **(C)** Defining the uses and parameters of the many types of psychotherapy has been a daunting task. Certain generalizations, however, have emerged. Most types of psychotherapy are brief, and the efficacy of these therapies has been easier to demonstrate than that of the more traditional, long-term therapies. Continual psychotherapy, ie, intermittent treatment for an extended period and having no planned end, can be effective in treating certain chronic conditions, and in this way is quite consistent with a medical model of care. The therapeutic value of consultation, which can even be a setting for the effective use of psychodynamic interventions, should not be overlooked. *(Hales and Frances, pp 410–412)*

612. **(A)** Although the eating disorders of bulimia nervosa and anorexia nervosa share many characteristics, there are two main distinguishing features. Changes in body weight in bulimic individuals, as opposed to anorectic individuals, are usually not severe enough to threaten life. The consumption of large quantities of food (binge eating) followed by purging is an essential feature of bulimia; it is also present, although less characteristic, in anorexia. Both disorders are associated with distortions in body image and dysphoria after eating. Antidepressant drugs have been used with some success in treating both disorders. *(APA, pp 539–550)*

613. (D)   The multiaxial system of diagnosis pioneered by the DSM includes five axes, or classes, of information, description, and diagnosis. Axis I describes major psychiatric disorders, including mood disorders, schizophrenia, mental retardation, and substance abuse. Personality disorders constitute axis II. Axis III lists physical disorders and disease. A listing of psychosocial stresses defines axis IV, and axis V describes level of adaptive functioning. *(APA, pp 25–32)*

614. (B)   The dexamethasone suppression test (DST) may provide additional evidence of the presence of endogenous major depression, but results must be interpreted with care. False-positive results (ie, nonsuppression *not* produced by biologic depression) can occur in association with obesity or pregnancy, as well as with serious illness such as anorexia. Medications that also can lead to false-positive DST results include carbamazepine, phenobarbital, indomethacin, estrogens, but not tricyclic antidepressants. Results in elderly individuals appear to be unaffected by their age; in contrast, DST results in children may have less validity. *(Hales and Frances, pp 188–190)*

615. (D)   Antisocial personality disorder represents a chronically maladaptive pattern of interaction and perception in which the rights of others are violated and in which social productivity (sustained job performance or intimate relationships) is impaired. Although an individual with antisocial personality disorder might engage in criminal acts, criminality as a socially defined behavior is determined by a variety of economic, cultural, and other environmental factors. Family studies have shown that antisocial personality is associated with several other psychiatric disorders, including histrionic personality disorder and alcoholism, which are diagnosable in first-degree relatives at higher rates than among the general population. These associations raise the possibility that the disorders may have common genetic as well as environmental determinants. Electroencephalographic studies reveal an increased preva-

lence of slow-wave activity, lowered thresholds for sedation, and slow cortical recovery from stimulation, suggesting that individuals with antisocial personality disorder manifest signs of cortical immaturity. Pharmacologic intervention has no proven efficacy in the treatment of antisocial personality. Early psychologic and behavioral interventions seem to improve long-term outcome. *(Kaplan and Sadock, vol 2, pp 1441–1444)*

616. (B)   Perhaps half or more of all women experience emotional disturbance in the early postpartum period. Symptoms usually appear between the third and seventh postpartum day and can include irritability, anxiety, fluctuating mood, feelings of inadequacy and shame, confusion and disorientation, and such psychotic disturbances as auditory hallucinations and nihilistic delusions. Both biologic and psychologic factors appear to be important etiologically in postpartum emotional illness. Choice of treatment depends on the type and severity of symptoms. *(Kaplan and Sadock, vol 1, pp 1059–1066)*

617. (B)   Recent lifetime prevalence studies have shown that social phobia ranks only behind major depression and alcohol dependence in the United States. Rather than being a variant of shyness, social phobia is a distinct neurobiological disorder with significant morbidity. Medications have been shown to be effective in many cases, with selective serotonin reuptake inhibitors and monoamine oxidase inhibitors showing the most promise. Persons with social phobia often also develop major depression or other anxiety disorders during the course of their lives. Social skills training can be an invaluable adjunct to treatment, allowing persons to feel more confident as they enter the world of social interaction, for what seems for many the first time in their lives. *(Lydiard and Falsetti)*

618. (E)   Methadone is an opioid that is widely used in treatment programs for heroin addicts. Substituted for heroin in maintenance programs, methadone itself can cause euphoria and depressive side effects and is associated with tolerance. The principle behind methadone maintenance is that if the drug can be obtained in legally sanctioned clinics linked with medical and rehabilitative facilities, then the addict has fewer incentives to obtain or remain on heroin. Other treatments, such as the use of narcotic antagonists, have yet to match the success of methadone maintenance in treating the large number of narcotic addicts in the United States. *(Kaplan and Sadock, vol 1, pp 857–860)*

619. **(B)** Disulfiram acts by inhibiting the breakdown of acetaldehyde, a major metabolite of alcohol. When a person on disulfiram therapy ingests alcoholic beverages (or absorbs alcohol from such sources as cosmetics), the subsequent accumulation of acetaldehyde causes a number of effects, including flushing, sweating, palpitations, nausea, and vomiting. These sudden, very unpleasant effects are generally safe in an otherwise healthy individual. Disulfiram therapy is absolutely contraindicated in the presence of heart disease and is potentially dangerous in many other conditions, including cirrhosis, nephritis, and pregnancy. Tolerance does not develop. In the past, when disulfiram was routinely used in large doses, as many as 20% of those treated developed a "disulfiram psychosis." The presentation of this organic mental disorder ranges from delirium to fullblown psychotic symptoms. This reaction is much less common today, but a history of psychosis continues to be a relative contraindication to disulfiram therapy. It is most important to emphasize that disulfiram therapy is properly used only in the context of a comprehensive alcoholism treatment plan, including counseling, group programs such as Alcoholics Anonymous, and careful medical supervision. *(Tupin et al, pp 136–140)*

620. **(A)** Extrapyramidal reactions, which can result from the use of antipsychotic medications, are divided into three classes. Akathisias are characterized by motor restlessness and inability to sit still. Acute dyskinesias, which produce sudden, often bizarre-appearing muscular contortions of the face

and upper body, can occur at very low dosages of antipsychotic medication; on the other hand, tardive dyskinesia is a late complication of long-term neuroleptic treatment. Parkinsonian syndromes, which can resemble Parkinson's disease in many of its manifestions, are the third class of extrapyramidal reactions. The agitation of akathisias, bizarre movements of dyskinesias, and bland affect of parkinsonian syndromes all can be mistaken for signs of worsening psychosis. Of the antipsychotic drugs, thioridazine produces few extrapyramidal side effects, whereas haloperidol is among the drugs producing the most. *(Tupin et al, pp 18–23)*

621. **(E)** Tricyclic antidepressants have atropine-like activity as a result of cholinergic blockade and, as a consequence, can produce such atropinic side effects as dry mouth, blurred vision, urinary retention, and postural hypotension. These drugs also enhance noradrenergic functioning by blocking the reuptake of norepinephrine, thus allowing the released neurotransmitter to stay longer at the receptor site. Because the site of antihypertensive action of guanethidine and related drugs is in noradrenergic neurons, drugs like tricyclic antidepressants that block norepinephrine reuptake will also block uptake of guanethidine, thus inhibiting its effectiveness. *(Tupin et al, pp 54–56)*

622. **(B)** Investigation of sociologic factors in suicide has led to the identification of "lower-risk" and "higher-risk" groups. In general, the risk of suicide increases proportionally with age, although the rate of teenage suicides has been accelerating in recent years. Men are at higher risk than women, and persons in professional occupations are at higher risk than blue-collar workers. Poor health, socioeconomic deprivation, marital breakdown, and history of alcohol abuse or chronic depression are all associated with higher suicide risk. Suicide risk appears to decline during periods of war or social persecution, for reasons that are unclear. *(Kaplan and Sadock, vol 2, pp 1739–1740,1748)*

623. **(D)** The limbic system consists of several structures of the brain linked by one common function: control or expression of emotional states and self-preservation behaviors. Specific areas of the brain that constitute the limbic system include the hippocampus and cingulate gyrus (which form part of the limbic lobe and are presumed to be active in determining emotional response) and the amygdala (which is thought to be involved with more primitive, instinctual behaviors related to self-preservation). The reticular formation is a region of the brain stem regulating arousal and inhibition of the peripheral motor system as well as other nonvoluntary physiologic functions. *(Kaplan and Sadock, vol 1, pp 19–23)*

624. **(E)** Symptoms of schizophrenia have been classified in a number of ways, beginning with Eugen Bleuler's "four A's": autism, ambivalence, associational difficulties, and affect disturbance. Kurt Schneider 30 years ago described what he termed "first rank" symptoms, which, if present and not associated with a known organic disorder, would indicate a diagnosis of schizophrenia. Among Schneider's first-rank symptoms are auditory hallucinations, somatic hallucinations, delusions, and the belief that thoughts either are being intruded on by others' thoughts or are being telegraphed to others and incorporated into their thoughts (thought insertion and thought broadcasting, respectively). Catatonia is not a first-rank symptom of schizophrenia. *(Kaplan and Sadock, vol 1, pp 889–890,970)*

625. **(D)** Paranoid schizophrenia is the most common subtype of schizophrenia in the United States. It tends to develop later in life than other schizophrenic subtypes, cause less cognitive impairment, and produce milder behavioral and social disorganization. Hallucinations and delusions characteristically are of a jealous, persecutory, or grandiose nature. *(Kaplan and Sadock, vol 1, pp 979–981)*

626. **(B)** Although the advent of antidepressant drugs has curtailed the use of electroconvulsive therapy (ECT), the procedure still is employed to treat persons with psychotic depression, medication-resistant depression, and florid mania. Protocols vary among treatment centers in regard to frequency and number of shocks, strength of shock, and method of administration (unilateral or bilateral). The use of pretreatment medication, including atropine to dry up secretions and succinylcholine to cause transient paralysis, has lowered the morbidity and mortality of ECT to levels less than those associated with antidepressant drug therapy. Transient memory loss usually occurs after each treatment. *(Kaplan and Sadock, vol 2, pp 2129–2140)*

627. **(E)** Acute amphetamine intoxication causes euphoria and restlessness, and acute overdose can lead to confusion, disorientation, psychotic symptoms (eg, persecutory and grandiose delusions and hallucinations that can mimic acute paranoid schizophrenia), convulsions, and coma. Chronic amphetamine abuse can produce psychosis and repetitive, compulsive behaviors such as bruxism (teeth gnashing); these symptoms may take months to disappear completely after withdrawal. Treatment of amphetamine intoxication is with benzodiazepines to produce sedation or with neuroleptic medications, particularly haloperidol to treat more serious cases. Withdrawal after chronic abuse can produce a depression of sufficient severity to warrant use of antidepressant drugs. *(Cassem, pp 25–26)*

628. **(B)** Mental retardation generally is divided into four levels of severity: mild (IQ 50 to 70), moderate (35 to 50), severe (20 to 35), and profound. Most retarded US citizens are in the mild range and thus can benefit from some education and often are able to live and work independently. Moderately retarded persons are considered trainable but not educable and frequently can care for themselves, especially in supervised environments. More severely retarded persons require custodial care. *(Herskowitz and Rosman, pp 512–514)*

629–632. **(629-B, 630-C, 631-D, 632-A)** Conversion disorder is a somatoform disorder in which an apparent physical deficit is actually an unconscious manifestation of a psychologic conflict. Affected individuals are unaware of the psychologic etiology of their symptoms. Conversion symptoms are thought to be a defense against intolerable feelings and a safeguard against carrying out indefensible actions.

Cyclothymic disorder can be thought of as subclinical bipolar disorder. Affected persons experience mood swings but of lower amplitude and severity than those characterizing manic–depressive illness. As a consequence, social and interpersonal functioning is less disrupted.

Social phobia is an anxiety disorder associated with avoidance of contact with other persons, especially groups, because of fear of humiliation. Often this fear is so intense that it affects judgment and attention to the point of interfering with even simple actions. When this scenario occurs, affected individuals can come away from a social encounter feeling even more convinced of their basic inadequacies and thus become even more avoidant and phobic.

One of the most dramatic of all psychiatric illnesses is dissociative identity disorder, or multiple personality disorder (MPD). Persons with MPD display two or more (sometimes many more) separable personalities. MPD is thought to arise as a result of extreme childhood trauma, such as physical or sexual abuse. *(APA, pp 363–366,411–417,452–457,484–487)*

633–640. (633-B, 634-H, 635-B, 636-A, 637-C, 638-E, 639-D, 640-B) Delusions and hallucinations are symptoms of psychosis. A delusion is a fixed, false, typically bizarre or improbable belief from which a person cannot be dissuaded. Delusions take several forms, including grandiose (eg, attributing great powers to oneself), nihilistic (eg, seeing oneself as a cause of universal misery), somatic, and paranoid. In contrast to delusions, obsessions are persistent thoughts that generally are plausible; affected persons are well aware of the abnormal preoccupation and can be quite distressed. A phobia is an extreme fear well

beyond the degree of actual threat posed by the feared object (eg, spiders) or experience (eg, heights).

Hallucinations are manufactured sensations without any basis in reality. Any of the five senses—sight, hearing, smell, taste, and touch—can be affected. Illusions, on the other hand, are misperceptions of an actual sensory stimulus. While hallucinations are associated with psychotic illnesses, illusions are associated with organic disorders.

Compulsions are repetitive, irresistible behaviors unconsciously designed to ward off or alleviate anxiety. These behaviors either are excessive or are not connected with the object of the anxiety in any discernible way.

A neurosis is a behavior pattern or set of beliefs that a person finds distressing or encumbering and generally not perceived as amenable to change. These beliefs and prejudices are nonpsychotic and stem from the effects of childhood experiences.

Persons experiencing a fugue have taken precipitous flight from their home environments, ending up in no particular place of meaning to them and with no recollection of how they got there or even of who they are. *(Kaplan and Sadock, vol 1, pp 464,637–668)*

641–647. (641-D, 642-A, 643-F, 644-A, 645-B, 646-C, 647-E). Fluoxetine is a serotonin blocker used widely in the treatment of major depressive episode. It also has proved effective in treating a number of other disorders, including obsessive–compulsive disorder. Alprazolam is a benzodiazepine drug most appropriate in the treatment of transient anxiety. Chronic use of alprazolam is discouraged because of its addictive potential. Triazolam is a triazolobenzodiazepine marketed as a hypnotic. In recent years this drug has become somewhat controversial because of case reports of confusion associated with its use.

Haloperidol and clozapine are antipsychotic drugs. Haloperidol is a high-potency, relatively nonsedating drug that is useful in rapid neuroleptization of agitated manic individuals. Because of the risk of agranulocytosis, use of clozapine is reserved for treatment of persons with chronic schizophrenia who have not responded well to other pharmacologic agents. Persons who develop extrapyramidal side effects from neuroleptic drugs often are given benztropine to alleviate these symptoms.

The most common use of lithium is the treatment of persons with bipolar disorder. However, it also has been helpful as an adjuvant to antidepressant treatment that has achieved less than optimal results. *(Kaplan and Sadock, vol 2, pp 2418–2427)*

REFERENCES

American Psychiatric Association (APA). *Diagnostic and Statistical Manual of Mental Disorders.* 4th ed. Washington, DC: American Psychiatric Association; 1994.

Cassem NH. *Massachusetts General Hospital Handbook of General Hospital Psychiatry.* 3rd ed. St Louis, Mo: Mosby Year Book; 1991.

Cummings JL, Benson DF. *Dementia: A Clinical Approach.* 2nd ed. Boston, Mass: Butterworth-Heinemann; 1992.

Goodwin JS, Goodwin JM, Vogel AV. Knowledge and use of placebos by house officers and nurses. *Ann Intern Med.* 1979;91:106–110.

Hales RE, Frances AJ, eds. *Psychiatry Update: American Psychiatric Association Annual Review.* Washington, DC: American Psychiatric Press Inc; 1987;6.

Halleck SL. *Law in the Practice of Psychiatry: A Handbook for Clinicians.* New York, NY: Plenum Medical Book Co, 1980.

Herskowitz J, Rosman NP. *Pediatrics, Neurology, and Psychiatry—Common Ground, Behavioral, Cognitive, Affective, and Physical Disorders in Childhood and Adolescence.* New York, NY: Macmillan Inc; 1982.

Kaplan HI, Sadock BJ. *Comprehensive Textbook of Psychiatry VI.* 6th ed. Baltimore, Md: Williams & Wilkins, 1995; 2 vols.

Lydiard RB, Falsetti SA. Treatment options for social phobia. *Psychiatric Annals.* 1995;25:570–576.

Mueller PS, Vester JW, Fermaglich J. Neuroleptic malignant syndrome. Successful treatment with bromocriptine. *JAMA.* 1983;249:386–388.

Salzmann C, Shader RI, Greenblatt DJ, et al. Long vs. short half-life benzodiazepines in the elderly. *Arch Gen Psychiatry.* 1983;40:293–297.

Schatzberg AF, Cole JO. *Manual of Clinical Psychopharmacology.* 2nd ed. Washington, DC: American Psychiatric Press Inc; 1991.

Tupin JP, Shader RI, Harnett DS. *Handbook of Clinical Psychopharmacology.* 2nd ed. Northvale, NJ: Jason Aronson Inc; 1992.

SUBSPECIALTY LIST: PSYCHIATRY

Question Number and Subspecialty

586. Nonpsychiatric illness
587. Psychopathology
588. Psychopathology
589. Psychopathology
590. Intervention
591. Intervention
592. Intervention
593. Assessment
594. Child psychiatry, assessment
595. Ethical and legal aspects
596. Psychopathology
597. Assessment
598. Assessment
599. Assessment
600. Ethical and legal aspects
601. Epidemiology
602. Child psychiatry, development
603. Child psychiatry, development
604. Child psychiatry, development
605. Nonpsychiatric illness
606. Epidemiology
607. Epidemiology
608. Intervention
609. Psychopathology
610. Ethical and legal aspects
611. Intervention
612. Assessment
613. Assessment
614. Assessment
615. Psychopathology
616. Assessment

617. Psychopathology
618. Intervention
619. Intervention
620. Intervention
621. Intervention
622. Assessment
623. Psychopathology
624. Assessment
625. Assessment
626. Intervention
627. Assessment
628. Psychopathology
629. Psychopathology
630. Psychopathology
631. Psychopathology
632. Psychopathology

633. Assessment
634. Assessment
635. Assessment
636. Assessment
637. Assessment
638. Assessment
639. Assessment
640. Assessment
641. Intervention
642. Intervention
643. Intervention
644. Intervention
645. Intervention
646. Intervention
647. Intervention

Preventive Medicine

Jocelyn C. White, MD

DIRECTIONS (Questions 648 through 699): Each of the numbered items or incomplete statements in this section is followed by answers or by completions of the statement. Select the ONE lettered answer or completion that is BEST in each case.

648. Which of the following is the major hazard at well-maintained sanitary landfill sites?

   (A) obstruction of drainage
   (B) objectionable odors
   (C) sea gulls
   (D) fire
   (E) rats

649. By which of the following processes is the most pure drinking water produced?

   (A) sedimentation
   (B) filtration
   (C) ion exchange resins
   (D) distillation
   (E) absorption

650. John Smith visits the physician at his place of work, complaining of testicular enlargement. The physician confirms the finding and refers the man for surgical treatment. The mass is discovered to be a seminoma. Appropriate treatment is given. A similar case occurred in this factory earlier in the year. The company physician should

   (A) inform the employer of the man's diagnosis
   (B) preserve the man's anonymity but indicate to management that this was the second case to occur in the past year

   (C) advise both management and the workers that two cases of testicular cancer have occurred in the past year
   (D) quietly begin a search for possible carcinogens but inform neither workers nor management
   (E) insist that information about the risk factors for testicular cancer be released to management and workers

651. The graph below represents a bimodal increase in numbers of death in London during the winter of 1952 to 1953 compared with the previous year. This phenomenon is most likely caused by

   (A) herd immunity
   (B) a propagated or progressive epidemic
   (C) two separate disease etiologies
   (D) application of specific control measures
   (E) ineffective case identification

Questions 652 through 656

In one day in a primary-care clinic, 15 persons with hypertension are evaluated. Some of them are already under treatment. Systolic blood pressure readings (mm Hg) are as follows: 132, 143, 150, 160, 170, 177, 146, 125, 144, 154, 143, 135, 210, 140, 143.

652. The mean systolic blood pressure reading (mm Hg) for the patient group described above is

   (A) 143
   (B) 144
   (C) 146
   (D) 151.5
   (E) 167.5

653. The modal reading of systolic blood pressures (mm Hg) in the group described is

   (A) 143
   (B) 144
   (C) 146
   (D) 151.5
   (E) 167.5

654. The median reading of systolic blood pressures (mm Hg) in the group described is

   (A) 143
   (B) 144
   (C) 146
   (D) 151.5
   (E) 167.5

655. In statistics, the term variance is used to describe

   (A) the sum of the differences of each reading from the mean, divided by the total number of readings ($\Sigma\, [x - \bar{x}]/n$)
   (B) the sum of the squares of the difference of each reading from the mean, divided by the total number of readings ($\Sigma\, [x - \bar{x}]^2/n$)
   (C) the sum of the squares of the difference of each reading from the mean, divided by one less than the total number of readings ($\Sigma\, [x - \bar{x}]^2/[n - 1]$)

   (D) the sum of the deviations in absolute values about the mean, divided by the total number of readings ($\Sigma\, |x - \bar{x}|\,/n$)
   (E) the sum of the logarithmic values of each reading, divided by the total number of readings ($\Sigma\, [\log x]/n$)

656. With each administration of a drug to a particular patient, there is an 8% chance of a toxic reaction. The patient requires five consecutive doses of the drug. The chance that this patient will have a toxic reaction is

   (A) 8%
   (B) 34%
   (C) 40%
   (D) 66%
   (E) 99%

Questions 657 and 658

A group of medical residents in an outpatient clinic start a screening program for diabetes. Of the 1000 individuals examined by blood glucose examination, 100 are found to be above the arbitrary cutoff value of 140 mg/dl. Of these 100 individuals, 50 are discovered to have diabetes on subsequent examination. Also, 50 individuals who did not have positive results on the screening test are discovered to have diabetes on further examination.

657. The sensitivity of the screening procedure described above is

   (A) 5%
   (B) 10%
   (C) 20%
   (D) 50%
   (E) 100%

658. The specificity of the screening procedure described above is

   (A) 5%
   (B) 10%
   (C) 50%
   (D) 95%
   (E) 100%

659. The randomized control trial is accepted as the most effective way of determining the relative efficacy and toxicity of a new therapy in comparison with an established method of treatment. Proper methodology includes all of the following EXCEPT

(A) careful planning before the trial begins

(B) randomized allocation of patients to treatment groups

(C) a null hypothesis stating that one treatment will be found superior to the other

(D) a double-blind protocol

(E) an acceptable definition of statistical significance

660. What is the source of payment for the majority of health care expenditures in the United States?

(A) health insurance

(B) health maintenance organization (HMO)

(C) self-pay

(D) government

(E) other

661. What proportion of health care expenditures in the United States do physicians receive?

(A) 10%

(B) 20%

(C) 30%

(D) 40%

(E) 50%

662. Deficiency of glucose-6-phosphate dehydrogenase (G6PD) is LEAST common among individuals whose ancestry is

(A) Northern European

(B) Sub-Saharan

(C) Mediterranean

(D) Near Eastern

(E) Central Asian

663. At present, the leading cause of death in the United States is:

(A) cerebrovascular disease

(B) heart disease

(C) cancer (all forms)

(D) injuries

(E) all others

664. In the age group 35 years and older, yearly death rates per 1000 persons from lung cancer are 0.07 for nonsmokers and 0.96 for cigarette smokers. Which of the following statements is true concerning interpretation of this finding?

(A) cigarette smokers are 14.7 times as likely to develop lung cancer as are nonsmokers

(B) the attributable risk measures the incidence or rate of recurrence

(C) the attributable risk measures the strength of an association, a high attributable risk leading to conclusions about etiology or causality

(D) the attributable risk of lung cancer caused by cigarette smoking is 93%

(E) in smokers, the overall rate of lung cancer death linked to cigarette smoking is 0.96

665. A recent advertisement for a drug that increases motility of the upper gastrointestinal tract says that it has been "used for 10 years" and that "1 billion doses have been used worldwide." The ad continues that the drug is "the logical treatment of choice to restore normal emptying and to relieve gas, bloating, nausea, vomiting, and heartburn." On the basis of this information, the claim that this drug is the "treatment of choice" is best described by which of the following statements?

(A) the claim is probably a sound one

(B) the claim is invalid because the comparison is not based on rates

(C) the claim is invalid because statistical significance is not mentioned

(D) the claim is invalid because no control or comparison group is reported

(E) the claim is invalid because a cohort effect may be operating

666. The prospective or cohort study is frequently used to test hypotheses about risk factors. In the determination of the value of a particular cohort study, which of the following conditions is most important?

(A) the study should be designed to yield accurate results quickly

(B) the study population should be large

(C) the study population should be carefully selected to preserve group characteristics

(D) the study should provide for periodic examination of cohort and control groups

(E) the study should allow the investigation of several risk factors simultaneously

Questions 667 and 668

667. Hypertension is known to have many sequelae and a highly significant morbidity. Utilizing the data given in the figure below for mild-to-moderate hypertension (diastolic blood pressure, 90 to 114 mm), if blood pressure is well controlled over a 3-year period, what is the likely percentage of diminution of all morbid events?

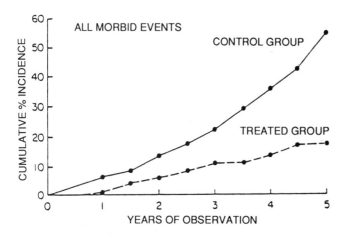

(A) 10%

(B) 20%

(C) 30%

(D) 40%

(E) 50%

668. In the same example, what is the percentage of effectiveness of the therapy?

(A) 10%

(B) 20%

(C) 30%

(D) 40%

(E) 50%

669. The population of the United States is growing older. In 1980, the percentage of the population over the age of 65 was 11.29%; by the year 2000, it is expected to rise to 13.11%. Which of the following statements is true?

(A) the section of the population that is increasing most rapidly is in the age range 65 to 75 years

(B) increased longevity is attributed to more effective cancer treatment

(C) men have higher expectation of longevity than women

(D) suicide is becoming increasingly evident in the older population

(E) increased longevity is attributed to reduction in cardiovascular disease

670. The use of coliform count as a measure of the safety of public water supplies is best explained by which of the following statements?

(A) it is an indicator of fecal contamination

(B) it is an indicator of industrial contamination

(C) coliform organisms are human pathogens

(D) coliform organisms accompany other, pathogenic water-borne organisms

(E) none of the above

671. All the following statements are true about the effects of cooking food EXCEPT

(A) food boiled in water seldom attains a temperature of 100°C (212°F)

(B) food baked at an oven temperature of about 175° to 205°C (350° to 400°F) rarely reaches this temperature

(C) food cooked at high altitude may contain live bacteria after cooking

(D) frying bacon may produce carcinogens

(E) cooking does not kill parasites in meat

672. The average per-person amount of solid waste produced yearly in towns and cities in the United States is

(A) 90 kg (200 lb)

(B) 450 kg (1000 lb)

(C) 900 kg (1 ton)

(D) 2700 kg (3 tons)

(E) 5400 kg (6 tons)

673. Epidemics of meningococcal disease are now rare in the United States. Sporadic cases do occur. Control has been attributed to

(A) increased herd immunity

(B) increased application of immunologic procedures

(C) increased bed space

(D) improved socioeconomic conditions

(E) lower community carrier rates

674. Sewage and water-borne industrial pollutants have affected many rivers, lakes, and streams. Fish are most likely to die as a result of this pollution because of

(A) changes in the pH of the water

(B) changes in the temperature of the water

(C) changes in the bacterial content of the water

(D) a drop in the oxygen content of the water

(E) the poisonous nature of some of the contaminants

675. Acoustic trauma occurs not only at work but also in the home. Sounds from 120 to 130 dBA are uncomfortably loud; 90 to 100 dBA, very loud; 70 to 80 dBA, moderately loud; 50 to 80 dBA, quiet; and 30 to 50 dBA, very quiet. Noise from which of the following domestic appliances is in the very loud range?

(A) food blender

(B) garbage disposal

(C) vacuum cleaner

(D) power mower

(E) clothes washer

676. Three of the major risk factors for coronary heart disease are hypercholesterolemia, hypertension, and cigarette smoking. When compared with persons with none of these risk factors, persons who have all three risk factors are how many times more likely to develop serious coronary heart disease?

(A) 2 times

(B) 5 times

(C) 8 times

(D) 12 times

(E) 20 times

677. Which of the following statements is true about the relationship between physicians and the many state laws regulating public health and medical practice?

(A) physicians are not liable for infractions against laws of which they were unaware

(B) by law, every state must collect relevant public health laws in a single publication

(C) by law, all state health rules and regulations are distributed to physicians

(D) physicians need to familiarize themselves only with the more common laws

(E) none of the above

678. The US Occupational Safety and Health Administration (OSHA) was formed in 1970 to encourage employers and employees to reduce hazards in the workplace. The primary emphasis of this agency is to

   (A) develop technical expertise to recognize occupational hazards

   (B) review state job safety and health standards

   (C) monitor compliance with job health and safety codes

   (D) maintain records of work-related illnesses

   (E) propose statutory changes or additions to job-related laws

679. Many women are playing vital roles in the workplace. There are now very few employment situations for which women are not considered entirely suitable. However, pregnancy does to some extent affect ability to perform certain tasks, and others are considered to increase risks for the mother or fetus, or both. According to current advice, which of the following job functions are indications to cease work or restrict that particular activity by 20 weeks of gestation?

   (A) lifting weights up to 14 kg

   (B) climbing stairs more than four times in an 8-hour shift

   (C) intermittent standing for periods greater than 30 minutes

   (D) repetitive stooping (more than 10 times per hour) and bending below knee level

   (E) intermittent climbing ladders four times in an 8-hour shift

680. A patient, previously unknown to you, says he had a prolapsed intervertebral disk 10 years ago. Since beginning to work as an automotive engineer in a shop that concentrates on electrical systems, at which he frequently has to lift automotive batteries, he claims he has experienced low-back pain with sciatic radiation. He requests you to certify that this work has disabled him. On examination, there is some restriction of flexion of the spine, straight leg raising on the right being limited to 45°. As a result of your examination, you should

   (A) recommend him for Social Security Disability Insurance (SSDI)

   (B) recommend him for Supplemental Security Income (SSI)

   (C) recommend him for Workmen's Compensation

   (D) advise him that he is unsuited for his present employment

   (E) recommend physical therapy and 4 days off work

681. Several substances to which parents may be exposed are known to be reproductive hazards. Which of the following substances are known to result in impairment of *both* paternal and maternal fertility?

   (A) ethylene oxide

   (B) infectious agents

   (C) anesthetic agents

   (D) inorganic lead

   (E) dibromochloropropane (DBCP)

682. In the United States, malnutrition is LEAST likely to occur among individuals in which of the following groups?

   (A) alcohol abusers

   (B) drug addicts

   (C) persistent self-medicators

   (D) vegetarians

   (E) persons with deficient general education

683. All the following statements are true about skin cancer, the most common form of cancer in light-skinned populations, EXCEPT

(A) dark-skinned populations are up to 50 times less likely to develop skin cancer than light-skinned populations

(B) the incidence of skin cancer increases with decreasing latitude

(C) the most common skin cancer is basal cell carcinoma

(D) predisposition to skin cancer is the major risk factor in one third of affected individuals

(E) in the United States, 40% of all cancers are skin cancers

684. Bladder cancer has been recognized as related to occupational exposure. Which of the following groups of workers are at greatest risk for developing bladder cancer?

(A) miners

(B) automotive brake and clutch mechanics

(C) insecticide makers and sprayers

(D) benzene and rubber-cement workers

(E) asphalt, coal tar, and pitch workers

685. All the following statements about prevention of and susceptibility to coccidioidomycosis are true EXCEPT

(A) persons with negative coccidioidin skin reactions are no longer susceptible

(B) persons living in the states of Maine or Washington are less susceptible than persons living in Arizona or New Mexico

(C) persons living in communities with rapidly changing populations are more susceptible than persons living in communities with a fixed population

(D) sowing grass seed in dusty lots can help prevent the spread of disease

(E) paving roads and recreation areas can help prevent the spread of disease

686. The most frequently occurring work-related infectious disease is

(A) brucellosis

(B) anthrax

(C) viral hepatitis type B

(D) leptospirosis

(E) tetanus

687. A human vaccine is available for which of the following arthropod-borne viral infections?

(A) Colorado tick fever

(B) eastern equine encephalitis

(C) dengue fever

(D) Venezuelan equine encephalitis

(E) yellow fever

688. In the United States, shigellosis is most likely to be spread by

(A) contaminated food

(B) contaminated water supplies

(C) case-to-case transmission

(D) contact with carriers

(E) none of the above

DIRECTIONS (Questions 689 through 699): Each group of items in this section consists of lettered headings followed by a set of numbered words or phrases. For each numbered word or phrase, select the ONE lettered heading that is most closely associated with it. Each lettered heading may be selected once, more than once, or not at all.

Questions 689 through 691

For each morbidity measurement below, select the statement that is most likely to be the correct definition.

   (A) the number of existing cases of a disease at a single moment in time, divided by the population at the same moment
   (B) the number of existing cases of a disease at a single moment in time, divided by the mean population for that year
   (C) the number of new cases of a disease diagnosed during a given period, divided by the mid-interval population
   (D) current cases of a disease, both new and old, during a given time period, divided by the mid-interval population
   (E) the number of new cases of a disease diagnosed during a given time period, divided by the mean of the population

689. Period prevalence rate

690. Incidence rate

691. Prevalence rate

Questions 692 through 694

For each mortality measurement below, select the proper definition.

   (A) deaths assigned to a specific disease, related to all deaths
   (B) all deaths reported, related to midyear population
   (C) deaths assigned to a specific disease, related to new and existing cases of that disease during the same year
   (D) deaths assigned to a specific disease, related to midyear population
   (E) unprocessed number of deaths in a given population

692. Crude death rate

693. Case fatality rate

694. Cause-specific death rate

Questions 695 through 699

For each function listed below, select the agency with which it is most likely to be associated.

   (A) the US Food and Drug Administration (FDA)
   (B) the US Department of Agriculture (USDA)
   (C) Environmental Protection Agency (EPA)
   (D) United Nations Food and Agriculture Organization (FAO)
   (E) World Health Organization (WHO)

695. Bans domestic marketing and use of the pesticide DDT

696. Monitors water pollution in the United States

697. Publishes an International Statistical Classification of Disease

698. Determines the level of diethylstilbestrol permissible in food products

699. Devoted to improvements of the health of agricultural workers

ANSWERS AND EXPLANATIONS

648. **(D)** No matter how well a sanitary landfill is maintained, fire is a perpetual hazard. Waste that is decomposing anaerobically reaches quite high temperatures, about 90°C (194°F). Spontaneous combustion and ignition may occur if the cover is thin and cracks, permitting the access of air. The other hazards listed in the question are also possible but do not provide such a major threat. *(Last, p 656)*

649. **(D)** Distillation is the artificial or engineered version of the process by which the natural hydrologic cycle is maintained. It is used for desalinization and other purposes in which special water purity is required. Naturally occurring spring or deep well water frequently tastes better, because taste is improved by small amounts of mineral deposits. Either of these sources, however, may be contaminated. Sedimentation, filtration, and absorption are possible methods of purification, but result in less purity from a bacteriologic or chemical standpoint. Ion exchange resins are used to remove specific ions, eg, reducing hardness. *(Last, p 632)*

650. **(D)** The code of ethical conduct for physicians providing occupational medicine services recommends that physicians should treat as confidential whatever is learned about individuals served. Information should be released only when required by law or because of overriding public health considerations. The occurrence of two similar cases of an illness in a year could be attributed to chance and does not at this stage indicate the risk of an overriding public health problem. Employers are entitled to advice regarding their worker's physical ability to perform their duties but are not entitled to diagnoses or details of a specific nature. Physicians employed in industry need to communicate to employers and employees, in an accurate yet wise and discreet manner, any information about health hazards. *(Levy and Wegman, p 185)*

651. **(C)** The shape of the graph that accompanies the question suggests different characteristics of the two peaks. In fact, the first peak coincided exactly with the great fog in London of December, 1952. The second peak in January through February coincided with an outbreak of influenza. If herd immunity had developed, a steady decline in the number of cases recorded could be expected. A propagated epidemic would normally produce a steadily increasing number of cases. Application of specific control measures is most likely to produce a steadily diminishing number of cases reported. Ineffective case identification normally leads to low levels of reporting, particularly at the outset of an epidemic. *(Last, pp 11–39,82)*

652. **(D)** The mean or average reading ($\bar{x}$) is the total of all readings ($\Sigma\,x$) divided by the number of readings (n), or $\bar{x} = (\Sigma\,x)/n$. In the question, the number of readings is 15 and the total of the readings is 2272. Therefore, the mean is

$$\frac{2272}{15} \cong 151.5$$

(Kramer, p. 126)

653. **(A)** The modal reading is the most frequently occurring observation. The mode is not readily adaptable to statistical calculation, and in small series of observations or readings there may be no modal reading at all. However, the determination of unimodal vs bimodal distribution within a given population may be useful in defining that population (eg, incidence of disease by age). *(Kramer, p 126)*

654. **(B)** The median is the observation that lies in the middle of a series: if the observations are tabulated in numerical order, half the observations are lower in numerical value and thus below the median, and the remainder are higher in numerical value and above the median. Clearly this value is easily identified if the series contains an odd number of readings. Although not very frequently used in statistics, the median has the advantage of not being as affected by extreme observations as the mean, which can be skewed by observations very much lower or higher than the majority. *(Kramer, p 127)*

655. **(C)** The statistical concept of variance takes into consideration the fact that the distribution of a sample may not represent accurately the distribution of the entire population. This potential difference may be measured by calculating the variance of both the sample and the true population. Variance is calculated as follows: the mean is subtracted from each value; this difference is squared, to make all these figures a positive number; then the sum of all squared differences is divided by one less than the total number of readings (variance = $\Sigma [x - \bar{x}]^2 / n - 1$). *(Kramer, p 127)*

656. **(B)** Probability is multiplicative, not additive. In the question presented, the chance that an administration of drug would *not* cause a toxic reaction is 0.92, making the chance of the patient being reaction-free for 5 consecutive doses $(0.92)^5 = 0.66 = 66\%$. Hence, the probability of at least one toxic reaction would be $1 - 0.66$, or 0.34. *(Colton, pp 70–71)*

657. **(D)** The sensitivity of a test is the percentage of people with the disease (true positives, TP) who are detected by the test. False negatives (FN) are those who have the disease but are not detected by the test. Percentage sensitivity is calculated as follows: [TP ÷ (TP + FN)] × 100. In the example given in the question the sensitivity is [50 ÷ (50 + 50)] × 100 = 50%. *(Last, pp 28–38)*

658. **(D)** The percentage specificity of a test is the percentage of those persons without the disease (true negatives, TN) who are correctly identified. False positives (FP) are those persons who are incorrectly labeled by the test as having the disease. The specificity is thus expressed as follows: [TN ÷ (TN + FP)] × 100. In the example given in the question, the specificity is [900 ÷ (900 + 50)] × 100 = 94.7% ≅ 95%. *(Last, pp 28–38)*

659. **(C)** Proper methodology of randomized control trials includes careful pretrial planning, random double-blind patient allocation, pretrial null hypothesis stating that the compared treatments are equally effective, and a clear definition of what constitutes statistical significance. Sample size has an effect on the efficiency of random control trials. Most studies have been found to include too few patients to ensure that a clinically meaningful difference in therapeutic effect would not be missed. In such studies, type I error (alpha error, significance error) occurs when a treatment is erroneously concluded to have an effect. Type II error (beta error) concludes that a treatment had no effect when in reality it did. These errors are statistical ways of examining false positive and false negative results. *(Kramer, pp 78–91)*

660. **(D)** In 1987 it was estimated that the government paid for 41% of health care expenditure through Medicare and Medicaid and other programs. This amounts to 212 billion dollars, of which 142 billion dollars are direct federal expenditure. Health insurance, including health maintenance organizations (HMOs), paid for 31% (155 billion dollars), whereas self-pay was 26% (128 billion dollars). *(Department of Health and Human Services Memorandum)*

661. **(B)** The rising costs of health care are a national problem: both the problem and the costs continually grow. Although health care now absorbs about 12% of the gross national product (GNP), most of it is attributed to physicians. While they order and are responsible for most of these costs, they only receive about 20% of the expenditure. Efforts are being made to curb all these costs. *(Last, pp 1074–1077)*

662. **(A)** About 12% of black Americans are deficient in glucose-6-phosphate dehydrogenase (G6PD). Several different forms of this genetically determined deficiency are found in persons of Mediterranean, Near Eastern, and Central Asian origin. G6PD deficiency is rare among Caucasians. *(Levy and Wegman, p 452)*

663. (B) Heart disease remains the most common cause of death. However, there has been a marked reduction of deaths attributable to heart disease in recent years (a reduction of 25% over the 10-year period 1968 to 1978). In overall mortality rates in 1980, there were 336 deaths per 100 000 population from heart disease. For ages 65 to 74, the rate was 1156; 75 to 84, 2801; 85 and up, 7342. Cancer overall mortality rate was 184; cerebrovascular disease, 75; injuries, 69. *(Last, pp 827–847)*

664. (D) Relative risk is the ratio of the incidence rate of those persons exposed to a certain condition or factor to the incidence rate of those persons not exposed. In the case described in the question, the relative risk is 0.96 divided by 0.07, or 13.7. Attributable risk measures the impact that removal of a certain factor may have on the incidence of the disease. Incidence or rate of recurrence is measured by the absolute risk. Relative risk measures the strength of an association, whereas absolute risk is used in actuarial situations. In the figures given, the overall rate of deaths from lung cancer in cigarette smokers is 0.96, of which 0.89 (0.96 − 0.07) is attributable to cigarette smoking. Thus, the percent attributable risk is 0.89 divided by 0.96 multiplied by 100, or 93%. *(Last, pp 28–30)*

665. (D) Extensive use of a substance may appear to have clinical significance for a physician, but statistical evidence demands comparison with control groups, even for long-established remedies. Continual prescription of a substance frequently leads to a situation in which the benefits of treatment are not compared with newer preparations, and the frequency of occurrence of side effects is not considered. Cohort effect is unlikely to be apparent if a large number of cases are reported on a worldwide basis (a cohort is a group of persons sharing a common experience within a defined time period). *(Last, pp 34–36)*

666. (D) Some cohort studies may yield quick results (eg, if respiratory irritants are being studied); in others, where the disease process is slow or the incidence is low, quick results are impossible to obtain (eg, investigations for leukemia). Only if the condition is rare is it essential for the study to include large numbers. Many studies of small groups of workers exposed to industrial risk have yielded very satisfactory results. Differences within the study group may confound the results; sometimes these difficulties may be overcome by stratifying the group, such as by age. Although personal habits and family history may be factors influencing the development of disease, they would not invalidate a cohort study. Ideally, the study should provide for periodic examination of both the cohort and the control groups. Not only does periodic examination permit more accurate diagnoses or determination of effects, but it also makes possible an estimation of the strength of the Hawthorne effect, which is the influence of the study itself on the group being studied (eg, British doctors who were being studied for the long-term effects of smoking were more likely than the rest of the population to improve their smoking habits). Some cohort studies do allow the simultaneous assessment of several risk factors, but this design is not necessary in every case. *(Last, pp 34–36; Levy and Wegman, pp 61–66)*

667–668. (667-A, 668-E) In the Veterans Administration Cooperative Study, from which the figure is extracted, the treated group was noted to have a cumulative percentage incidence of 10% as compared with 20% in the controls. Thus, the cumulative reduction of incidence of all morbid events was reduced by 10%. It is important in epidemiologic studies to be very clear about such comparisons. For this reason, by convention, percentages of percentages are never used. The treatment regimen may, however, be described to be 50% effective by this measurement, as the cumulative incidence is reduced from 20 to 10%. In this comparison, a different parameter is introduced. No longer is there comparison of incidence, but a different concept, "effectiveness," is introduced. It is very easy to make exaggerated claims about effectiveness of a particular therapy. Caution clearly needs to be applied to understand statements and comparisons. *(Last, pp 849–858)*

669. **(E)**   The section of the population increasing most rapidly is at the higher age range: by the year 2000, those over 80 years will constitute 28.8% of those aged 65 years and over as against 20.2% in 1980. There has been some increase in deaths in the elderly attributed to cancer, but there is a reduction in those attributed to heart disease. Suicide has decreased in the population over age 65 in recent years. Life expectation for men is lower than for women. *(Last, pp 973–975)*

670. **(A)**   Coliform organisms are present in the gastrointestinal tract of humans and other animals. Some coliform organisms in water supplies are of nonfecal origin and are not necessarily pathogenic; thus, the presence of coliform organisms does not signify the existence of a definite health hazard. However, from a bacteriologic point of view, coliform organisms should not be present in significant numbers in any public water supply from which drinking water is obtained. *(Last, pp 629)*

671. **(E)**   Cooking is still the best way of controlling parasite disease contracted through eating meat. Parasites are heat-labile and thus are destroyed by adequate cooking. In addition, cooking garbage before feeding it to pigs has proved to be an effective method of controlling trichinosis. During boiling (especially at high altitudes), baking, and cooking, food may not reach temperatures sufficiently high to kill contaminating bacteria. Recent evidence has suggested that frying bacon preserved with nitrite may produce nitrosamine, which is carcinogenic. *(Last, p 610)*

672. **(C)**   The amount of solid waste produced per capita in US cities is approximately 2.5 kg (5.6 lb) daily. This waste is composed of 0.7 kg (1.5 lb) of postconsumer waste (ie, waste including household waste and waste generated as a result of retailing), 0.7 kg (1.5 lb) of street and road litter, and 1.2 kg (2.6 lb) of industrial waste. Yearly, the amount of solid waste produced is approximately 1 ton per person; the cost of disposing of 1 ton of waste is $60. In addition, large quantities of agricultural and animal waste are produced, as well as a considerable amount of mining waste. *(Last, pp 649–698)*

673. **(D)**   Crowded or impoverished groups of the population seem to be highly susceptible to epidemics of meningococcal disease. Although there is poverty in the United States, and individual families may live in crowded conditions, this is not as generalized as in some other countries. Naturally occurring (herd) immunity does not seem to be responsible for the reduced number of outbreaks. Immunologic precautions have not been generally applied to whole populations. Epidemics have not been demonstrated to be more frequent in populations with higher carrier rates. The biologic reasons for reduction seem to be obscure. *(Last, pp 157–158)*

674. **(D)**   Industrial wastes and municipal sewage flowing untreated into a natural collection of water results in an increase both in growth and decomposition of algae. The activity of the algae reduces the oxygen content of the water, which is measured as the biochemic oxygen demand (BOD). A decrease in BOD is generally indicative of successful waste-water treatment and is accompanied by a reduction of other pollutants. *(Clark and MacMahon, pp 764–765)*

675. **(D)**   Household noises can be loud enough to cause acoustic damage. A power mower is rated at a sound level of 96 on the dBA scale (an arbitrary measure of intensity on a sound meter), placing it clearly in the very loud scale. Use of ear muffs or plugs for anyone using a power mower regularly for long periods is advisable. Food blenders are at a sound level of 88 dBA, which is nearly at the sound level of shouting (90 dBA). The sound values for other household appliances are garbage disposal, 80 dBA; clothes washer, 78 dBA; and vacuum cleaner, 70 dBA. *(Levy and Wegman, pp 247–261)*

676. **(B)** Prospective epidemiologic studies have shown the quantitative effect that three of the major risk factors for coronary heart disease—hypertension, hypercholesterolemia, and cigarette smoking—have on risk. In the US Pooling Project, the increase was twofold when one risk factor was present. When any two or all three risk factors were present, the probability of developing fatal coronary heart disease was increased fourfold to five-fold. The impact of other risk factors that have been identified is being studied. *(Clark and MacMahon, p 201)*

677. **(E)** Each state has a unique set of public health laws. Although the majority of relevant, current state laws are distributed to physicians, this practice rarely applies to long-established laws. Most states do not have current, complete sets of health rules and regulations available to the public, in part because these laws are continually changing. Every practitioner should obtain copies of all relevant laws through the state department of health or attorney general's office. For physicians and other citizens, ignorance of the law is no defense. *(Warren, p 19)*

678. **(C)** In 1970, Congress passed the Occupational Safety and Health Act, which created the Occupational Safety and Health Administration (OSHA) "to assure so far as possible every working man and woman in the nation safe and healthful working conditions to preserve our human resources." In the agency's first years, emphasis was placed on developing technical expertise and processing of scientific information, but since 1981 the emphasis has been mainly on encouraging voluntary compliance with safety codes, rather than on code enforcement. This change in emphasis has been controversial: many experts believe that enforcement is required to significantly improve the health and safety of workers. *(Levy and Wegman, p 135)*

679. **(D)** Some employers, under the guise of protecting the fetus from hazardous exposure, have developed policies that exclude women from certain jobs or otherwise restrict their activities in the workplace. Of all the activities listed, only stooping and bending below knee level carry specific hazards. In general, if a woman wishes to do so, she should be permitted to continue employment until the onset of labor. *(Last, pp 575–576)*

680. **(E)** SSDI and SSI require the treating physician to determine only the degree of the patient's impairment. The determination of ability to work is made by an administrative body. The physician should concentrate on medical advice and treatment. Causality is difficult to determine. In advising a patient, it is generally important to avoid attribution of cause, since the exact working conditions and other circumstances may affect the subjective experience of pain. *(Last, p 563)*

681. **(D)** The timing of an exposure to a toxic agent is a significant determinant of its effect. Relatively few substances affect both male and female fertility adversely. Lead does do so, in addition to causing many other blood and organ defects. In the mother, lead may have other untoward effects during pregnancy, such as causing spontaneous abortion, giving rise to behavioral or developmental disabilities for the fetus, and contaminating breast milk. *(Last, p 575)*

682. **(D)** Alcoholics and drug addicts, especially if they live alone and are not part of an intact family or household, are likely to miss meals or exist on foods lacking in nutrition. Many over-the-counter and prescription drugs can promote nutritional deficiency if taken over long periods of time. Persons of limited general education often are ignorant of essential information regarding nutrition. Long-time vegetarians of the vegan type, who eat no animal products, may suffer deficiencies in vitamin B_{12}, iron, and protein. Vegetarians less strict with their diet are not as affected, and, of course, those many vegetarians watchful of their health also generally escape nutritional problems. *(Clark and MacMahon, pp 514–516)*

683. **(D)** Skin cancer is the most common form of cancer in light-skinned populations and accounts for 40% of all cancer in the United States. Light-skinned populations are up to 50 times as likely as dark-skinned populations to develop skin cancer. The major risk factor is exposure to ultraviolet radiation over a period of time; therefore, workers in outdoor occupations, dedicated sunbathers, and persons who live in low latitudes are especially at risk. Sensitivity to ultraviolet radiation is not a major risk factor. Basal cell carcinoma is the most common skin cancer in the United States, accounting for 65% of all skin cancer. *(Last, p 514)*

684. **(E)** Bladder cancer has been related to occupational exposure to coal products (not coal itself), aromatic amines, and leather dusts. Coal miners and automotive brake and clutch mechanics are more at risk for developing malignant disease of the lungs, pleura, and peritoneum, caused by the inhalation of asbestos and other carcinogenic inhalants. Benzene is associated with bone marrow disease. Insecticide makers and sprayers have a higher-than-normal incidence of skin cancer. *(Levy and Wegman, p 220)*

685. **(A)** Coccidioidomycosis is due to an endemic infection. Incidence of coccidioidomycosis is highest in the arid southwestern area of the United States and declines to the north and east. States in the northwest, extreme northeast, and southeast are largely unaffected. Persons who have negative skin reactions to coccidioidin are susceptible to the disease, and living in a region of rapidly changing population is considered a risk factor. Sowing grass seed and paving roads and recreation areas have been recommended as preventive measures, because both would reduce dust, in which the organisms are carried. *(Last, p 287)*

686. **(C)** In 1980, 15 318 cases of viral hepatitis, type B, were reported to the Centers for Disease Control. Hepatitis B is by far the most common work-related infectious disease and continues to be a major problem for health professionals. The major source of infection is blood and blood products. Other infectious diseases that can be work-related include leptospirosis, brucellosis, tetanus, and the rarely occurring anthrax. These conditions can occur in farmers, in workers who come into contact with sewage, and in other occupations. *(Levy and Wegman, pp 282–286)*

687. **(E)** A vaccine against yellow fever is available for human use. Yellow fever is endemic in the region of the world between 15° north and 15° south latitude; vaccination is required for all airline personnel and passengers entering the area. To date, a vaccine has been produced for only one other arthropod-borne virus infection, Rift Valley fever. This condition had been of minor importance until several years ago, when an outbreak of 20 000 cases occurred in the Nile River area of Africa. *(Last, pp 60,219–220,225–226)*

688. **(C)** Person-to-person spread is the most common mode of transmission of shigellosis, and secondary attack rates are high. Outbreaks of food-borne and water-borne infection occur rarely. Water-borne infection generally only occurs from inadequately chlorinated, semipublic water supplies. Food may be primarily infected (eg, turkeys infected by tainted feed) or, like salad, infected as a result of poor hygiene of food handlers. Carrier states rarely last more than a year after contact with infection. *(Last, pp 175–176)*

689–691. **(689-D, 690-C, 691-A)** Incidence and prevalence frequently are confused with each other. Incidence measures the number of *new* cases of a particular disease related to the population at risk, which is normally defined in terms of the population at the middle of the period under study. Prevalence is calculated on the basis of the number of *existing* cases at a given time related to the population at risk at that same time, not to a hypothetical population. For this reason prevalence rate often is referred to as the point prevalence rate. Period prevalence rate combines both point prevalence and incidence. It is of limited usefulness because it is generally preferable to separate new cases from existing or chronic cases.

Because incidence is the number of new cases of a disease, it would be an especially helpful indicator of infectious diseases, which may occur in epidemics. In other situations, it may be more important to study the prevalence, which would be a way of estimating the amount of care (ie, the nature and number of medical services) needed in any community. For example, knowing the prevalence of certain types of renal failure could determine the need for renal dialysis units in a community. *(Clark and MacMahon, pp 39–40,56)*

692–694. (692-B, 693-C, 694-D) Death rates are frequently calculated and reported for all causes and ages, or in many combinations of age, sex, race, and geographic area. Frequently the population base is a political or census division because residence or population at risk can be determined easily. The period of calculation is usually one year, but the population base may be 1000 to 100 000.

Crude death rate is the number of all deaths reported, related to midyear population. It is of value in comparing the health of one locality or country with another and can be a general measure of health care. Case fatality rate is not generally related to a standard 1-year period but frequently reflects the duration of an acute episode of illness or length of hospitalization. In an acute epidemic, it is sometimes defined as the number of deaths divided by the number of new cases, all the cases in such an epidemic being new. Otherwise, case fatality rate refers to both new and existing cases of a disease. Cause-specific death rate is valuable in studying the incidence, virulence, and effectiveness of treatment. It is defined as the number of deaths from a specified disease, related to a midyear population. *(Clark and MacMahon, pp 38–39)*

695–699. (695-C, 696-C, 697-E, 698-A, 699-D) In the United States, the organizational responsibility for monitoring food and water safety is complex. Among the federal control agen-

cies, the Environmental Protection Agency (EPA) is the most recent and in many ways the most active and powerful. This agency has now set up an elaborate system of regulation and control of the use of pesticides and has banned the commercial marketing of DDT. The EPA also monitors water pollution in general, but other agencies are involved, too. The Food and Drug Administration (FDA) has defined action levels in fish of polychlorinated biphenyls (PCBs), a toxin that presumably is water borne. The FDA retains the authority to remove from the market food containing excess pesticides or other toxic substances and sets levels of diethylstilbestrol (DES) permissible in food products (especially poultry) at the time of marketing. The US Department of Agriculture (USDA) determines wholesomeness standards for the production and sale of meat.

International control is assisted by the World Health Organization (WHO). This agency has mounted control programs for the eradication of communicable disease, with conspicuous success in eradicating smallpox. It also publishes an International Statistical Classification of Disease (ICD). The United Nations Food and Agriculture Organization (FAO) is devoted to the improvement of the health of agricultural workers all over the world. *(Last, pp 43,486–487,592,647)*

REFERENCES

Ahlbom A, Norell S. *Introduction to Modern Epidemiology.* Chestnut Hill, Mass: Epidemiology Resources, Inc; 1990.

Clark DW, MacMahon B. *Preventive and Community Medicine.* 2nd ed. Boston, Mass: Little, Brown & Co; 1981.

Colton T. *Statistics in Medicine.* Boston, Mass: Little, Brown & Co; 1974.

Kelley WN. *Textbook of Internal Medicine.* Philadelphia, Penn: J.B. Lippincott Co; 1989.

Kramer MS. *Clinical Epidemiology and Biostatistics. A Primer for Clinical Investigators and Decision-Makers.* Berlin, Germany: Springer-Verlag; 1988.

Last JM. *Maxcy-Rosenau Public Health and Preventive Medicine.* 13th ed. Norwalk, CT: Appleton & Lange; 1992.

Levy BS, Wegman DH. *Occupational Health: Recognizing and Preventing Work Related Disease.* 2nd ed. Boston, Mass: Little, Brown & Co; 1995.

Mausner JS, Bahn AK. *Epidemiology: An Introductory Text.* Philadelphia: WB Saunders Co; 1985.

Warren DG. *A Legal Guide for Rural Health Programs.* Cambridge, Mass: Ballinger Publishing Co; 1979.

Wyngaarden JB, Smith LM. *Cecil's Textbook of Medicine.* 18th ed. Philadelphia: WB Saunders Co; 1996.

SUBSPECIALTY LIST: PREVENTIVE MEDICINE

Question Number and Subspecialty

648. Disease control
649. Disease control
650. Ethical, legal
651. Epidemiology
652. Biostatistics
653. Biostatistics
654. Biostatistics
655. Biostatistics
656. Biostatistics
657. Biostatistics
658. Biostatistics
659. Biostatistics
660. Health services
661. Health services
662. Biostatistics
663. Epidemiology
664. Biostatistics
665. Biostatistics
666. Biostatistics
667. Biostatistics
668. Biostatistics
669. Disease control
670. Disease control
671. Disease control
672. Disease control
673. Disease control
674. Disease control
675. Disease control
676. Disease control
677. Disease control
678. Health services
679. Ethical, legal
680. Ethical, legal
681. Disease control
682. Epidemiology
683. Epidemiology
684. Epidemiology
685. Disease control
686. Disease control
687. Disease control
688. Disease control
689. Epidemiology
690. Epidemiology
691. Epidemiology
692. Epidemiology
693. Epidemiology
694. Epidemiology
695. Ethical, legal
696. Ethical, legal
697. Ethical, legal
698. Ethical, legal
699. Ethical, legal

Clinical Competence Review
Questions

DIRECTIONS (Questions 700 through 817): Each of the numbered items or incomplete statements in this section is followed by answers or by completions of the statement. Select the ONE lettered answer or completion that is BEST in each case.

Questions 700 through 702

The basal body temperature chart shown below is from a 28-year-old woman (gravida 0, para 0).

700. The data from the basal body temperature chart shown above support which of the following conclusions?

   (A) the woman appears to have had an ovulatory cycle
   (B) progesterone production peaks just before the temperature drop on about day 14
   (C) luteinizing hormone (LH) peaks only after the temperature rise has been sustained
   (D) the time from the anticipated LH surge to menses in this cycle is normal
   (E) in this cycle follicle-stimulating hormone (FSH) would achieve maximum levels on day 23

701. The most likely diagnosis of the condition represented in the chart is

   (A) luteal-phase defect
   (B) Stein–Leventhal syndrome (polycystic ovaries)
   (C) salpingitis isthmica nodosa
   (D) müllerian agenesis
   (E) Asherman's syndrome

702. All the following statements are true about the diagnosis and treatment of this condition EXCEPT

   (A) it can be a cause of habitual abortion or infertility
   (B) endometrial biopsy performed 2 days before the onset of menstruation can confirm the diagnosis
   (C) administration of ethinyl estradiol has been a successful treatment of this condition
   (D) the aim of therapy is to raise the number of LH receptors on the granulosa cells of the ovarian follicle
   (E) affected women may show abnormally low postovulatory serum progesterone levels

Questions 703 through 707

A 24-year-old woman (gravida 2, para 1) registers at a local prenatal clinic at 26 weeks' gestation. Her hematocrit is 28%.

703. The most likely cause of the woman's low hematocrit is

    (A) Cooley's anemia
    (B) pernicious anemia
    (C) folic acid deficiency
    (D) glucose-6-phosphate dehydrogenase deficiency
    (E) iron deficiency

704. The most useful combination of laboratory tests to confirm the correct diagnosis would be

    (A) stool culture for ova and parasites and hemoglobin electrophoresis
    (B) complete blood cell count with indices and serum iron concentration
    (C) serum vitamin B_{12} and serum iron concentrations
    (D) reticulocyte count and complete blood cell count
    (E) mean corpuscular volume and reticulocyte count

705. Regarding the iron requirements of pregnancy, all of the statements below are true, EXCEPT

    (A) pernicious anemia is the most common anemia of pregnancy
    (B) 300 mg of iron goes to the fetus
    (C) 500 mg of iron is used to expand maternal hemoglobin
    (D) 200 mg of iron is shed through the gut
    (E) the hemoglobin level of most healthy women at term is 11 g/dL

706. Regarding this type of anemia in pregnancy, which of the following statements is true?

    (A) fetal blood sampling should be done to see if this anemia has affected the fetus
    (B) this type of anemia seldom affects the fetus

    (C) genetic counseling should be provided to this woman before her next pregnancy
    (D) treatment of this type of anemia with iron is commonly associated with hemosiderosis
    (E) packed red blood cell transfusion is the only successful way to treat this type of anemia, but should be withheld until the hematocrit is less than 24

707. The laboratory test that would *first* reflect response to treatment in the case presented would be

    (A) serum iron concentration
    (B) hematocrit
    (C) reticulocyte count
    (D) total iron-binding capacity
    (E) smear of peripheral blood

Questions 708 through 712

A 26-year-old woman (gravida 3, para 2) is 28 weeks pregnant. She seeks medical attention because of urinary frequency and urgency, and a diagnosis of urinary tract infection is made.

708. Which of the following statements about urinary tract infection associated with pregnancy is true?

    (A) most women with this disorder have symptoms
    (B) fever is common
    (C) many symptomatic women do not have bacteriuria
    (D) pregnant women are less likely than nonpregnant women to develop urinary tract infection
    (E) age and parity do not affect the incidence of this condition

709. Regarding the accurate diagnosis of urinary tract infection during pregnancy, which of the following statements is true?

(A) the clinical picture of fever, chills, dysuria, and frequency may be the most sensitive indicators of urinary tract infection

(B) 100 000 colonies of bacteria per milliliter of collected clean-catch urine are the best indicator of urinary tract infection in pregnancy

(C) in high-risk women, 100 to 1000 colonies of bacteria per milliliter of collected clean-catch urine may be significant

(D) bladder washout techniques are the best available techniques for diagnosis of urinary tract infection in pregnancy

(E) radiography of the urinary tract in pregnancy need not be postponed in any patient with recurrent infection

710. Which of the following statements describing treatment for this disorder is true?

(A) bacteriostatic drugs are preferable to bactericidal drugs

(B) the use of sulfonamides is contraindicated

(C) catheterization is necessary to determine the effectiveness of treatment

(D) laboratory testing should be repeated 1 to 2 weeks after treatment

(E) long-term chemoprophylaxis should be instituted for the duration of the pregnancy if recurrent infection occurs

711. The organism or type of organism most commonly causing this condition is

(A) *Mycoplasma*

(B) RNA viruses

(C) enterobacteria

(D) group B streptococci

(E) anaerobes

712. All the following statements about the relationship between urinary tract infection and pregnancy are true EXCEPT

(A) there is a higher rate of perinatal sepsis in the offspring

(B) there is a higher rate of postpartum endometritis in the mother

(C) relapse after antibiotic therapy may indicate the presence of an anatomic abnormality

(D) endocervical cultures often reveal the same organism

(E) a history of urinary tract infection before pregnancy does not increase the risk of pregnancy-related urinary tract infection

Questions 713 through 719

A 22-year-old woman goes to the local emergency room because of fever, a rash, and malaise associated with menstruation. A diagnosis of toxic shock syndrome (TSS) is considered.

713. Which of the following symptoms would be LEAST likely to be associated with TSS?

(A) constipation

(B) myalgia

(C) syncope

(D) headache

(E) oliguria

714. Of the following microorganisms, the one isolated most commonly from women with TSS is

(A) *Chlamydia*

(B) *Streptococcus*

(C) *Staphylococcus aureus*

(D) *Escherichia coli*

(E) herpes simplex virus, type 2

715. TSS is most likely to be associated with which of the following laboratory findings?

    (A) elevated SGOT and SGPT levels
    (B) elevated platelet count
    (C) decreased blood urea nitrogen level
    (D) decreased serum creatine phosphokinase level
    (E) decreased serum uric acid level

716. The most likely cause of the tissue damage associated with TSS is

    (A) bacteremia
    (B) viremia
    (C) nonenteric toxin production
    (D) hyperthermia
    (E) alteration in blood clotting control

717. The characteristic rash in women with TSS is best described as

    (A) papular and nonpruritic
    (B) macular, diffuse, and red
    (C) vesicular and occurring in a dermatomal distribution
    (D) rarely desquamative
    (E) desquamative but sparing the palms of the hands and soles of the feet

718. The most effective therapy for the woman described in this case would be

    (A) massive fluid replacement therapy
    (B) oxacillin or a cephalosporin
    (C) dopamine
    (D) massive doses of corticosteroids
    (E) naloxone

719. Which of the following statements regarding prognosis and management of TSS is true?

    (A) appropriate drug therapy prevents recurrence
    (B) recurrence rate in women who have not received antibiotic therapy is 90%
    (C) tampon use is still not proven to be safe even if posttreatment cultures are negative

    (D) the use of "regular"-size tampons is not associated with recurrence
    (E) less frequent tampon changing causes less vaginal irritation and, therefore, less chance of recurrence

Questions 720 through 723

A 33-year-old woman (gravida 1, para 0) is in the 35th week of pregnancy. She goes to the local emergency room because of uterine pain and vaginal bleeding. Her blood pressure, which had been 110/70 mm Hg last month, is now 150/100 mm Hg.

720. The most likely reason for the woman's vaginal bleeding is

    (A) placenta previa
    (B) abruptio placentae
    (C) ruptured Gartner's cyst
    (D) incompetent cervix
    (E) fibroid uterus

721. Which of the following laboratory values would be LEAST consistent with the diagnosis of preeclampsia?

    (A) an elevated hematocrit
    (B) platelet count of less than $100\,000/mL^3$
    (C) elevated fibrin degradation products
    (D) elevated plasma uric acid concentration
    (E) dramatically shortened prothrombin time

722. Vaginal blood loss caused by the disorder described in the case is often

    (A) associated with uterine atony
    (B) a combination of fetal and maternal blood loss
    (C) less than the true blood loss because of maternal intra-abdominal hemorrhage
    (D) less than the true blood loss because of concealed retroplacental hemorrhage
    (E) none of the above

723. Regarding placental abruption, which of the following statements is true?

(A) there is no indication for cesarean section in these cases

(B) oxytocin stimulation of labor is contraindicated

(C) blood loss is seldom of significance because of myometrial tamponade

(D) amniotomy plays a key role in correct management of this complication of labor

(E) the uterus may be persistently hypertonic

Questions 724 through 726

A 3-week-old male infant, who has been in good health after an uncomplicated pregnancy, labor, and delivery, begins to feed very poorly. His temperature is 38.9°C (102°F). His mother calls the infant's pediatrician, and the boy is subsequently hospitalized. Cultures are obtained from blood, urine, and cerebrospinal fluid, which is cloudy. A diagnosis of meningitis is made.

724. The bacterial agents most likely to be responsible for this infant's meningitis are

(A) *Haemophilus influenzae, Streptococcus pneumoniae,* and *Neisseria meningitidis*

(B) *Haemophilus influenzae, Streptococcus pneumoniae,* and *Staphylococcus aureus*

(C) *Staphylococcus aureus* and group A *Streptococcus*

(D) group B *Streptococcus, Escherichia coli,* and *Listeria monocytogenes*

(E) group B *Streptococcus* and *Staphylococcus aureus*

725. Of the following, which would be appropriate therapy for this patient?

(A) penicillin alone or oxacillin alone

(B) penicillin and chloramphenicol or ampicillin and chloramphenicol

(C) ampicillin and gentamicin or ampicillin and cefotaxime

(D) ampicillin alone or gentamicin alone

(E) chloramphenicol alone or cefotaxime alone

726. Which of the following is most likely to occur as a complication of this child's meningitis?

(A) hearing loss

(B) visual impairment

(C) brain abscess

(D) kernicterus

(E) quadriplegia

Questions 727 and 728

A 2-year-old girl is brought to the emergency room because of a cough that has been worsening during the past 3 days. Her temperature is 38.3°C (101°F), and she has mild inspiratory stridor. A roentgenogram of the neck is taken, but because of the child's movement only an anteroposterior view is satisfactorily obtained. This roentgenogram is shown on page 208.

727. The most likely diagnosis in the case presented is

(A) epiglottitis

(B) infectious laryngotracheitis

(C) spasmodic croup

(D) angioneurotic edema

(E) foreign-body aspiration

728. The next step in the treatment of this child should be to

(A) administer cefotaxime intravenously

(B) administer racemic epinephrine by aerosol or intermittent positive-pressure breathing

(C) administer theophylline intravenously

(D) endotracheal intubation

(E) endoscopy

Figure for use with questions 727 and 728.

Questions 729 through 731

For the past day, a 16-year-old girl has had fever, vomiting, and watery diarrhea. She also complains of intermittent abdominal pain and generalized myalgia. On physical examination she is noted to be slightly lethargic. Temperature is 39.7°C (103.5°F), pulse is 154 beats/min, and blood pressure is 80/46 mm Hg. Her conjunctivae and pharynx are hyperemic, and she has a generalized erythematous maculopapular rash that spares her wrists.

729. The most likely diagnosis in the case described above is

(A) scarlet fever

(B) Kawasaki's disease

(C) ruptured appendix

(D) Rocky Mountain spotted fever

(E) toxic shock syndrome

730. The cause of the girl's disease is

(A) group A beta-hemolytic *Streptococcus*

(B) *Staphylococcus aureus*

(C) *Rickettsia rickettsii*

(D) fecolith impaction

(E) unknown

731. Recommended treatment for the disease process described above is

(A) tetracycline

(B) gentamicin and clindamycin

(C) oxacillin

(D) penicillin

(E) surgery

Questions 732 and 733

A 6-year-old boy is seen by a pediatrician for routine physical examination. On physical examination the pediatrician notes the presence of dark, coarse pubic hair, enlargement of the penis and testes, and acne of the face and upper back. Upon questioning, the mother relates that the child often has a body odor similar to that of her teenage son after a baseball game. A graph of the child's height during the last few years is shown below.

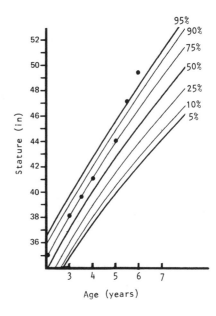

732. Which of the following tests is most likely to reveal the cause of this child's problem?

(A) computed tomography (CT) scan of the head

(B) abdominal ultrasound examination

(C) surgical exploration of the abdomen

(D) skin biopsy

(E) chromosomal analysis

733. The most likely diagnosis in this child is

(A) idiopathic precocious puberty

(B) a hypothalamic tumor

(C) McCune–Albright syndrome

(D) Klinefelter's syndrome

(E) XYY syndrome

Questions 734 through 737

A 15-month-old boy who developed an upper respiratory tract infection yesterday had a generalized tonic–clonic seizure earlier today. According to his parents, who took their son to the hospital, his eyes rolled backward and the seizure lasted 30 seconds. Temperature on arrival at the hospital is 40°C (104°F), respiratory rate is 22/min, and blood pressure is 90/60 mm Hg. The boy is alert, smiling, and walking from room to room. On physical examination, his anterior fontanel is almost closed, he has rhinorrhea, and his neck is supple. The child has bruises below both knees. The rest of the physical examination is unremarkable.

734. The most likely diagnosis in the case described is

(A) idiopathic epilepsy

(B) meningitis

(C) simple febrile seizure

(D) complex febrile seizure

(E) child abuse

735. At this point, the boy's physician should

(A) order a complete blood cell count

(B) order serum electrolyte and blood glucose levels

(C) obtain a CT scan of the head

(D) perform a lumbar puncture

(E) schedule electroencephalography for the following day

736. The correct therapeutic response to the boy's seizure would be to

(A) prescribe oral phenobarbital

(B) administer intravenous phenytoin

(C) administer intravenous antibiotics

(D) reassure the parents

(E) notify the local child protection agency

737. The prognosis associated with the boy's condition is best described as

(A) poor

(B) fair

(C) excellent

(D) difficult to assess

(E) dependent on the adjustments made in the child's environment

Questions 738 through 740

A 2-month-old boy is being evaluated for the growth pictured on page 210. At birth his skin was clear, but when he was 1 month old his mother noted a light red growth on his arm. During the last month, it increased in size and turned bright red.

738. The most likely diagnosis of the skin lesion pictured is

(A) melanoma

(B) osteochondroma

(C) nevus flammeus

(D) cavernous hemangioma

(E) strawberry hemangioma

739. The treatment of choice of this disorder is

(A) surgery

(B) radiation therapy

(C) argon laser therapy

(D) topical corticosteroids

(E) observation

Figure for use with questions 738 through 740.

Figure for use with questions 741 through 743.

740. Response to treatment is best described by which of the following statements?

(A) recovery will be total, with no evidence of scar

(B) recovery will be poor, with probable malignant transformation

(C) recovery will be poor, with metastasis to regional lymph nodes

(D) recovery will be favorable, but other lesions of the same type are likely to develop

(E) there is not enough information to predict outcome

Questions 741 through 743

An 8-year-old boy has the scalp rash shown above at right. Two weeks ago the rash was quite small and very scaly, but since then it has slowly enlarged. The rash now is 2 cm by 2 cm in size; it is raised, has small vesicles and pustules on its surface, and is indurated and boggy. The boy is afebrile.

741. The most likely diagnosis of the skin lesion described is

(A) seborrheic dermatitis

(B) impetigo

(C) alopecia areata

(D) herpetic skin lesion

(E) kerion

742. The etiology of the skin disease presented above is

(A) genetic

(B) fungal

(C) bacterial

(D) viral

(E) unknown

743. The treatment of choice of the underlying skin disease is

(A) topical steroids

(B) intralesional steroids

(C) griseofulvin

(D) adenosine arabinoside (ara-A)

(E) dicloxacillin

Questions 744 through 746

A 7-year-old boy who has been in excellent health complains of intermittent palpitations. He states that the palpitations begin and end abruptly and last from 30 minutes to 2 hours. Between episodes he is asymptomatic. Physical examination is unremarkable. His electrocardiogram is shown on page 211.

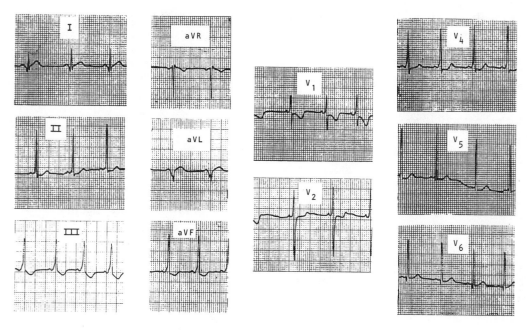

Figure for use with questions 744 through 746.

744. The most likely diagnosis in the case described is

(A) psychoneurosis

(B) Wolff–Parkinson–White syndrome

(C) Lown–Ganong–Levine syndrome

(D) sinus tachycardia

(E) nodal tachycardia

745. The boy's palpitations are most likely due to

(A) anxiety

(B) supraventricular tachycardia

(C) atrial fibrillation

(D) ventricular fibrillation

(E) wandering pacemaker

746. The most effective first-line therapy for the boy's disorder would be

(A) antianxiety medications

(B) psychotherapy

(C) digoxin

(D) quinidine

(E) electrical cardioversion

Questions 747 through 749

A 12-year-old boy with sickle cell disease is hospitalized because of severe pain in both legs. The child is afebrile and physical examination is within normal limits except for pallor, a grade 2/4 systolic ejection murmur, and mild generalized tenderness of both lower extremities. Hemoglobin concentration is 7.5 g/dL.

747. Appropriate initial therapy should include

(A) intravenous fluids

(B) intravenous antibiotics

(C) blood transfusion

(D) withholding pain medications

(E) withholding oral fluids

748. Complications of sickle cell disease include all of the following EXCEPT

(A) sequestration crisis

(B) vasoocclusive crisis

(C) aplastic anemia

(D) pulmonary edema

(E) hand–foot syndrome

749. Children with sickle cell anemia are at increased risk for developing bacteremia with

   (A) *Streptococcus pneumoniae*
   (B) beta-hemolytic *Streptococcus*
   (C) *Escherichia coli*
   (D) *Staphylococcus aureus*
   (E) *Klebsiella pneumoniae*

Questions 750 and 751

A 58-year-old man develops a syndrome consisting of a "shade" falling smoothly over his left field of vision and numbness of his right hand and face lasting between 5 and 10 minutes. He has had two episodes recently.

750. The most likely diagnosis of the man's disorder is

   (A) recurrent cerebral embolism
   (B) Adams–Stokes attacks
   (C) epileptic seizure
   (D) migrainous accompaniments
   (E) transient cerebral ischemic attacks

751. Treatment of this man's disorder might include

   (A) ergot preparations
   (B) beta-blockers
   (C) antiplatelet drugs
   (D) antiarrhythmic drugs
   (E) antiseizure drugs

Questions 752 and 753

For the last 6 months, a 30-year-old man has had low back pain associated with morning stiffness and lessened with exercise. Roentgenograms of his back are shown on page 213.

752. The most likely diagnosis for the man's disorder is

   (A) rheumatoid arthritis
   (B) ankylosing spondylitis
   (C) herniated nucleus pulposus
   (D) pseudogout
   (E) Reiter's syndrome

753. Systemic complications of this disease include all of the following EXCEPT

   (A) peripheral vasculitic lesions
   (B) aortitis with aortic insufficiency
   (C) cardiac conduction defects
   (D) iritis
   (E) apical pulmonary fibrosis with cavities

Questions 754 and 755

A 44-year-old man has chronic headaches, rhinorrhea, earache, low-grade fever, arthralgias, and anorexia. Sinus roentgenograms reveal bilateral maxillary sinusitis. He is treated with antibiotics but then develops cough, chest pain, and hemoptysis. Physical examination reveals a saddle-nose deformity and a nasal mucosal ulceration. Chest roentgenography demonstrates cavitary infiltrates. Urinalysis shows 10 to 12 RBC/HPF. Blood urea nitrogen concentration is 35 mg/dL, and serum creatinine concentration is 2.0 mg/dL. Sputum examination shows no acid-fast organisms, fungi, or malignant cells.

754. The most likely diagnosis in the case described is

   (A) polyarteritis nodosa
   (B) tuberculosis
   (C) sarcoidosis
   (D) Wegener's granulomatosis
   (E) pulmonary abscess

755. Long-term treatment of this man's disease should consist of

   (A) prednisone
   (B) cyclophosphamide
   (C) penicillin
   (D) isoniazid and rifampin
   (E) isoniazid, streptomycin, and *p*-aminosalicylic acid (PAS)

Figures for use with questions 752 and 753.

756. A 25-year-old woman complains of epigastric pain. She has a long history of bronchial asthma, which has been treated with a long-acting theophylline drug and beta-adrenergic aerosol. An upper gastrointestinal series reveals a hiatal hernia and reflux. She is started on cimetidine, 300 mg four times daily. Within a week she develops nausea. Her physician now should order which of the following tests?

(A) esophagogastroduodenoscopy
(B) stool examination for occult blood
(C) repeat upper gastrointestinal series
(D) serum theophylline level
(E) CT scan of the abdomen

Questions 757 and 758

A 48-year-old man has developed calcium oxalate kidney stones on 12 occasions, despite following a diet free of dairy products and drinking large amounts of fluid. Urinalysis reveals a normal pH, and 24-hour calcium, uric acid, and oxalate levels are normal. Blood testing reveals normal levels of calcium, phosphorus, uric acid, and urea nitrogen. Urine cultures produce no growth. Intravenous pyelography shows opaque calculi in both kidneys.

757. Initial treatment of this man's disorder should be with

(A) a thiazide drug
(B) allopurinol
(C) cellulose phosphate
(D) nephrolithotomy
(E) increased fluid intake and dietary restriction

Figure for use with questions 762 and 763.

758. Despite proper treatment the man continues to form and pass new stones. Treatment now should consist of

(A) a thiazide drug and allopurinol in combination

(B) cellulose phosphate in higher concentration

(C) orthophosphate as the neutral salt

(D) parathyroidectomy

(E) nephrolithotomy

Questions 759 and 760

A 35-year-old man suddenly develops a generalized pruritic macular erythematous rash and fever. Four days ago, he saw his physician because of a sore throat that started the day before, and he was started on penicillin, 250 mg four times daily, after a throat culture grew out beta-hemolytic streptococci. Laboratory studies now reveal a blood urea nitrogen level of 35 mg/dL. Urinalysis shows no casts, 2+ protein, 50 RBC/HPF, and 50 WBC/HPF. Complete blood cell count is normal except for eosinophilia (12%). Urine protein concentration is 650 mg/24 h.

759. The most likely diagnosis in the case described is

(A) acute poststreptococcal glomerulonephritis

(B) membranous glomerulonephritis

(C) polyarteritis nodosa

(D) Schönlein–Henoch purpura

(E) drug-induced interstitial nephritis

760. The treatment of choice for the man's disorder would be to

(A) stop the penicillin

(B) increase the dosage of penicillin

(C) prescribe methicillin

(D) prescribe prednisone

(E) prescribe azathioprine and prednisone

761. A 15-year-old boy with chronic bronchial asthma has severe wheezing and pain in his shoulders. Auscultation reveals a "crunching" sound over his precordium, and palpation of his neck reveals subcutaneous emphysema. Initial treatment should consist of

(A) intermittent positive-pressure breathing and a beta-adrenergic agent

(B) intravenous aminophylline

(C) positive end-expiratory pressure therapy

(D) insertion of a chest tube

(E) bronchoscopy

Questions 762 and 763

A 25-year-old black woman has tender red nodules on both shins. Her chest roentgenogram is shown on page 214. She is otherwise asymptomatic.

762. The most likely diagnosis is

(A) herpes simplex disease

(B) Hodgkin's disease

(C) lymphoma

(D) coccidioidomycosis

(E) sarcoidosis

763. The best treatment for the woman described would be

(A) reassurance and no drugs

(B) prednisone

(C) idoxuridine

(D) amphotericin B

(E) radiation therapy

Questions 764 through 766

For the past several years, a 52-year-old woman has felt fatigued and has had symmetrical swelling, redness, and tenderness of the proximal interphalangeal joints of her hands. Physical examination reveals swelling of the proximal interphalangeal and metacarpophalangeal joints of her hands and wrists. Nodules are found over the extensor surfaces of her elbow. Roentgenograms of her hands are shown above at right.

Figures for use with questions 764 through 766.

764. The most likely diagnosis for the woman described is

(A) systemic lupus erythematosus

(B) rheumatoid arthritis

(C) osteoarthritis

(D) gout

(E) Reiter's syndrome

765. Laboratory findings would include all of the following EXCEPT

   (A) anemia
   (B) elevated sedimentation rate
   (C) rheumatoid factor
   (D) anti-DNA antibodies
   (E) antinuclear antibodies

766. Initial therapy for the woman described should consist of

   (A) methotrexate 7.5 mg weekly
   (B) prednisone, 7.5 mg daily
   (C) allopurinol, 300 mg daily
   (D) aspirin, 12 tablets daily
   (E) gold compound injections

Questions 767 through 769

A 51-year-old man has been well since a myocardial infarction 2 years ago. His nonfasting cholesterol level is 245 mg/dL.

767. The first step in his management would be

   (A) no further action; his cholesterol is not high enough for concern
   (B) obtain a cholesterol after a 12-hour fast
   (C) obtain a lipid profile (cholesterol, triglycerides, and HDL cholesterol) after a 12-hour fast
   (D) initiate a cholesterol-lowering diet
   (E) lipoprotein electrophoresis

768. If dietary treatment is initiated in this patient, measures would include all of the following EXCEPT

   (A) weight loss if the patient is obese
   (B) limit alcohol intake to one drink per day
   (C) increase intake of water-soluble fiber
   (D) restrict saturated fat to < 10% of total calories
   (E) restrict cholesterol to 300 mg per day

769. Drug treatment should be considered for this patient if

   (A) his serum cholesterol exceeds 200 mg/dL after 2 months of an appropriate diet
   (B) his serum cholesterol exceeds 200 mg/dL after 6 months of an appropriate diet
   (C) his LDL cholesterol exceeds 160 mg/dL after 2 months of an appropriate diet
   (D) his LDL cholesterol exceeds 160 mg/dL after 6 months of an appropriate diet
   (E) his LDL cholesterol exceeds 190 mg/dL after 6 months of an appropriate diet

Questions 770 through 772

A 32-year-old woman has migratory arthritis of her wrists and ankles and a vesiculopustular skin eruption. She is afebrile. Physical examination reveals tenosynovitis of her wrists.

770. The most likely diagnosis for the woman described is

   (A) gonococcal arthritis
   (B) Reiter's syndrome
   (C) rheumatoid arthritis
   (D) systemic lupus erythematosus
   (E) meningococcemia

771. Laboratory findings associated with this disease usually include

   (A) positive culture of synovial fluid for gonococci
   (B) HLA-B27 haplotype
   (C) rheumatoid factor
   (D) anti-DNA antibodies
   (E) none of the above

772. The treatment of choice of the woman's disease would be

   (A) ceftriaxone, 1 g daily
   (B) prednisone, 40 mg daily
   (C) aspirin, 12 tablets daily
   (D) ibuprofen, 600 mg three times daily
   (E) erythromycin, 250 mg four times daily

Questions 773 and 774

A 40-year-old woman has episodic headaches that last 30 minutes and are associated with sweating, palpitations, and feelings of apprehension. She has lost 6.8 kg (15 lb) over the past 3 months. Physical examination reveals a thin woman with a pulse of 112 beats/min and a blood pressure of 150/100 mm Hg lying and 130/80 mm Hg standing.

773. The most likely diagnosis in the case described is

   (A) pheochromocytoma
   (B) hyperaldosteronism
   (C) posterior fossa tumor
   (D) renal artery stenosis
   (E) carcinoid syndrome

774. The most helpful diagnostic test would be

   (A) CT scan of the brain
   (B) hypertension intravenous pyelography
   (C) 24-hour urinary 5-hydroxyindoleacetic acid (5-HIAA) levels
   (D) 24-hour urinary aldosterone levels
   (E) 24-hour urinary vanillylmandelic acid (VMA) and catecholamine levels

Questions 775 through 778

A 70-year-old man, previously known to be normotensive with atrial fibrillation, is brought to the emergency room with a history of sudden onset of abdominal pain of 2 hours duration. On examination he is found to have a blood pressure of 120 mm Hg systolic and 80 mm Hg diastolic, heart rhythm irregular, and abdominal examination unremarkable.

775. The most likely diagnosis is

   (A) superior mesenteric artery embolism
   (B) superior mesenteric artery thrombosis
   (C) superior mesenteric vein thrombosis
   (D) low-flow syndrome
   (E) dissecting aneurysm of the aorta

776. The most likely metabolic abnormality in this patient is

   (A) metabolic acidosis
   (B) metabolic alkalosis
   (C) respiratory acidosis
   (D) respiratory alkalosis
   (E) none of the above

777. The diagnostic procedure of choice is

   (A) plain roentgenography of abdomen
   (B) blood gas determination
   (C) mesenteric angiography
   (D) CT scan of abdomen
   (E) diagnostic peritoneal tap

778. In the management of this patient all of the following are indicated EXCEPT

   (A) analgesics
   (B) heparin
   (C) papavarin
   (D) antibiotics
   (E) observation until more definite signs develop

Questions 779 and 780

779. A 41-year-old woman has an asymptomatic breast mass. All of the following features in the history would increase the risk of carcinoma EXCEPT

   (A) history of carcinoma in the other breast
   (B) history of breast cancer in blood-related family members
   (C) history of infertility
   (D) pregnancy before the age of 18 years
   (E) total hysterectomy and bilateral salpingo-oophorectomy at the age of 38 years

780. The woman described undergoes mammographic examination. All of the following features on mammogram are suggestive of a malignant mass EXCEPT

(A) presence of microcalcification in the mass
(B) smooth, sharp, circumscribed border
(C) spiculated edges
(D) thickening and retraction of the skin over the mass
(E) ductal dilatation

Questions 781 through 784

781. A 42-year-old man with cirrhosis has esophageal varices. The preferred initial measure for controlling esophageal variceal hemorrhage is

(A) esophageal balloon tamponade
(B) systemic intravenous vasopressin infusion
(C) mesenteric arterial vasopressin infusion
(D) gastric hypothermia
(E) esophogogastroduodenoscopy

782. The procedure that would afford the greatest protection against a recurrence of esophageal variceal bleeding is

(A) portacaval shunt
(B) conventional splenorenal shunt
(C) ligation of esophageal varices
(D) transection of the esophagus and staple anastomosis
(E) none of the above

783. Distal splenorenal shunt (Warren shunt) has been used to control hemorrhage from esophageal varices. All of the following statements concerning this procedure are true EXCEPT

(A) portal pressure is not decreased
(B) encephalopathy occurs less frequently than with portacaval shunt
(C) rebleeding occurs with the same frequency as with portacaval shunt

(D) five-year survival rate is similar to that following portacaval shunt
(E) coronary vein ligation is an integral part of the operation

784. Concerning sclerotherapy for bleeding varices all of the following statements are correct EXCEPT

(A) indicated in gastric varices
(B) indicated in esophageal varices
(C) may cause esophageal stricture
(D) multiple sessions may be required
(E) preferably performed in nonemergent situation

785. A 19-year-old man is transported to an emergency room after being involved in an automobile accident. Apparently he was driving the car and hit a telephone pole, sustaining a blunt injury to the anterior chest wall. A CT scan is obtained and is shown on page 219. Which of the following abnormalities is a sequela of the lesion depicted on the CT scan?

(A) pancreatic pseudocyst
(B) hemobilia
(C) splenic pseudocyst
(D) perinephric hematoma
(E) none of the above

Questions 786 and 787

A 20-year-old construction worker accidentally sustained blunt injury to his right temple. Soon after the injury he was dazed but was able to resume his work. Four hours later, when he returned home, his relatives noticed him to be slightly confused. Subsequently he became progressively lethargic and was brought to the emergency room. He was found to be very drowsy, responding to painful stimuli. His right pupil was dilated.

Figure for use with question 785.

786. The most useful diagnostic procedure in this patient is

(A) skull roentgenogram
(B) spinal tap
(C) ultrasonography
(D) electroencephalography
(E) CT scan

787. In the management of this patient all of the following maneuvers are beneficial EXCEPT

(A) deliberate hypocapnia (Pco_2 25 to 30 Torr)
(B) osmotic diuresis
(C) spinal tap
(D) intravenous barbiturates
(E) temporal craniotomy

Questions 788 through 791

A man is hospitalized for evaluation of abdominal pain. A flat-plate abdominal roentgenogram is obtained and shown on page 220.

788. The abnormality visualized on this roentgenogram is the result of

(A) excess bile salt
(B) excess cholesterol
(C) excess lecithin
(D) excess calcium
(E) a suppurative infection

Figure for use with questions 788 through 791.

789. The man whose roentgenogram is shown develops sudden, severe epigastric pain with nausea, vomiting, and diaphoresis. Laboratory testing shows leukocytosis and amylasemia. Poor prognostic features would include all of the following EXCEPT

(A) serum amylase concentration greater than 500 Somogyi units/dL

(B) serum calcium concentration less than 8 mg/dL

(C) serum glutamic oxaloacetic transaminase concentration greater than 250 sigma frankel units/dL

(D) P_{O_2} less than 60 mm Hg on arterial blood–gas determination

(E) a drop in hematocrit of more than 10 percent

790. Other complications of the lesion seen on the roentgenogram presented include all of the following EXCEPT

(A) acute cholangitis

(B) intestinal obstruction

(C) obstructive jaundice

(D) carcinoma of the liver

(E) hydrops of the gallbladder

791. The man described above is operated on. During the operation, the common bile duct is accidentally transected, involving the entire circumference at the level of cystic duct insertion. The most appropriate step for managing this complication would be

    (A) ligation of the proximal end so that the duct can dilate, which would facilitate a subsequent anastomosis

    (B) anastomosis of the proximal end to a Roux-en-Y limb of the jejunum

    (C) end-to-end anastomosis of the transected ends and drainage of the area with a rubber drain

    (D) end-to-end anastomosis of the transected ends over a T-tube

    (E) end-to-side choledochoduodenostomy

Questions 792 and 793

A 10-month-old baby is brought to the emergency room with 6-hour history of bilious vomiting, passage of pink jellylike material from the rectum, and intermittent episodes of severe crying. On physical examination a sausage-shaped mass is felt on the right side of the abdomen.

792. The most likely diagnosis is

    (A) congenital hypertrophic pyloric stenosis

    (B) intestinal volvulus

    (C) intussusception

    (D) necrotizing enterocolitis

    (E) acute pyelonephritis

793. The next step in the management of the patient is

    (A) administration of atropine

    (B) exploratory laparotomy

    (C) barium enema

    (D) administration of antibiotics

    (E) intravenous pyelography

Questions 794 and 795

A first-born male child develops projectile vomiting at the age of 5 weeks. Vomitus is free of bile. The child remains hungry and vomits after taking feedings. Examination reveals visible peristalsis in the upper abdomen along with a palpable nodule in the right upper quadrant.

794. The most likely diagnosis for the boy described above is

    (A) esophageal atresia

    (B) hypertrophic pyloric stenosis

    (C) duodenal web

    (D) midgut volvulus

    (E) incarcerated inguinal hernia

795. Treatment of choice for the condition described above is

    (A) Heller's myotomy

    (B) pyloromyotomy

    (C) gastrojejunostomy

    (D) duodenojejunostomy

    (E) esophageal dilation

Questions 796 through 798

A 40-year-old man who has had chronic duodenal ulcer disease comes to the emergency room because he has been vomiting for 5 days and cannot retain any food.

796. Metabolic derangements in the man described above would likely include all of the following EXCEPT

    (A) dehydration

    (B) azotemia

    (C) acidosis

    (D) hypernatremia

    (E) acid urine

797. The operation LEAST acceptable for the treatment of the condition described above is

(A) truncal vagotomy
(B) truncal vagotomy and pyloroplasty
(C) truncal vagotomy and gastrojejunostomy
(D) truncal vagotomy and antrectomy
(E) subtotal gastrectomy

798. Which of the following operative procedures for the management of chronic duodenal ulcer is associated with the *lowest* incidence of recurrent ulceration?

(A) bilateral truncal vagotomy and antrectomy
(B) bilateral truncal vagotomy and pyloroplasty
(C) bilateral truncal vagotomy and gastrojejunostomy
(D) bilateral truncal vagotomy and gastroduodenostomy
(E) proximal gastric vagotomy

799. A man known to have cirrhosis comes to the hospital because he has been vomiting blood. The diagnostic study most useful in identifying the source of bleeding is

(A) esophagogastroduodenoscopy
(B) upper gastrointestinal series
(C) splenoportography
(D) hepatic wedge-pressure measurement
(E) celiac angiography

Questions 800 through 802

A 22-year-old graduate student is brought by his family to the local emergency room. They say that ever since he returned home for a 3-week Christmas vacation he has been restless, irritable, and sleeping poorly. They have never seen him like this before, although it has been 8 months since he last was home. He refuses a physical examination and tells you in pressured speech, "I've never been better. Nobody understands the important work I'm engaged in right now. I have to leave—they'll find me here." He is fully conscious and alert.

800. On the basis of the information available, the LEAST likely diagnosis for the man described would be

(A) bipolar I disorder
(B) schizophrenia, paranoid type
(C) brief psychotic disorder
(D) cyclothymic disorder
(E) substance abuse

801. Which of the following organic disorders would be most likely to produce a clinical picture like the one described?

(A) Addison's disease
(B) Cushing's disease
(C) hypokalemia
(D) hypothyroidism
(E) multiple sclerosis

802. Appropriate laboratory tests performed for the man described show normal values. The medication most likely to be of *immediate* benefit would be

(A) lithium carbonate
(B) fluoxetine
(C) clomipramine
(D) valproate
(E) chlorpromazine

803. Sleep disruption is a common symptom of major depression. All the following polysomnographic findings would likely be found in a person with major depression EXCEPT

(A) altered REM architecture
(B) increased REM latency
(C) decreased stage 3 sleep
(D) decreased stage 4 sleep
(E) early-morning awakening

804. A psychiatric consultation is requested because a 23-year-old primiparous woman admitted last night for hyperemesis has in the past hour begun to display bizarre, catatonic-like behavior. Friends and family members say she has never acted like this before, although she has always been "high-strung" and has been in counseling for the past 6 months. Complete physical examination, including vital signs, shows no abnormalities. Findings from all admission laboratory tests are normal. The only medications she has received since admission have been acetaminophen for a headache last night and prochlorperazine 4 hours ago for nausea. On the basis of this information, the consultant should recommend a trial of which of the following medications?

(A) phenobarbital

(B) benztropine

(C) oxazepam

(D) haloperidol

(E) methylphenidate

Questions 805 and 806

A 62-year-old man has been treated for anxiety by his family physician for the past 10 years. At first he received diazepam, but for the past 3 years he has been taking thioridazine, 75 mg daily. In the past 6 months the man has begun to develop facial tics and darting tongue movements. His physician seeks a consultation.

805. The most likely explanation for the development of the man's symptoms is

(A) chronic thioridazine overdosage

(B) tolerance to thioridazine

(C) noncompliance with thioridazine therapy

(D) tardive dyskinesia

(E) early dementia

806. The man's physician should be advised to

(A) discontinue thioridazine

(B) increase the dosage of thioridazine

(C) add an anticonvulsant drug

(D) prescribe an anticholinergic drug

(E) seek a neurologic consultation

807. A 41-year-old man seeks psychiatric consultation because he has been unable to sleep well in the 4 weeks since his wife died in an automobile accident. His appetite is poor, and he has lost 2.3 kg (5 lb); in addition, he feels guilty about not having gone with his wife on the day of her death. He is not suicidal, though he questions his deeply held religious beliefs. He has returned to work, but only part-time. He reports that he cried quite a lot the first week after his wife's death and still cries now, though less often.

After his visit to the psychiatrist the man feels better. Two days later, however, he returns asking for medication to help him sleep. The best treatment at this point would consist of

(A) amitriptyline, 150 mg at bedtime

(B) phenelzine, 30 mg in the morning and 30 mg at bedtime

(C) diazepam, 10 mg every 6 hours

(D) oxazepam, 30 mg at bedtime

(E) hospitalization

808. A 31-year-old woman reports that for the past 3 weeks she has had occasional episodes of sudden and overwhelming anxiety. Between attacks she is nervous and worried about when the next attack will occur. She cannot recall a precipitating stress before the episodes, which do not seem to be associated with particular events or time of day. All the following could be recommended treatment for this woman's disorder EXCEPT

(A) alprazolam, 1 mg tid

(B) desipramine, 100 mg daily

(C) haloperidol, 2 mg daily

(D) relaxation therapy

(E) psychotherapy

809. Treatment with electroconvulsive therapy (ECT) would be most appropriate for which of the following individuals?

(A) a 68-year-old woman with medication-resistant psychotic depression

(B) a 47-year-old woman with medication-resistant delusional disorder

(C) a 38-year-old man with acute lithium-resistant mania

(D) a 28-year-old woman with severe catatonic schizophrenia

(E) a 21-year-old man in a hallucinogen-induced delirium

810. A 56-year-old man develops acute renal failure after surgery for ruptured aortic aneurysm. However, he refuses dialysis. His internist, who tries unsuccessfully to persuade him to accept treatment, seeks an immediate psychiatric consultation. Mental-status testing reveals the man to be fully alert and oriented, cognitively intact, and not psychotic. He says he is refusing dialysis because he has "lived a full life" and does not want to be "tied to a machine, even if this means I'll die." The man's family urgently wants him treated. The psychiatrist should tell the man's internist that the man

(A) is temporarily incompetent to decide on treatment, so treatment should be started

(B) is competent to decide on treatment, but his refusal should be overruled because of the existence of a medical emergency

(C) is competent to decide on treatment, so his refusal of dialysis must be respected

(D) is behaving in a self-destructive manner, so he should be committed for treatment against his will

(E) shows no evidence of a major psychiatric illness and is aware of the consequences of his decision

Questions 811 and 812

A 74-year-old woman, widowed last year, says she has "depression." For the past 3 months she has been increasingly weepy and has been sleeping more fitfully. Her appetite is reduced, and she has lost several pounds. A recent complete physical examination showed mild hypertension, for which she takes a diuretic, and osteoarthritis, for which she takes aspirin.

811. Which of the following mental status changes would be LEAST compatible with a diagnosis of major depression?

(A) agitation

(B) fluctuating state of consciousness

(C) poor short-term memory

(D) paranoid delusions

(E) refusal to cooperate

812. The woman described above is started on imipramine, at an initial daily dosage of 50 mg, raised to 100 mg, and then to 150 mg after 4 days. After initially reporting better sleep and perhaps a slightly less depressed mood, she reports 10 days later that she cannot sleep more than 2 hours per night and is now so "confused" she nearly missed the appointment "because I thought today was tomorrow!"

The best course of action now would be to

(A) stop the imipramine

(B) order an imipramine blood level and increase the dosage

(C) order an imipramine blood level and decrease the dosage

(D) prescribe a low dosage of haloperidol at bedtime

(E) schedule an emergency CT scan of the head

Questions 813 and 814

A 36-year-old computer salesman is brought into the local emergency room by ambulance. He is sweating, very anxious, and has a tremor of the hands and eyelids; his blood pressure and body temperature are mildly elevated, and his pulse is rapid. He has been vomiting, the last time producing blood-tinged vomitus. When questioned he says he is a heavy drinker but has not had a drink in 36 hours. He says he has never had delirium tremens, though he has had "blackouts."

813. All the following admission orders would be appropriate in the case described EXCEPT

(A) vital signs every hour

(B) liquid diet

(C) intramuscular thiamine, 100 mg

(D) oral chlordiazepoxide, 50 mg every 4 hours

(E) oral chlorpromazine, 100 mg as needed for severe agitation

814. In 2 days the man's vital signs have returned to normal, and all signs of alcohol withdrawal have disappeared. The man's physician should now

(A) discontinue all current medications and discharge the man from the hospital

(B) discontinue all current medications and observe

(C) discontinue all current medications and begin disulfiram

(D) taper medications over the next 5 days

(E) maintain the current regimen for 2 weeks

815. A 45-year-old woman is hospitalized for psychiatric treatment after 6 weeks of worsening insomnia, anorexia, and obsessive thoughts of worthlessness. She has had three hospitalizations in the past 12 years for similar illnesses and has been treated successfully with the tricyclic antidepressant drug imipramine on all three occasions. A work-up for organic disease is unrevealing, and imipramine therapy is begun, with the dosage reaching 150 mg daily after 3 days. Two weeks later she appears only minimally improved. The explanation LEAST likely to account for her lack of therapeutic response would be that

(A) the dosage is too low

(B) the dosage is too high

(C) she has not been swallowing her medication

(D) treatment is still in the "lag period" of therapeutic response

(E) she has become a nonresponder to imipramine

816. A 41-year-old depressed man has been treated for 6 weeks with therapeutic dosages of a tricyclic antidepressant drug. His psychiatrist has noted some clinical improvement but less than hoped. To potentiate the effect of the antidepressant, the psychiatrist could add which of the following preparations to the man's treatment regimen?

(A) lithium carbonate

(B) monoamine oxidase inhibitor

(C) thyroxine

(D) niacin

(E) amphetamine

817. Brief psychotherapy can be described by all the following statements EXCEPT

    (A) the setting of a strict time limit for treatment can itself be therapeutic
    (B) initially unmotivated persons often respond well to the short-term model
    (C) focus on a specific crisis facilitates short-term treatment
    (D) brief therapeutic interventions often lead to permanently better functioning
    (E) intrapsychic conflict often can be resolved in short-term treatment

DIRECTIONS (Questions 818 through 824): Each group of items in this section consists of lettered headings followed by a set of numbered words or phrases. For each numbered word or phrase, select the ONE lettered heading that is most closely associated with it. Each lettered heading may be selected once, more than once, or not at all.

Questions 818 through 824

For each clinical situation described below, select the most likely therapeutic drug of choice.

    (A) desipramine
    (B) methylphenidate
    (C) haloperidol
    (D) clomipramine
    (E) alprazolam

818. Childhood obsessive–compulsive disorder

819. Tourette's syndrome

820. Bulimia nervosa

821. Extremely aggressive behavior associated with conduct disorder or mental retardation

822. Enuresis

823. Attention-deficit hyperactivity disorder (first-line treatment)

824. Attention-deficit hyperactivity disorder (if first-line treatment cannot be used or has not been successful)

DIRECTIONS (Questions 825 through 835): Each of the numbered items or incomplete statements in this section is followed by answers or by completions of the statement. Select the ONE lettered answer or completion that is BEST in each case.

825. A definite association has been established between the development of cardiovascular abnormalities and exposure to

    (A) aromatic hydrocarbons
    (B) methanol
    (C) fluorocarbons
    (D) xylene
    (E) carbon tetrachloride

826. Which of the following statements about the epidemiology of poliomyelitis is true?

    (A) females are more frequently affected than males
    (B) most infected individuals produce recognizable symptoms
    (C) water supplies have conclusively been established as a source of infection
    (D) the most common mode of spread is by airborne infection
    (E) paralytic disease appears to be on the increase in certain parts of the world

827. A married man, aged 35, the father of three children, visits his physician stating that for the last 3 weeks he has felt increasingly tired, that he has a painless cough that is "like an ordinary cold," but it keeps him awake. On examination, he has a temperature of 37.2°C (99°F), the throat appears normal apart from a clear mucus droplet on the posterior wall of the oropharynx, and examination of the chest reveals no abnormality. Which of the following organisms may be responsible for the condition?

    (A) rhinovirus
    (B) coronavirus
    (C) parainfluenza
    (D) respiratory syncytial virus
    (E) *Mycoplasma pneumoniae*

828. In the above case, which of the following medications is likely to be most effective, assuming the patient does not have sensitivity to any?

(A) ascorbic acid

(B) phenylephrine nose drops

(C) amantadine

(D) vidarabine

(E) erythromycin

829. Tetanus toxoid has proved to be one of the most effective immunizing agents. Current indications for its use include all of the following EXCEPT

(A) routine immunization every 10 years

(B) a deep, dirty wound in a person who has had repeated immunizations

(C) a wound in a person with an uncertain history of immunization

(D) in combination with diphtheria toxin in pediatric practice

(E) a clean wound in a person whose last dose was less than 5 years ago

830. In the routine health care of children, a blood lead level should ideally be checked at

(A) 6 months to 1 year of age

(B) 1 to 2 years of age

(C) 2 to 5 years of age

(D) 5 to 11 years of age

(E) yearly intervals

831. Informed consent is now recognized as a very important component in the practice of medicine. Written consent is advisable in all of the following situations EXCEPT

(A) the physician records oral consent in the notes for a minor ambulatory surgical procedure

(B) the procedure is quite common (eg, sigmoidoscopy)

(C) the patient is a minor, there is an element of urgency, and the parents give permission by telephone

(D) the physician has a good relationship with the patient and the procedure is minor, carrying minimal risk

(E) the treatment clearly is minor, nonhazardous, and routine

832. Under certain circumstances, it may be legitimate to detain individuals in an institution against their wishes. This situation would arise for which of the following persons?

(A) a person who has bizarre fantasies and actions

(B) a person who is mentally incompetent and unable to manage personal affairs

(C) a person about whom a close relative has submitted a petition that the person is actually and presently insane

(D) a person whose continued liberty poses a danger

(E) a person who has visual and auditory hallucinations

833. The causative organism of cholera, *Vibrio cholerae*, has been recognized for 100 years. Outbreaks of cholera often reach epidemic proportions; the history of seven pandemics can now be traced. The most recent only now appears to be subsiding. The spread of infection, enhanced by modern transportation, is most likely by

(A) fomites

(B) mosquitoes

(C) infected food sources

(D) person-to-person transmission

(E) flies

834. Cytomegalovirus (CMV) infections have attracted increasing attention since their discovery in 1956. Prevalence rates are high throughout the world. Regarding infection with these viruses, which of the following statements is true?

 (A) a woman who sheds this virus from her cervix during pregnancy is likely to produce an infected baby

 (B) once a mother is affected, she is likely to infect future pregnancies

 (C) if virus affects the placenta, the fetus will also be affected

 (D) an infected infant who does not shed virus at the age of 6 months may be considered free of CMV

 (E) institutionalized children are more likely to excrete the virus and have antibodies in their serum

835. Which of the following statements correctly describes the administration of chelating agents, such as ethylenediaminetetraacetic acid (EDTA) and penicillamine, for the treatment of heavy metal poisoning?

 (A) it is advised for asymptomatic persons suspected of having ingested the toxin

 (B) it quickly counteracts the toxic effects of the metal poisoning

 (C) it should be reserved only for persons with symptomatic exposure

 (D) it reduces absorption of the metal from the gastrointestinal tract

 (E) it counteracts the effects of future exposure to the toxin

DIRECTIONS (Questions 836 through 849): Each group of items in this section consists of lettered headings followed by a set of numbered words or phrases. For each numbered word or phrase, select the ONE lettered heading that is most closely associated with it. Each lettered heading may be selected once, more than once, or not at all.

Questions 836 and 837

Several groups of organic compounds have recently been associated with serious toxic effects. For each of the following descriptions of occurrence and use of a substance, choose the group of compounds with which it is most closely associated.

 (A) nitrosamines
 (B) epoxy compounds
 (C) polychlorinated biphenyls
 (D) polybrominated biphenyls
 (E) organophosphorus compounds

836. Because they do not conduct electricity and can withstand high temperatures, they were used extensively in electrical transformers

837. Widely used as insecticides, they are responsible for more deaths on a worldwide basis than any other group of substances

Questions 838 through 849

One of the main aims of current preventive medicine is to identify those persons who are in high-risk categories for disease and to screen them regularly and appropriately. This is frequently more cost-effective than indiscriminate screening of large populations. For each of the high-risk categories of adults aged 40 to 64 listed below, identify the specific screening procedure, listed A through L, which should be performed for a related condition.

- (A) fasting blood glucose
- (B) VDRL and gonorrhea testing
- (C) urinalysis for bacteriuria
- (D) chlamydial testing
- (E) gonorrhea testing
- (F) tuberculin skin test
- (G) electrocardiogram (ECG)
- (H) sigmoidoscopy
- (I) colonoscopy
- (J) hepatitis B vaccine
- (K) pneumococcal and influenza vaccine
- (L) influenza vaccine annually

838. Homosexually active men

839. The markedly obese

840. Prostitutes

841. Those with multiple sexual partners

842. Stable diabetic individuals

843. Recent immigrants or refugees

844. Men with two or more cardiac risk factors

845. Residents of chronic care facilities

846. Persons with chronic pulmonary disease

847. Persons aged 50 and over who have a personal history of endometrial, ovarian, or breast cancer

848. Persons with a family history of polyposis coli

849. Persons who attend clinics for the treatment of sexually transmitted disease

ANSWERS AND EXPLANATIONS

700–702. (700-A, 701-A, 702-C) Evidence of ovulation is provided indirectly from the 0.4 to 0.6°F rise in temperature secondary to progesterone secretion and its thermogenic effect. The maximum secretion of progesterone will occur in the second half of the cycle, and LH surges at midcycle just before ovulation. From the time of ovulation until the next menses is usually fairly constant at 14 days in fertile women. FSH peaks just before ovulation.

Luteal phase defect demonstrates itself as a decreased length of the luteal phase or decreased levels of progesterone in the serum during the luteal phase. Accepted as a cause of infertility and habitual abortion, this diagnosis is confirmed by luteal phase endometrial biopsy showing a developmental lag of more than 2 days when compared with the menstrual calendar.

This condition has been treated with clomiphene citrate, human menopausal gonadotropins, and exogenous progesterone with varying rates of success. *(Gant, pp 186–187; DeCherney, pp 1000–1001)*

703–707. (703-E, 704-B, 705-A, 706-B, 707-C) The most commonly seen anemia in pregnancy is a physiologic anemia secondary to an increase in plasma volume proportionately greater than the concomitant increase in red blood cell mass. This can usually be averted by providing adequate intake of oral iron (dietary or supplemental) from early on in pregnancy. Iron-deficiency anemia seldom affects the fetus, even in severe cases, and is neither genetic nor difficult to treat.

The diagnosis is confirmed by a low hematocrit, a hypochromic and microcytic peripheral blood smear, decreased serum iron concentrations, abnormal red cell indices, and normal iron-binding capacity. The earliest sign of therapeutic success is the appearance of reticulocytosis on the peripheral smear. *(Gant, pp 444–445; Cunningham, pp 1172–1173)*

708–712. (708-C, 709-C, 710-E, 711-C, 712-E) Although many women who have urinary symptoms may not be infected, there are probably a greater number of asymptomatic yet infected patients. The 100 000 colonies of bacteria per milliliter was a standard developed nearly 30 years ago and is clearly not the best diagnostic standard for the pregnant patient. More sophisticated diagnostic techniques are either too invasive or cumbersome or expensive for routine use.

Regarding the prevention and therapy of urinary tract infection in pregnancy, the primary goal is to prevent pyelonephritis and preterm birth associated with perinatal maternal infections. Patients with urinary tract abnormalities or a history of previous infections when not pregnant are even more at risk than other gravidas. Patients with pyelonephritis should be hospitalized for intravenous therapy. Recurrent infection is probably best treated with antibiotic prophylaxis during pregnancy and further evaluation can be performed postpartum. The simple lower urinary tract infection can be treated with any of a number of antibiotics depending on sensitivity studies. The most common causative organism is *Escherichia coli*. *(Cunningham, pp 1128–1132)*

713–719. (713-A, 714-C, 715-A, 716-C, 717-B, 718-A, 719-C) Toxic shock syndrome is associated with all the clinical features of circulatory shock plus muscle damage and neurologic symptoms. *Staphylococcus aureus* is the most commonly associated organism, but the disease itself is caused by the endotoxin and, therefore, not amenable to therapy with antibiotics. The mainstay of therapy is massive fluid replacement. The diagnosis is made from the multisystem involvement in combination with the diffuse red maculopapular rash associated with desquamation of the palms and soles in the convalescent pe-

riod. The use of tampons predisposes to both the initial episode and to reinfections. *(DeCherney, pp 780–782)*

720–723. (720-B, 721-E, 722-D, 723-E) Preeclampsia is associated with maternal hypertension, decreased plasma volume, and therefore, a falsely elevated hematocrit. It is also strongly associated with abruption of the placenta. Painful third trimester bleeding is the key to diagnosis here. Red cell destruction (microangiopathic hemolytic anemia) is also taking place, elevating uric acid and consuming platelets. In its most severe forms, this disease may be accompanied by disseminated intravascular coagulation with consumption of coagulation factors, elevation of clotting times, increased levels of fibrin split products, and decreased levels of coagulation associated proteins.

Blood may accumulate behind the placenta (concealed hemorrhage) and cause violent labor or persistent hypertonus. Despite this fact, atony is also possible. When the "cure" becomes delivery, in the absence of fetal distress, there is no contraindication to stimulation of labor. *(Gant, pp 433–434)*

724–726. (724-D, 725-C, 726-A) The most common causes of bacterial meningitis during the neonatal period are organisms that are found in the mother's vaginal flora, most specifically group B *Streptococcus, Escherichia coli* and other gram-negative enteric bacilli, and *Listeria monocytogenes*. In the child beyond the first 1 or 2 months of life, the most common organisms are *Haemophilus influenzae, Streptococcus pneumoniae*, and *Neisseria meningitidis*.

There are several combinations of antibiotics that will effectively and safely provide coverage for the neonatal group of organisms. This includes ampicillin and an aminoglycoside or ampicillin and cefotaxime. The ampicillin not only broadens the gram-negative coverage, but also provides coverage for *L. monocytogenes,* which generally is not sensitive to either aminoglycosides or cephalosporins. Complications of meningitis are numerous and common. In most series, hearing loss has been the most common permanent sequela. Other complications include visual impairment, seizures, and mental retardation. Brain abscess is rare. Hemiparesis is occasionally seen as a complication of bacterial meningitis, but quadriplegia usually results from a spinal cord lesion and would be extremely unlikely as a sequela of meningitis. Kernicterus is a complication of neonatal hyperbilirubinemia and is not related to meningitis. (*Rudolph et al, pp 536–544*)

727–728.   (727-B, 728-B)   A 3-day history of worsening cough and the development of fever and mild inspiratory stridor are consistent with a diagnosis of infectious laryngotracheitis, which usually is caused by parainfluenza virus. Chest x-ray typically reveals subglottic swelling. In the differential diagnosis, epiglottitis typically develops more acutely, with affected children having severe stridor on the first day of the illness. Although spasmodic croup is quite similar to infectious laryngotracheitis, it is not associated with fever. The roentgenographic findings and history presented in the case are not consistent with a diagnosis of either angioneurotic edema or aspiration of a foreign body.

A variety of measures have been used in the treatment of viral laryngotracheitis. Cool mist has been used for decades and is assumed to be helpful. Racemic epinephrine by either aerosol or intermittent positive-pressure breathing has been shown to provide symptomatic relief, presumably by vasoconstriction and reduction of local edema. Corticosteroids are used frequently and there is some data to support this, although the use of these agents remains controversial. Theophylline is useful in treating bronchospasm but is of no value in the treatment of croup. (*Rudolph et al, pp 674–676*)

729–731.   (729-E, 730-B, 731-C)   Toxic shock syndrome, recognized only in the last decade, requires prompt diagnosis and treatment. The syndrome usually occurs in women using highly absorbent tampons. Typical historical and physical findings include sudden onset of fever and gastrointestinal symptoms, abdominal pain and myalgias, tachycardia, hypotension, hyperemia, and generalized erythematous maculopapular rash that spares the wrists. *Staphylococcus aureus* usually can be grown from blood or vaginal cultures. Treatment of choice is with the antibiotics oxacillin or nafcillin.

Scarlet fever and Kawasaki's disease resemble toxic shock syndrome, but they are not typically associated with watery diarrhea, myalgias, or abdominal pain. Acute onset of symptoms and the presence of a rash and conjunctival erythema make ruptured appendix an unlikely diagnosis. The rash of Rocky Mountain spotted fever typically begins on the extremities (especially the wrists) and spreads to the trunk. (*Feigin and Cherry, pp 1277–1295*)

732–733.   (732-A, 733-B)   The child in question presents signs of isosexual precocious development. The fact that the testes are large rather than small indicates that the problem is of central origin with the precocious release of gonadotropins. If the problem were due to androgen-secreting tumor or some other ectopic source of androgenic hormones, such as untreated congenital adrenal hyperplasia, one would expect the central release of gonadotropins to be shut off and the testes, therefore, small. Although most cases of isosexual precocious puberty in girls are idiopathic, this is not the case in boys, in whom a hypothalamic tumor can be found in an appreciable percentage of cases.

Klinefelter's syndrome (XXY) is a common cause of primary hypogonadism rather than precocious puberty. The XYY syndrome occurs in about 1 in 1000 male births and is associated with tall stature and acne. Precocious puberty, however, is not a feature of this syndrome and, indeed, a few of the patients have presented with undescended testes, or hypogonadism, or both. (*Rudolph et al, pp 1795–1799*)

734–737.   (734-C, 735-D, 736-D, 737-C)   Evaluation of a child having a generalized convulsion requires great care. The most frequent cause of a short generalized tonic–clonic seizure is simple febrile seizure. It is important to rule out the possibility of meningitis, which can present with seizures along with the more common signs of acute illness and irritability. Idiopathic epilepsy usually occurs in children older than 5 years of age. Short, generalized convulsions are not typical of complex febrile seizures. The presence of bruises below the knees is common in children and, especially in a child with signs and symptoms of a febrile illness, need not suggest the possibility of child abuse.

Although the use of lumbar puncture in diagnosing a simple febrile seizure is controversial, it is essential so that a diagnosis of meningitis can be ruled out. (Fontanel size is difficult to assess, and neck examination may not be a reliable guide in diagnosing meningitis.) Blood count and serum electrolytes and blood glucose levels may be helpful, but they are not essential. Electroencephalography would only confirm the occurrence of a seizure and would not clarify the patient's status or diagnosis. A CT scan of the head would not be indicated in the case presented.

Present recommendations for the treatment of febrile seizures include the use of antipyretics during febrile illnesses. Phenobarbital should not be used to treat children having a first simple febrile seizure. Prognosis is usually excellent; rarely does a seizure disorder later develop. (*Rudolph et al, pp 1965–1967*)

738–740. (738-E, 739-E, 740-A) Strawberry hemangiomas arise when vascular tissue fails to communicate with adjoining vascular elements. This tissue enlarges and creates the typical appearance of a raised erythematous tumor. Strawberry hemangiomas develop after birth and have a relatively benign course if left alone. They enlarge through the first year of life, then slowly regress in size. By the time affected children are 9 years old, 90% of strawberry hemangiomas have undergone complete resolution. If a hemangioma is impinging on a vital structure, argon laser therapy may be needed. However, any intervention should be avoided if at all possible.

Nevus flammeus is a flat, vascular rash

that is also called a "stork bite." Cavernous hemangiomas involve deeper tissue layers than do strawberry hemangiomas and do not have a raised red appearance. Osteochondromas may be raised tumors, but they tend to have the color of the surrounding skin. (*Rudolph et al, pp 917–919*)

741–743. (741-E, 742-B, 743-C) Tinea capitis is a common fungal infection in prepubertal children. It typically is a well-circumscribed rash with scaly raised borders. The hair shafts may be irregularly broken. This lesion may develop an inflammatory appearance and become a kerion, which is a raised tumor that is boggy and indurated. The treatment of choice is griseofulvin. Systemic steroids are sometimes needed if the lesion does not resolve.

Seborrheic dermatitis and impetigo should be considered in the differential diagnosis of kerion, although they do not attain such a large size. Herpetic lesions are vesicular but also do not reach the size or have the appearance of a kerion. Alopecia areata, the loss of hair in sharply demarcated circular or oval patches, should not be confused with tinea capitus and kerion. (*Rudolph et al, pp 933–934*)

744–746. (744-B, 745-B, 746-C) The boy presented in the question has the typical electrocardiographic findings of Wolff–Parkinson–White syndrome. Wolff–Parkinson–White syndrome is due to muscular connections between the atrium and ventricle. Electrical impulses can travel through these connections instead of through the atrioventricular node. Lead III reveals a short interval and a slow upstroke of the QRS wave (a delta wave). Abrupt episodes of palpitations with no symptoms between episodes are typical of this syndrome. Affected persons develop supraventricular tachycardia because of a re-entry mechanism. This tachycardia, which is intermittent, usually can be prevented by administration of digoxin. Unresponsive cases may require radiofrequency ablation of aberrant pathways.

Lown–Ganong–Levine syndrome is similar to Wolff–Parkinson–White syndrome but the PR interval is not shortened. There is no evidence of sinus or nodal tachycardia, ventricular fibrillation, or wandering pacemaker. (*Rudolph et al, pp 1452–1453*)

747–749. (747-A, 748-D, 749-A) The child with sickle cell disease described in the question is having a vasoocclusive crisis. This is a painful condition caused by bone ischemia, resulting from diminished blood flow secondary to intravascular sickling of red blood cells. Appropriate therapy includes generous hydration to reduce blood viscosity and sickling. Intravenous fluids are helpful, but there is no reason to restrict oral intake of fluid or a regular diet. Because the kidneys of these patients tend to have an impaired concentrating ability, fluid maintenance generally should be estimated at one and a half to twice the usual volume. Because the patient described is afebrile and without signs of localized infection, such as osteomyelitis, intravenous antibiotics are not required. Blood transfusion is not used routinely in the initial management of vasoocclusive crises. Patients with sickle cell disease ordinarily have hemoglobin levels of 7 to 8 g/dL. Although addiction to narcotics is a concern in patients with sickle cell disease, adequate pain medication is an important part of therapy. Attempts to withhold medication or undermedicate the patient often result in apprehension and an increased need for such medication.

Other complications of sickle cell disease include aplastic anemia, sequestration crisis (the accumulation of a large volume of blood in the spleen, which can lead to peripheral hypovolemia), and hand–foot syndrome, probably as a result of infarction of the small bones of the hands and the feet and characterized by pain and swelling. Although pulmonary function may be impaired in sickle cell disease, pulmonary edema is not a recognized complication in children. Bacteremia is a potentially life-threatening complication. Children with sickle cell disease have impaired resistance to encapsulated organisms, specifically *Streptococcus pneumoniae*, *Haemophilus influenzae*, and *Salmonella*. (*Rudolph et al, pp 1203–1207*)

750–751. (750-E, 751-C) Transient cerebral ischemic attacks typically last from a few seconds up to 5 to 6 minutes. In the carotid system, the ocular disturbance is ipsilateral and the sensorimotor disturbance is contralateral. Unlike an epileptic seizure or an Adams–Stokes attack, consciousness is maintained. Migraine is an unlikely diagnosis in the case described, because it usually develops earlier in life and the ocular disturbance is bilateral. Treatment for transient cerebral ischemic attacks include antiplatelet drugs, anticoagulants, or surgical endarterectomy. (*Isselbacher, pp 2228–2244*)

752–753. (752-B, 753-A) Ankylosing spondylitis should be suspected in any man younger than 40 years of age who has had an insidious onset of low back pain that has persisted for at least 3 months, is associated with morning stiffness, and eases with exercise. The diagnosis is established by the finding of symmetrical sacroiliitis on roentgenogram. Spinal complications include vertebral fracture, resulting from rigidity of the spine, and the cauda equina syndrome. Systemic complications of ankylosing spondylitis include cardiac conduction defects, iritis, aortitis with aortic insufficiency, and apical pulmonary fibrosis with cavities resembling tuberculous lesions. Nearly all white patients with ankylosing spondylitis, but only half of all black patients, are HLA-B27 positive. Therapy consists of nonsteroidal antiinflammatory drugs and physical therapy. (*Isselbacher, pp 1664–1667*)

754–755. (754-D, 755-B) The presence of chronic sinusitis, otitis media, cavitating pulmonary lesions, and renal disease suggests a diagnosis of Wegener's granulomatosis. Polyarteritis and sarcoidosis are not associated with pulmonary cavities. Pulmonary abscess and tuberculosis are unlikely in the case described because of the patient's other symptoms and lack of sputum pathology. The use of cytotoxic drugs, such as cyclophosphamide, has greatly improved the prognosis of persons with Wegener's granulomatosis. The vast majority of patients go into long-term remission when treated with these drugs. Treatment should be carried on for a year after remission begins. *(Isselbacher, pp 1674–1676)*

756. **(D)** It has been shown that cimetidine decreases the clearance of theophylline, thereby elevating theophylline blood levels. Theophylline blood levels above 20 µg/mL often are associated with nausea. If cimetidine is to be prescribed for persons also requiring a theophylline preparation, the dose of theophylline should be reduced. *(Isselbacher, p 402)*

757–758. **(757-A, 758-C)** The man described in the question has idiopathic calcium oxalate nephrolithiasis. He formed stones despite maintaining a high fluid intake and avoiding dairy products. Thiazide treatment, the next logical step in therapy, decreases the frequency of stone formation in a significant percentage of patients. Unfortunately, the patient presented continued to form kidney stones. Administration of orthophosphate as the neutral salt has been shown to be effective in preventing recurrent stone formation in patients who do not respond to thiazide therapy. Allopurinol is not likely to help in the absence of uricosuria. Cellulose phosphate is a treatment for absorptive hypercalcemia. Surgery would not be indicated in the case described. *(Isselbacher, pp 1329–1333)*

759–760. **(759-E, 760-A)** In the case described the diagnosis of penicillin-induced interstitial nephritis is supported by the presence of skin rash, eosinophilia, proteinuria of less than 1 g/24 h, and the absence of casts in the urine. The onset of renal disease in poststreptococcal glomerulonephritis typically occurs 1 to 3 weeks after infection of skin or pharynx with a nephritogenic strain of *Streptococcus*. The treatment of choice is to stop the penicillin and, when necessary, start temporary dialysis. A short course of corticosteroids in high doses has been used in patients who have significant systemic symptoms. The prognosis for recovery is excellent. *(Isselbacher, pp 410, 1269)*

761. **(B)** In the question, the boy with bronchial asthma has developed pneumomediastinum and subcutaneous emphysema, two conditions that rarely require therapy. The use of intermittent positive-pressure breathing or positive end-expiratory pressure therapy is contraindicated in the presence of pneumomediastinum. Bronchoscopy is contraindicated in the presence of severe wheezing. Aminophylline should be administered to the boy described as primary treatment of the asthma. *(Isselbacher, p 1233)*

762–763. **(762-E, 763-A)** The most likely diagnosis in the case described is sarcoidosis. Erythema nodosum would be an unusual manifestation of Hodgkin's disease and malignant lymphoma. Because the woman is otherwise asymptomatic, coccidioidomycosis is unlikely, and the presence of hilar adenopathy would help to rule out a diagnosis of herpes simplex infection. Eighty percent of patients who present with the stage of sarcoidosis described in the question show regression of lung disease within 2 years; thus, no specific therapy is needed. Common indications for corticosteroid therapy include progressive pulmonary involvement, ocular involvement, involvement of the central nervous system, and persistent hypercalcemia. The other therapies listed in the question are not used to treat sarcoidosis. *(Isselbacher, pp 1679–1684)*

764–766. **(764-B, 765-D, 766-D)** Persons who have rheumatoid arthritis frequently seek initial medical attention because of symmetrical polyarthritis involving the hands, wrists, and feet. Morning stiffness lasting at least an hour also is common. Rheumatoid nodules are seen in 20% of affected persons and are located most commonly over the exterior surfaces of the elbows. Unlike rheumatoid arthritis, osteoarthritis usually involves the distal interphalangeal joints of the hands. Reiter's syndrome and systemic lupus erythematosus are associated with other symptoms in addition to rheumatologic ones, and gout is rare in women. Laboratory findings indicative of rheumatoid arthritis include normocytic, normochromic anemia; elevated sedimentation rate; and positive latex-fixation test for rheumatoid factor. Antinuclear antibodies are present in 20 to 60% of patients, but anti-DNA antibodies are not produced. The best initial therapy for most patients is aspirin or a nonsteroidal anti-inflammatory agent, plus a judicious combination of exercise and rest. *(Isselbacher, pp 1648–1655)*

767. **(C)** The National Cholesterol Education Program recommended that all cholesterol levels exceeding 240 mg/dL are high and require further evaluation by obtaining a lipid profile, consisting of cholesterol, triglycerides, and HDL cholesterol, after a 12-hour fast. Because recent food intake has little impact on the cholesterol level, the screening test need not be done in the fasting state. It would be inappropriate to initiate any form of treatment before determining the LDL cholesterol level as this patient's high cholesterol could be due to an elevated HDL cholesterol and not a high LDL cholesterol. Lipoprotein electrophoresis is rarely indicated, certainly not in a patient with normal triglyceride levels. *(Report of the National Cholesterol Education Program Expert Panel on Detection, Evaluation, and Treatment of High Blood Cholesterol in Adults)*

768. **(B)** Although there may be other good reasons to limit alcohol intake, it need not be severely restricted in patients with an elevated cholesterol unless they also have high triglycerides. Weight loss will often, but not always, lower cholesterol levels in obese patients. Weight reduction is always worthwhile in obese individuals because of its other health benefits. Water-soluble fiber does lower LDL cholesterol levels. The Step 1 diet of the National Cholesterol Education Program includes restrictions of dietary total fat to <30% of calories, saturated fat to <10% of calories, and cholesterol to 300 mg/day. If needed, the Step 2 diet further limits saturated fats to <7% of calories and cholesterol to 200 mg/day. *(Isselbacher, pp 1100–1113)*

769. **(D)** The National Cholesterol Education Program recommended that decisions on drug treatment be based on the LDL choles-

terol level. Medications are indicated for high-risk patients when their LDL cholesterol exceeds 160 mg/dL. This patient is at high risk because of his prior myocardial infarction. In general, dietary measures should be continued for at least 6 months before considering the use of any medications. Because of the modest elevation in cholesterol levels in this patient, there is a good chance that his LDL level can be lowered adequately with appropriate dietary measures. In patients with extremely high cholesterol levels, medications may be started earlier in the course of dietary treatment as it would be highly unlikely that diet alone would lower the LDL cholesterol to an acceptable range. Drugs are recommended in low-risk patients when the LDL cholesterol is greater than 190 mg/dL after a 6-month dietary regimen. *(Isselbacher, pp 1100–1113)*

770–772. **(770-A, 771-E, 772-A)** The gonococcal arthritis–dermatitis syndrome is the most common form of acute arthritis in sexually active adults. The combination of vesiculopapular skin eruptions on an erythematous base and an acute arthritis that is migratory, is associated with significant tenosynovitis, and changes from polyarticular in small joints to monoarticular should suggest this diagnosis.

In persons with gonococcal arthritis-dermatitis syndrome, cultures of the synovial fluid frequently show no growth, even when gonococci are cultured from other sites. Recommended treatment is intravenous ceftriaxone 1 g daily, until clinical improvement is seen, followed by oral ciprofloxacin 500 mg twice a day, cefuroxime axetil 500 mg twice a day, or amoxicillin 500 mg with clavulanic acid 125 mg three times a day, to complete a 7-day to 10-day course of antibiotic therapy.

Reiter's syndrome, which usually affects men, is associated with arthritis, conjunctivitis or uveitis, and mucosal lesions. Rheumatoid arthritis and systemic lupus erythematosus do not usually produce the type of skin eruption associated with gonococcal arthritis-dermatitis syndrome. Persons with meningococcemia are usually febrile. *(Isselbacher, pp 554–558)*

773–774. (773-A, 774-E) Pheochromocytomas are catecholamine-producing tumors that are usually benign. Hypertension is the most common clinical sign in patients with pheochromocytoma. Sustained hypertension is present in 60% of patients, and paroxysms, which occur in more than 50% of patients, consist of headaches, sweating, palpitations, and a sense of impending doom. Other clinical signs include postural hypotension and tachycardia. Elevated urine levels of vanillylmandelic acid (VMA), catecholamine, and metanephrine are diagnostic of pheochromocytoma. Phenoxybenzamine, an alpha-adrenergic antagonist, is most effective in controlling blood pressure. Subsequently, beta-blocking drugs may be added to control tachycardia or arrhythmias. Preoperative volume expansion with a high-sodium diet is also beneficial. After adequate preparation, surgical removal of the tumor should be undertaken; careful monitoring is crucial because of the danger of arrhythmias, hypertensive crisis during removal of the tumor, and severe hypotension after removal is accomplished. *(Isselbacher, pp 1976–1979)*

775–778. (775-A, 776-A, 777-C, 778-E) Acute mesenteric ischemia is increasing in frequency. The causes of acute mesenteric ischemia include superior mesenteric artery (SMA) thrombosis and embolism, superior mesenteric venous thrombosis, low-flow syndrome, and dissecting aneurysm of the aorta when the mesenteric arterial lumen is occluded. SMA embolism manifests as sudden onset of pain with minimal or no abdominal findings in the early stages. Embolism should be suspected in patients with atrial fibrillation and recent myocardial infarction who suddenly develop abdominal pain. Occlusion of SMA results in ischemia of the bowel. The resultant anaerobic metabolism leads to an accumulation of lactic acid and metabolic acidosis. Clinical exam is often not as helpful since patient's pain is often more severe than suggested by the clinical findings. Mesenteric angiography is the diagnostic procedure of choice. This procedure can confirm the diagnosis and provides information concerning the level of occlusion, associated vasospasm, and the extent of collateral circulation. Plain roentgenograms of the abdomen in early stages show nondiagnostic features and in late stages may demonstrate air in bowel wall and in the liver. Blood gas determination shows metabolic acidosis that is not pathognomonic of the condition. SMA occlusion decreases intestinal blood flow by mechanical obstruction and by inducing vasoconstriction. Unless diagnosed early and treated promptly the prognosis is poor. One should not wait for definite peritoneal signs to develop. Peritoneal signs are an indication of necrosis, which is an advanced stage of the condition. Heparin is administered to prevent propagation of the thrombus and further occlusion of the collateral vessels; papavarin is administered to overcome vasospasm and improve blood flow, analgesics to relieve pain, and antibiotics to counteract colonization of ischemic bowel by bacteria. *(Hardy, pp 912–916)*

779. (D) The incidence of breast cancer is higher in women who have a family history of breast carcinoma or who have had breast carcinoma in the past. Early pregnancy and castration before the age of 35 years decrease the risk of breast cancer. Infertile women are at a greater risk of developing breast carcinoma than are fertile women. *(Sabiston, pp 541–544)*

780. (B) Mammographic examination is a useful method of breast examination for detecting early lesions. A mass containing microcalcification and having irregular borders is likely to be malignant. Skin thickening over the mass and duct or vessel dilatation also are suggestive features of malignancy. Benign lesions are characterized by sharp, well-circumscribed margins and homogeneous density. *(Sabiston, p 536)*

781. (E) This is the initial methodology preferred by most physicians. Control of variceal bleeding is crucial in allowing complete evaluation of a patient and beginning preparation for definitive treatment. Systemic intravenous infusion of vasopressin is an effective method of controlling variceal hemorrhage. It is as effective as intraarterial vasopressin infusion into the superior mesenteric artery and is associated with fewer complications. Systemic intravenous somatostatin has also proven efficacious in treating variceal hemorrhage with fewer cardiovascular side effects when compared to vasopressin. Gastric hypothermia is not readily available and has not been demonstrated to be superior to vasopressin treatment. Esophageal tamponade is effective in controlling bleeding but is associated with serious complications, such as rupture of the esophagus. *(Sabiston, pp 1101–1103; Greenfield, pp 1048–1049)*

782. **(A)** Portacaval shunt effectively decompresses the portal system. It is associated with a low rate of recurrent variceal bleeding but a high incidence of encephalopathy. The other procedures listed in the question do not decompress the portal bed as effectively as portacaval shunt and have a higher incidence of recurrent bleeding; however, they are associated with a lower incidence of encephalopathy. *(Sabiston, pp 1103–1112)*

783. **(C)** Distal splenorenal shunt (Warren shunt) was devised to selectively decompress esophageal varices without decreasing portal blood flow. The procedure does not decrease portal pressure. It is associated with a lower incidence of encephalopathy and a higher incidence of recurrent bleeding compared to portacaval shunt. Coronary and left gastroepiploic veins are transected after ligation to isolate varices from the rest of the portal bed. *(Sabiston, pp 1106–1110)*

784. **(A)** Sclerotherapy has become popular in controlling bleeding from esophageal varices because of low mortality and efficacy approaching that of operative treatment in stopping the bleeding. The procedure is contraindicated in gastric varices as they are difficult to tamponade and bleeding from the needle puncture site is a problem. Multiple sessions are required to obliterate the varices. Complications include esophageal ulceration, localized perforation, mediastinitis, pulmonary ef-

fusion, sepsis, and stricture. *(Sabiston, pp 1110–1111)*

785. **(B)** Complications for liver laceration include hemorrhage, abscess formation, and hemobilia, which is bleeding into biliary passages. Communication between branches of the hepatic artery and biliary ducts results in hemobilia, which typically produces colicky abdominal pain and upper and lower gastrointestinal tract bleeding. Treatment consists of occluding the communicating vessel. *(Schwartz and Shires, p 323; Feliciano, pp 510–515)*

786–787. **(786-E, 787-C)** A complication of head injury is intracranial bleeding, which may be epidural, subdural, or intracerebral in location. Arterial epidural hematoma is frequently the result of a middle meningeal tear. The typical presentation of epidural hemorrhage includes momentary loss of consciousness, followed by a lucid interval, terminating in loss of consciousness. Ipsilateral pupillary dilatation with contralateral hemiparesis may be seen. CT scan demonstrates skull fracture, localizes the mass, and demonstrates brain displacement and concomitant cerebral injury.

Resuscitative measures include osmotic diuresis and deliberate hypocapnia to decrease intracranial tension. Barbiturates decrease cerebral metabolism and cerebral blood flow. Spinal tap, which can precipitate herniation of brain, is contraindicated. Temporal craniotomy, which allows decompression of the brain and permits control of bleeding, is the treatment of choice. When performed early, the results are excellent. *(Schwartz et al, pp 1833–1835; Feliciano, pp 267–278)*

788. **(B)** The radiographic abnormality seen in the roentgenogram presented is gallstones. Cholesterol, which is insoluble in water, becomes soluble in lecithin-bile salt micelles. However, when cholesterol saturation exceeds the limits of micellar ability to keep cholesterol in solution, stone formation takes place. Excess secretion of cholesterol into bile as well as decreased secretion of bile salts and lecithin can cause cholesterol gallstone formation. *(Schwartz et al, pp 1376–1383)*

789. (A) Assessing the severity of acute pancreatitis can be difficult. Hypocalcemia, elevated SGOT concentration, a drop in hematocrit, and hypoxia are indicative of poor prognosis, especially if three or more of these findings are present simultaneously. Serum amylase level does not correlate with the severity of the disease. *(Greenfield, pp 791–804)*

790. (D) Biliary calculi can cause acute cholecystitis, hydrops of the gallbladder, intestinal obstruction (gallstone ileus), and obstructive jaundice (from choledocholithiasis). There are data to imply that the incidence of gallbladder carcinoma is increased by the presence of gallstones. No evidence indicates that gallstones cause carcinoma of the liver. *(Schwartz et al, pp 1380–1383)*

791. (D) The appropriate step for correcting common duct injury recognized at operation depends on the site of injury and the extent of loss of the duct. If the injury is at the level of cystic duct insertion and has not caused loss of duct substance, end-to-end anastomosis with T-tube decompression of the bile duct is the preferred procedure. The T-tube is used to prevent bile leakage and subsequent fibrosis. If the duct is injured close to the duodenum, end-to-side choledochoduodenostomy is preferred. If the proximal duct is injured or if the length of a lost segment of duct is greater than 1 cm, a Roux-en-Y procedure (anastomosis of the distal end of the divided jejunum to the duct and implantation of the proximal end into the side of the jejunum) is recommended. Ligation of the proximal duct should be avoided except when the duct is so small that a primary repair is not possible. Ligation allows the duct to dilate, facilitating subsequent repair. *(Hardy, pp 689–690)*

792–793. (792-C, 793-C) Intussusception frequently affects children between 5 and 12 months. The usual presenting features consist of a triad of abdominal pain, vomiting, and passage of "red currant jelly" stools. In between the episodes of abdominal pain the child will remain symptom-free. The intussuscepted segment of the bowel may be felt as a sausage-shaped mass when the abdominal muscle is relaxed and the mass is not under the cover of the liver. Barium enema establishes the diagnosis and is helpful in reducing the intussusception. Contraindications for barium enema include signs of peritoneal irritation, duration of symptoms longer than 24 hours, and features of bowel obstruction on plain roentgenograms. *(Sabiston, pp 1282–1284)*

794. (B) Congenital hypertrophic pyloric stenosis is not an infrequent condition. It has a predilection for male infants, and peak incidence is at 4 to 6 weeks of life. The etiology is unknown. Presenting features include projectile vomiting of nonbilious material, visible peristalsis in the upper abdomen, and presence of a palpable mass (an "olive") in the right upper quadrant. *(Hardy, pp 1140–1141)*

795. (B) Treatment of choice for hypertrophic pyloric stenosis is pyloromyotomy. Before surgery, fluid and electrolyte imbalances must be corrected. Prognosis is excellent. *(Hardy, p 1140–1141)*

796. (C) In the case described, the man has lost water, hydrogen ion, chloride, and potassium. Bicarbonate, a by-product of gastric acid secretion, accumulates and causes metabolic alkalosis. Renal compensation—excretion of bicarbonate as sodium bicarbonate—is affected by the potassium deficit, which limits sodium–potassium exchange. In order to conserve potassium, the kidneys exchange sodium with hydrogen, resulting in paradoxic aciduria. Azotemia is the result of dehydration. *(Schwartz, p 71)*

797. (A) Many operative procedures are available for treating chronic duodenal ulcer. Vagotomy produces gastric stasis. Thus, unless a superselective vagotomy is performed (in which the branches of the vagus to the body and the fundus are transected, preserving the hepatic and celiac branches along with those supplying the pylorus), vagotomy should be combined with a drainage procedure, such as gastrojejunostomy. In patients with gastric outlet obstruction, vagotomy alone is contraindicated because it does not relieve obstruction and it aggravates stasis. *(Schwartz and Ellis, pp 221–239)*

798. **(A)** In a person with chronic duodenal ulcer, the incidence of recurrent ulceration following vagotomy and antrectomy is approximately 1%. The incidence associated with proximal vagotomy is 15%. Vagotomy and drainage procedures have recurrence rates of about 10%. *(Schwartz et al, p 1138)*

799. **(A)** Although most instances of hematemesis associated with cirrhosis are due to esophageal varices, in approximately 20 to 25% of persons with cirrhosis upper gastrointestinal tract bleeding is due to other lesions. These lesions include gastritis, peptic ulcer, hiatus hernia, and gastric cancer. The best procedure to locate the bleeding site is esophagogastroduodenoscopy, which has the potential of not only locating a lesion but also demonstrating bleeding from the lesion. Although a gastrointestinal barium series may demonstrate a lesion, it may not identify the source of bleeding. Angiography only shows active bleeding at the time of examination. Splenoportography only is useful in demonstrating varices. Hepatic wedge pressure determines portal pressure but does not identify sites of bleeding. *(Sabiston, pp 1101–1103)*

800. **(D)** Restlessness, irritability, insomnia, and pressured speech are all features of mania. Frequent accompanying psychotic symptoms include flight of ideas and grandiose delusions. The differential diagnosis of a first episode of mania would include the following: bipolar I disorder, especially in the presence of a positive family history; brief psychotic disorder commonly known as "stress psychosis"; schizophrenia, which typically is characterized by a prodromal phase of declining function; and substance abuse, notably with amphetamines. Cyclothymic disorder is a condition of mood swings that are less exaggerated than those in bipolar disorder. *(APA, pp 350–355)*

801. **(B)** Although all the diseases listed in the question can produce psychiatric symptoms, Cushing's disease (or syndromes of steroid excess) would be most likely to cause a severely psychotic presentation. Depression, including psychotic depression, is the most typical psychiatric presentation of Cushing's disease, but affected persons also can display paranoid delusions, auditory hallucinations, and agitation in a symptom complex that can resemble schizophrenia or mania. Addison's disease and hypothyroidism most often produce symptoms reminiscent of a major depressive episode. Multiple sclerosis can present as a psychotic disorder, but the incidence of such a presentation is thought to be quite low. *(Lishman, pp 429–440,595–596)*

802. **(E)** In the pharmacotherapy of a person with severe acute mania, most authorities recommend treatment with neuroleptic drugs. Chlorpromazine and thioridazine are prescribed commonly because of their sedative side effects, although nonsedating neuroleptics such as haloperidol also can be effective. Benzodiazepines such as lorazepam can be useful in cases of mild manic agitation. Lithium is the most appropriate drug in the treatment of the manic phase of bipolar disorder, but its onset of action takes several days. Fluoxetine and clomipramine are antidepressants. Valproic acid is also used to control bipolar disorders. *(Kaplan and Sadock, vol 1, pp 1169–1171)*

803. **(B)** Sleep disruption is a cardinal symptom of major depressive illness. Clinically, common sleep changes include early-morning awakening, mid-cycle awakenings, and difficulty falling asleep. Polysomnographic changes include decreased stage 3 and stage 4 sleep, short REM latency, and other disturbances in REM architecture. Investigators have had some success treating depressive illness by altering sleep patterns, such as by sleep deprivation or more specific REM deprivation. *(Hales and Frances, pp 249–254)*

804. **(B)** Drugs related to antipsychotic medications are used to treat some nonpsychiatric

conditions and, thus, can cause side effects more often associated with antipsychotic therapy. For example, prochlorperazine (Compazine) is a popular antiemetic that is related to chlorpromazine. Extrapyramidal reactions can accompany prochlorperazine therapy and are best treated by antiparkinsonian medications, such as benztropine. *(Kaplan and Sadock, vol 2, pp 2003–2007)*

805. **(D)** Tardive dyskinesia is a potentially irreversible side effect of antipsychotic drug therapy. Typically, it develops after several years of significant use of antipsychotic medications, although it can arise in association with short-term treatment and fairly low dosages. Early symptoms include facial tics and unusual movements of the tongue; later symptoms include bizarre jaw movements, torticollis, choreoathetosis of the extremities, and labored respiration. The cause of tardive dyskinesia is not clear. *(Kaplan and Sadock, vol 2, p 1913)*

806. **(A)** The usual first step in treating tardive dyskinesia, especially early in the course of the disorder, is to stop the antipsychotic drug. For many patients, symptoms recede significantly or even disappear; but for others, symptoms will persist or may even worsen transiently. Switching drug treatment to the neuroleptic clozapine may be beneficial, although this drug can cause other serious side effects. Several medications, including lithium, reserpine, and diazepam, have been tried in the treatment of tardive dyskinesia, but none has emerged as clearly effective. *(Kaplan and Sadock, vol 2, pp 2005–2006)*

807. **(D)** Simple grief (bereavement) is not considered a psychiatric disorder. Symptoms include manifestations of depression: sleep and appetite disturbances, feelings of guilt, and lassitude. However, use of antidepressant medications is not advised unless more florid symptoms develop (eg, significant psychomotor retardation or obsessional thoughts of guilt or worthlessness) or symptoms persist for several months. In the case

presented in the question, the use of a short-acting antianxiety agent for sleep would be beneficial, especially if combined with supportive psychotherapy. *(APA, pp 684–685; Kaplan and Sadock, vol 2, pp 1723–1728)*

808. **(C)** Panic disorder, a syndrome occurring most typically in young women, is characterized by recurring sudden attacks of severe anxiety or fear that are not clearly precipitated by identifiable life events or stresses. (However, if attacks occur coincidentally with the same event, such as shopping, a phobic association may develop.) A variety of treatments have been recommended, including relaxation therapy, psychotherapy, and drug therapy. Medications commonly prescribed at present to treat panic disorders include the benzodiazepine, alprazolam, and antidepressants in a wide range of dosages; the use of neuroleptic drugs is not indicated. *(APA, pp 397–403; Cassem, pp 175–177)*

809. **(A)** Electroconvulsive therapy (ECT) is an effective treatment of severe depression, especially in the elderly. In this age group, risks of drug toxicity are increased, and the time required for antidepressants to act may compromise metabolic status. In general practice, ECT is reserved for the treatment of delusional depressions that resist a reasonable trial of drug therapy. *(Hales and Frances, pp 415–416)*

810. **(E)** A patient's refusal of life-saving treatment poses vexing legal and ethical problems for physicians. In the situation described in the question, treatment could be instituted in most states if a medical emergency were deemed present, if the man were suicidal by virtue of a major psychiatric disorder, or if the man were judged to be incompetent to make the decision to refuse treatment. However, competency or lack of competency can be determined by legal authority only. The role of psychiatrists in determining competency is solely advisory. Psychiatrists must carefully assess a person's mental status for evidence of cognitive or psychologic impairment, as well as document the person's abil-

ity to engage in rational decision making and to understand the consequences of decisions made. *(Cassem, pp 627–632)*

811. **(B)** Differential diagnosis of depression in the elderly must include dementia, metabolic and neoplastic disease, and medication effects. Mental status changes can include psychomotor agitation (or retardation), impaired short-term memory and concentration, and, in psychotic depression, delusions and hallucinations. Fluctuating state of consciousness defines delirium, not depression. Refusal to cooperate with a mental status evaluation may, at times, cause depression to be mistaken for dementia, in a condition called pseudodementia. *(APA, pp 100–103,222–224)*

812. **(C)** Because of slower rates of drug metabolism, elderly individuals often require lower dosages of medications than would be true in younger persons. Although the average daily dosage of imipramine and related antidepressants is 150 mg, this amount of drug in some older persons can cause insomnia, memory disturbance, delusions, and delirium. Although blood levels can establish drug toxicity, the clinical picture in the question is so suggestive of a toxic reaction that dosage should be lowered empirically while test results are pending. Symptoms of drug toxicity remit spontaneously as blood level falls. *(Wood et al)*

813. **(E)** In the treatment of alcohol withdrawal syndromes, close observation is mandatory to guard against seizures and delirium. A benzodiazepine—chlordiazepoxide commonly is used—is prescribed to control symptoms; the drug can be given on an as-needed basis or in a regularly administered regimen. Thiamine is given to prevent development of Wernicke–Korsakoff syndrome, and multivitamin supplementation is encouraged. Diet at first should be aimed at supplying fluids and nutrition while minimizing the danger of aspiration. Chlorpromazine should not be given to persons in alcohol withdrawal because it lowers seizure threshold. *(Cassem, pp 12–17)*

814. **(D)** The danger period for alcohol withdrawal is said to last a full 7 days. Prophylactic therapy discontinued too quickly can lead to recrudescence of withdrawal symptoms. Disulfiram can be started 24 hours after the last drink. *(Cassem, pp 12–17)*

815. **(E)** In the case described in the question, perhaps the most likely explanation for the woman's poor clinical response to imipramine therapy is the relatively brief time she has been on the drug (older antidepressant drugs, such as imipramine, take from 2 to 6 weeks to show full clinical effect). Other possible explanations include noncompliance, undermedication, and *over*medication (tricyclics are believed to have a "therapeutic window" of effectiveness); detection of all three of these phenomena would be aided by obtaining serum imipramine levels. The chances are very good that, given her history of response to imipramine in the past, the woman described will ultimately respond again to imipramine therapy. *(Cassem, pp 541–555)*

816. **(A)** Both lithium and triiodothyronine (T_3) have been used as adjunctive therapies to potentiate the action of tricyclic antidepressant drugs. With lithium, this effect usually appears at a blood level less than that required in treating bipolar disorder. Similarly, a low T_3 dosage is used in augmenting tricyclic action. As a general therapeutic principle, tricyclic and monoamine oxidase inhibitor (MAOI) antidepressants should not be given concurrently. *(Hales and Frances, pp 199–200,417–419)*

817. **(B)** The usefulness of brief dynamic psychotherapy has become more recognized in recent years. Persons who present with an identified conflict or problem and who demonstrate motivation for change and ability to tolerate the stress of self-examination can achieve significant, often permanent improvement. Short-term treatment has proven able to examine intrapsychic issues effectively and usefully. Setting a specific, brief course of therapy often can enhance motiva-

tion and thus by itself increase the likelihood of treatment success. It should be noted that how brief is "brief" is not at all established; brief psychotherapy can range from a half-dozen to 40 or more appointments. *(Hales and Frances, pp 406–408)*

818–824. **(818-D, 819-C, 820-A, 821-C, 822-A, 823-B, 824-A)** Tricyclic antidepressant drugs have been very useful in treating a variety of psychiatric disorders in children and adolescents. Clinical trials and clinician experience have shown that desipramine, especially when combined with behavioral intervention, is an effective treatment for many individuals suffering from bulimia nervosa as well as from enuresis. Desipramine has also been helpful in treating children who have attention-deficit hyperactivity disorder and who have not responded well to first-line drug treatment with a psychostimulant agent, such as methylphenidate, dextroamphetamine, or pemoline. Ironically, tricyclic antidepressants have not had a successful track record in the treatment of childhood depression.

Like desipramine, haloperidol, an antipsychotic agent, has found a place in the treatment of a number of childhood psychiatric disorders. Haloperidol has been a long-standing drug treatment of choice for children with Tourette's syndrome, a disorder characterized by the presence of multiple tics, most notably vocal ones. Extremely aggressive behavior associated with conduct disorder or with mental retardation also can be treated with haloperidol, as can the psychosis produced by childhood schizophrenia.

It is now recognized that obsessive–compulsive disorder affects a significant number of children. Psychopharmacologic treatment is the same as with adults—namely clomipramine or fluoxetine. *(Shaffer, pp 1–28,69–130,150–154,174–176)*

825. **(C)** Fluorocarbons have been shown to induce arrhythmias in workers involved in their use in several industries. They have been used as theoretically inert propellants in aerosols, as solvents for use in dry cleaning,

and in fire extinguishers. The other substances listed in the question have not been demonstrated to be linked to the development of cardiovascular abnormalities. However, such abnormalities are of sufficiently frequent occurrence in the United States to merit an active search for other possible associations. *(Levy and Wegman, pp 432–436)*

826. **(E)** Poliomyelitis has a reservoir of infection among humans, who shed the virus in pharyngeal secretions and feces. The most common mode of spread is by the oral route. Neither flies nor water supplies have been conclusively established as sources of infection. Males are more frequently affected than females. Minor cases may exist in a community without being recognized by symptoms other than those caused by nonspecific virus infections. Poliomyelitis remains highly endemic in many developing countries. Statistics from these countries are not always reliably available. The disease is chiefly recognized in its paralytic form. *(Last, pp 80–81)*

827. **(E)** The incubation period of rhinovirus and coronavirus colds is 48 to 72 hours. Parainfluenza virus and respiratory syncytial virus (RSV) cause bronchiolitis, croup, and pneumonia in young children but usually result in uncomplicated colds in adults. Mycoplasma infections characteristically have a longer incubation period and more protracted symptoms. They occur in adults especially when they are in contact with children who have frequent persistent coughs and colds. *(Kelley, pp 121,1756–1757)*

828. **(E)** In spite of strong assertions from some quarters, notably from the Nobel Prize winner Linus Pauling, evidence is not conclusive that ascorbic acid (vitamin C) has therapeutic activity in colds. Phenylephrine nose drops may diminish nasal secretion, and be good symptomatic therapy. The antiviral agents amantadine and vidarabine are unlikely to be effective in illness that is of longer duration than the usual virus infection. Erythromycin has some effect in diminishing symptoms in mycoplasma infections, especially if given early. This medication should be continued for 10 days in this condition. *(Kelley, pp 121, 1756–1757)*

829. **(E)** A complete primary series of immunizations with tetanus toxoid conveys long-lasting protection (10 years or more) in most recipients. It is therefore assumed that in the emergency care of clean wounds, when the last immunization is known to have been given within the last 10 years and have been a full immunizing course, a boosting dose is not essential. However, because a small proportion of vaccines do not maintain an effective level of immunization for 10 years, in the treatment of wounds that are other than clean and minor, a booster dose is advised if there is no clear history of toxoid administration in the previous 5 years. Where there is such a history, and the wound is clean and minor, it is now generally accepted that no further booster dose is necessary. *(Last, pp 76–78)*

830. **(B)** The age at which children most frequently ingest the largest amounts of lead is during the crawling and walking stage, which is also the oral–anal stage of development. Thus, the children most at risk are between the ages of 1 and 2 years. Until children are mobile, they are unlikely to come into contact with objects that might have been coated with lead-based paint. After 2 years of age, children normally have less tendency to put unusual objects in their mouths. *(Clark and MacMahon, p 545)*

831. **(E)** Oral consent may be a valid form of authorizing some medical procedures. However, in the case of any surgical procedure or in the use of an instrument, such as a sigmoidoscope, to which there must be attributed minimal risk, a written form of consent is highly desirable. When the patient is a minor and away from home, even in emergency situations written consent should be sought from someone who is prepared to act as guardian with parental permission. In most children's camps, for example, a responsible

official should have received prior authorization from the parents to give such consent. Most difficulties have arisen when physicians have felt that their explanation of the situation is sufficient, in view of prior knowledge of the patient. No matter how minor the procedure, if there is any attached risk it is always advisable to have a written statement of informed consent. Only when the treatment is indeed minor, is not hazardous, and is routine is oral consent to be regarded as sufficient. Even under these circumstances, the oral consent should be recorded in the notes at the time. *(Warren, p 104)*

832. **(D)** Before a person can be confined to an institution, a competent professional must decide that the person is actually or at present insane and that there is a danger of injury to the patient or others. A person who is mentally incompetent is more appropriately protected by the legal appointment of a guardian to make the necessary decisions and manage property, rather than by confining that person. A person who merely has strange fantasies may be neither mentally incompetent nor a danger to self or others. Auditory and visual hallucinations do not necessarily pose a threat of danger or injury to self or others and therefore are not in themselves grounds for confinement. *(Warren, p 130)*

833. **(C)** *Vibrio cholerae* has its only reservoir in humans and tolerates exposure and drying poorly. It survives longer in water, especially if the water is at temperatures of 18 to 23°C (60 to 70°F). It therefore does not spread on infected clothing (fomites). Direct person-to-person transmission probably does not occur. Contaminated water is the main source of infection; frequent exposure to polluted surface water through bathing, food preparation, and utensil washing are major sources of infection. Although flies may transport small numbers of vibros from excreta to food, lack of multiplication makes it unlikely that flies play an important part in transmission. Mosquitoes are not vectors. *(Last, pp 176–178)*

834. (E) It has been reported that 28% of pregnant women shed cytomegalovirus (CMV) from the cervix at some time during pregnancy. The percentage of infants affected is not as high as this. It is therefore assumed that there must be some effective mechanisms that prevent fetal infection when the mother is excreting CMV. The virus may affect the placenta and not the fetus. A congenitally infected infant may shed the virus intermittently for years. Close contact with body secretions containing the virus seems to be responsible for the higher incidence among institutionalized children. *(Last, pp 144–145)*

835. (C) Chelating drugs are given as treatment for symptomatic poisoning by lead and other heavy metals. They should not be given prophylactically, since the agents themselves have some possible toxic side effects. These toxic effects may add to those already caused by ingestion of the metals and may actually increase absorption of the metal. For these reasons, advice should be given to workers to seek employment away from exposure to the offending agent while therapy continues. *(Levy and Wegman, pp 206–207)*

836–837. (836-C, 837-E) Polychlorinated biphenyls (PCBs) were extensively used in the manufacture of electrical transformers until production was halted in the mid-1970s. Workers who have been exposed to the substances have been noted to have an acnelike eruption with inflammatory pustules. Other effects are eye irritation and gastrointestinal disturbance. The substances are persistent, and more than 25% of the population in the United States is thought to have residues of greater than one part per million in adipose tissue. Dietary exposure of the general population has been alleged to occur through milk, eggs, cheese, meat, and fish.

Organophosphorus compounds have been widely used since the 1950s as insecticides, both in national pest control programs and domestically. They have been responsible for more deaths on a worldwide basis than have any other groups of compounds. From the point of view of the environmental

toxicologist, it was perhaps fortuitous that many pests began to develop resistance to the substances fairly early in the use of these compounds. More recently, concern for environmental control has further limited their use; studies have attributed carcinogenic properties to several of these pesticides.

Nitrosamines are highly toxic and dangerous to handle. Toxic amounts may be absorbed without warning, because danger signals such as specific odor or irritant effects are lacking. The manufacture of electrical products and of rubber, dyes, lubricating oils, explosives, insecticides, and fungicides all have been associated with these substances. They may be used as solvents as well as agents in the manufacturing process. Nitrosamines have carcinogenic properties and have been transmitted transplacentally.

Epoxy compounds are used in the production of resins. They cause irritation of the skin and mucosa. Experimental studies have indicated such possible effects as testicular atrophy and defective spermatogenesis. Although the substances are irritants, more serious toxicity has so far not been demonstrated. *(Last, pp 431–433,442–444,481–482,606)*

838–849. (838-J, 839-A, 840-B, 841-E, 842-C, 843-F, 844-G, 845-L, 846-L, 847-H, 848-I, 849-D) The list of recommendations for preventive services come from the US Preventive Services Task Force. The list is neither exhaustive nor final. Clinicians frequently wish to add other preventive measures after considering a patient's history or other clinically relevant individual circumstances. The list concentrates on those tests that have been proven to be cost-effective in the population risk groups noted. For each risk group, other tests may and should be done. The wording of the question is important for the student to notice. It requests appropriate tests for the *related* conditions, not for the disease from which the population group may be derived. Thus, for example, it is assumed that a diabetic population would have serial fasting glucose serum levels as a part of the treatment for the condition. Hence the correct screening procedure for a related condition in the known diabetic population is urinalysis for bacteruria, which may reveal a urinary tract infection in a population that has polyuria and therefore might be "asymptomatic," or at least overlooked by the physician.

Homosexually active men are at high risk for numerous infections. It is well recognized that a major risk is HIV infection, but apart from the use of protective condoms and restricting the number of partners, no preventive measures have been demonstrated to be effective. In common with IV drug abusers, this group is also at high risk for hepatitis B infection, for which immunization is effective.

Markedly obese individuals are at high risk for diabetes. This association may be stronger than a risk factor, in that a high proportion of obese individuals who are treated by effective weight reduction may require neither insulin nor oral hypoglycemic agents to control diabetes. A fasting blood glucose may detect a condition that is treatable by dietary measures, and this may be the reinforcement necessary to persuade some individuals to adhere to dietary advice.

Prostitutes and persons with multiple sex partners are especially at risk for gonorrhea. Syphilis is more common in prostitutes, possibly because their lifestyle may continue for many years. Prostitutes should therefore be screened for both diseases. Otherwise, gonorrhea is principally diagnosed because of presenting symptoms, when treatment with antibiotics is relatively easy and short, in spite of the development of strains of the organism that are resistant to some antibiotics. Syphilis has a longer latent period, and it is therefore frequently advisable to screen for it.

In patients with diabetes, polyuria is a common symptom. In a well-controlled diabetic, a physician may attribute the frequency of urination to polyuria, missing a bacteruria. Infections of all kinds are more frequent in diabetics and are often reasons for suddenly poor control of the disease. Infections are always serious for a diabetic and should therefore be treated early.

Tuberculosis is becoming more frequent once again. The reservoir of infection seems to be in nations where low socioeconomic conditions prevail and in the immunocompromised population, which includes those infected with HIV. Potential immigrants are tested, but the physician should bear in mind that infection may be dormant or latent at the time immigration is sought.

Men with two or more cardiac risk factors—high blood pressure, high blood cholesterol levels, cigarette smoking, diabetes mellitus, or a family history of coronary artery disease—should have a preventive ECG performed at every routine physical examination.

Pandemics of influenza from any strain of virus are particularly devastating for populations of individuals in nursing homes. These persons should receive immunization against the predicted strains of influenza (which are made commercially available each year) as a routine. Little ongoing immunity is achieved by this vaccination, which should therefore be repeated annually.

Patients who suffer from any condition that increases the risk of pneumococcal infection, which includes any patient with chronic cardiac or pulmonary condition and several other conditions, such as sickle cell disease, should receive initially a combined pneumococcus and influenza vaccine. The immunity conveyed by the pneumococcal vaccine is relatively permanent, so subsequent immunization may be performed with influenza vaccine alone.

Persons aged 50 or over who have first-degree relatives with colorectal cancer or who have a personal history of endometrial, ovarian, or breast cancer or a previous history of inflammatory bowel disease or polyps should have annual fecal occult blood investigations and sigmoidoscopy.

Persons with a family history of polyposis coli should have regular fecal occult blood tests and regular colonoscopy. The interval between colonoscopies depends on the individual patient and the recommendation of the gastroenterologist. The latter depends on the findings and the confidence of the success of the procedure.

Persons who attend clinics for the treatment of sexually transmitted disease and those attending other high-risk clinics such as adolescent and family planning clinics should be regularly tested for concomitant chlamydial infection. This infection is also more prevalent in those who have multiple sexual partners. More common in women, it may give rise to symptoms in men, who are frequently carriers. *(Last, pp 6–7)*

REFERENCES

Internal Medicine

Isselbacher KJ, Braunwald E, Wilson JD, et al, eds. *Harrison's Principles of Internal Medicine.* 13th ed. New York, NY: McGraw-Hill Book Co; 1994.

Report of the National Cholesterol Education Program Expert Panel on Detection, Evaluation, and Treatment of High Blood Cholesterol in Adults.

Obstetrics and Gynecology

Cunningham FG, MacDonald PC, Gant NF. *Williams Obstetrics.* 19th ed. East Norwalk, Conn: Appleton & Lange; 1993.

DeCherney AM, Pernoll ML. *Current Obstetric & Gynecologic Diagnosis & Treatment.* 8th ed. East Norwalk, Conn: Appleton & Lange; 1994.

Gant NF, Cunningham FG. *Basic Gynecology and Obstetrics.* East Norwalk, Conn: Appleton & Lange; 1993.

Pediatrics

Feigin RD, Cherry JD. *Textbook of Pediatric Infectious Diseases.* 3rd ed. Philadelphia, Pa: WB Saunders Co; 1992.

Fleischer GR, Ludwig S. *Textbook of Pediatric Emergency Medicine.* Baltimore, Md: Williams & Wilkins; 1993.

Rudolph AM, Hoffman JIE, Rudolph CD. *Pediatrics.* 20th ed. Norwalk, Conn: Appleton & Lange; 1996.

Psychiatry

American Psychiatric Association (APA). *Diagnostic and Statistical Manual of Mental Disorders.* 4th ed. Washington DC: American Psychiatric Association; 1994.

Cassem WH. *Massachusetts General Hospital Handbook of General Hospital Psychiatry.* St. Louis, Mo: Mosby Year Book; 1991.

Hales RE, Frances AJ, eds. *Psychiatry Update: American Psychiatric Association Annual Review.* Washington DC: American Psychiatric Press Inc; 1987;6.

Kaplan HI, Sadock BJ. *Comprehensive Textbook of Psychiatry VI.* 6th ed. Baltimore, Md: Williams & Wilkins; 1995; 2 vols.

Lishman WA. *Organic Psychiatry. The Psychological Consequences of Cerebral Disorder.* 2nd ed. Oxford, England: Blackwell Scientific Publications; 1987.

Shaffer D, ed. *The Psychiatric Clinics of North America: Pediatric Psychopharmacology.* Philadelphia, Pa: WB Saunders Co; 1992.

Wood KA, Harris MJ, Morreale A, et al. Drug-induced psychosis and depression in the elderly. *Psychiatr Clin North Am.* 1988;11:167–193.

Preventive Medicine

Ahlbom A, Norell S. *Introduction to Modern Epidemiology.* Chestnut Hill, Mass: Epidemiology Resources, Inc; 1990.

Clark DW, MacMahon B. *Preventive and Community Medicine.* 2nd ed. Boston, Mass: Little, Brown & Co; 1981.

Kelley WN. *Textbook of Internal Medicine.* Philadelphia, Pa: JB Lippincott Co; 1989.

Last JM, Wallace R. *Maxcy-Rosenau-Last Public Health and Preventive Medicine.* 13th ed. Norwalk, Conn: Appleton & Lange; 1992.

Levy BS, Wegman DH. *Occupational Health: Recognizing and Preventing Work Related Disease.* Boston, Mass: Little, Brown & Co; 1995.

Luft HS. Assessing the evidence of HMO performance. *Milbank Memorial Fund Quarterly; Health and Society.* 1980; (Oct-Dec):501–536.

Mausner JS, Bahn AK. *Epidemiology: An Introductory Text.* Philadelphia: WB Saunders Co; 1985.

Morton RF, Hebel JR. *A Study Guide to Epidemiology and Biostatistics.* Baltimore, Md: University Park Press; 1996.

Warren DG. *A Legal Guide for Rural Health Programs.* Cambridge, Mass: Ballinger Publishing Co; 1979.

Wyngaarden JB, Smith LM. *Cecil's Textbook of Medicine.* 18th ed. Philadelphia: WB Saunders Co; 1996.

Surgery

Aaron RK, Ciombor D. Venous thromboembolism in orthopedic patients. *Surg Clin North Am.* 1983; 63:529–537.

Antip RG, Burke JF. Skin coverage. *Curr Probl Surg.* 1983;20:637–640.

Bartlett RH, Whitehouse WH, Turcotte JS. *Life Support Systems in Intensive Care.* Chicago, Ill: Year Book Medical Publishers Inc; 1984.

Braverman. LE, Utinger RD, eds. *Werner & Ingbar's The Thyroid: A Fundamental Clinical Text.* 6th ed. Philadelphia, Pa: Lippincott; 1991.

Browse NL. *An Introduction to the Symptoms and Signs of Surgical Disease.* Chicago, Ill: Year Book Medical Publishers Inc; 1978.

Condon RE, Nyhus LM, eds. *Manual of Surgical Therapeutics.* 6th ed. Boston, Mass: Little, Brown & Co; 1992.

Conley JJ, ed. *Complications of Head and Neck Surgery.* Philadelphia, Pa: WB Saunders Co; 1979.

Cummings CW, et al ed., *Otolaryngology—Head and Neck Surgery,* 2nd ed. St. Louis, Mo: Mosby–Year Book; 1993.

David JA. *Wound Management.* Springhouse, Pa: Springhouse Corp; 1986.

Feliciano DV, Moore EE, Mattox KL, eds. *Trauma.* 3rd ed. Stamford, Conn: Appleton & Lange; 1996.

Gitnick GL. *Current Gastroenterology.* Boston, Mass: Houghton Mifflin Professional Publishers; 1980;1.

Greenfield LJ, Mulholland MW, Oldham KT, Zelenock GB. *Surgery Scientific Principles and Practice.* Philadelphia, Pa: Lippincott; 1993.

Greenfield LJ, Wakefield TW. *Prevention of Venous Thrombus and Pulmonary Embolism Advances in Surgery.* Chicago, Ill: Year Book Medical Publishers Inc; 1989; 22.

Hardy JD, ed. *Hardy's Textbook of Surgery.* Philadelphia, Pa: JB Lippincott Co; 1988.

Juhl JH. *Paul and Juhl's Essentials of Roentgen Interpretation.* New York, NY: Harper & Row Publishers Inc; 1993.

Marini JJ. *Respiratory Medicine and Intensive Care for the House Officer.* Baltimore, Md: Williams & Wilkins; 1987.

Moore FA, Haenel JB, Moore EE. Alternatives to Swan-Ganz cardiac output monitoring. *Surg Clin N Am.* 1991;71:699–717.

Rosenthal LE, Mobley HLT. *Contemp Gastroenterol.* 1988;1:9–13.

Sabiston DC, ed. *Davis-Christopher Textbook of Surgery.* 13th ed. Philadelphia, Pa: WB Saunders Co; 1981.

Schwartz SI, Ellis H, eds. *Maingot's abdominal operations,* 9th ed. Norwalk, Conn: Appleton & Lange; 1990.

Schwartz SI, Shires GT, Spencer FC, eds. *Principles of Surgery.* 5th ed. New York, NY: McGraw-Hill Book Co; 1994.

Skinner DG, deKernion JB. *Genitourinary Cancer.* Philadelphia, Pa: WB Saunders Co; 1978.

Tanagho EA, McAninch JW. *Smith's General Urology.* 13th ed. Norwalk, Conn: Appleton & Lange; 1992.

Vander AJ. *Renal Physiology.* 5th ed. New York, NY: McGraw-Hill Book Co; 1995.

SUBSPECIALTY LIST: CLINICAL COMPETENCE REVIEW

Question Number and Subspecialty

Obstetrics and Gynecology

700. Endocrinology, infertility
701. Endocrinology, infertility
702. Endocrinology, infertility
703. Clinical obstetrics, abnormal
704. Clinical obstetrics, normal
705. Primary care
706. Primary care
707. Clinical obstetrics, normal
708. Clinical obstetrics, abnormal
709. Clinical obstetrics, normal
710. Clinical obstetrics, abnormal
711. Clinical obstetrics, abnormal
712. Clinical obstetrics, abnormal
713. Clinical gynecology
714. Clinical gynecology
715. Clinical gynecology
716. Clinical gynecology
717. Clinical gynecology
718. Clinical gynecology
719. Clinical gynecology
720. Clinical obstetrics, abnormal
721. Clinical obstetrics, abnormal
722. Clinical obstetrics, abnormal
723. Clinical obstetrics, abnormal

Pediatrics

724. Infection
725. Infection
726. Infection
727. Ear, nose, and throat
728. Ear, nose, and throat
729. Infectious disease
730. Infectious disease
731. Infectious disease
732. Endocrinology
733. Endocrinology
734. Neurology
735. Neurology
736. Neurology
737. Neurology
738. Neoplastic disease
739. Neoplastic disease
740. Neoplastic disease
741. Infectious disease
742. Infectious disease
743. Infectious disease
744. Structure, genetic
745. Structure, genetic
746. Structure, genetic
747. Hematology
748. Hematology
749. Hematology

Internal Medicine

750. Neurology
751. Neurology
752. Rheumatology
753. Rheumatology
754. Pulmonology
755. Pulmonology
756. Pulmonology
757. Nephrology
758. Nephrology
759. Nephrology
760. Nephrology
761. Allergy and immunology
762. Allergy and immunology
763. Allergy and immunology
764. Rheumatology
765. Rheumatology
766. Rheumatology
767. Cardiology
768. Cardiology
769. Cardiology
770. Infectious disease

771. Infectious disease
772. Infectious disease
773. Endocrinology
774. Endocrinology

Surgery

775. Vascular surgery
776. Vascular surgery
777. Vascular surgery
778. Vascular surgery
779. Breast
780. Breast
781. Gastrointestinal bleeding
782. Gastrointestinal bleeding
783. Liver
784. Gastrointestinal tract
785. Trauma
786. Trauma
787. Trauma
788. Biliary surgery
789. Biliary surgery
790. Biliary surgery
791. Biliary surgery
792. Gastrointestinal tract
793. Gastrointestinal tract
794. Pediatric gastrointestinal surgery
795. Pediatric gastrointestinal surgery
796. Fluids and electrolytes
797. Gastrointestinal tract
798. Gastrointestinal tract
799. Gastrointestinal bleeding

Psychiatry

800. Assessment
801. Psychopathology
802. Intervention
803. Psychopathology
804. Assessment
805. Assessment
806. Intervention
807. Intervention
808. Intervention
809. Intervention
810. Ethical and legal aspects
811. Assessment
812. Intervention
813. Intervention
814. Intervention
815. Assessment
816. Intervention

817. Intervention
818. Child psychiatry, intervention
819. Child psychiatry, intervention
820. Child psychiatry, intervention
821. Child psychiatry, intervention
822. Child psychiatry, intervention
823. Child psychiatry, intervention
824. Child psychiatry, intervention

Preventive Medicine
825. Disease control
826. Disease control
827. Disease control
828. Disease control
829. Disease control
830. Disease control
831. Ethical and legal
832. Ethical and legal

833. Disease control
834. Disease control
835. Disease control
836. Disease control
837. Disease control
838. Disease control
839. Disease control
840. Disease control
841. Disease control
842. Disease control
843. Disease control
844. Disease control
845. Disease control
846. Disease control
847. Disease control
848. Disease control
849. Disease control

Practice Test

Carefully read the following instructions before taking the Practice Test.

1. This examination consists of 120 single-item questions and 60 case study questions organized according to the clinical-encounter settings.
2. The questions are presented with subjects integrated; however, questions are grouped by type.
3. The Practice Test mimics one booklet of the actual *Step 3* examination by presenting the exact number of questions in exam-type format. Content and question-type breakdown are similar to those you will encounter on the examination.
4. You are allotted approximately 48 seconds per item, which is approximately 2 hours for this test. Be sure to time yourself accordingly.
5. Be sure you have extra pencils and erasers, a clock, a comfortable setting, and an adequate amount of undisturbed, distraction-free time. Relax!
6. Remove and fill out the answer sheet as instructed. (The answer sheet is on pages 317–318.)
7. Once you have completed the Practice Test, check your answers and assess your areas of weakness against the subspecialty list on pages 312 through 314.

DIRECTIONS (Questions 1 through 49): Each of the numbered items or incomplete statements in this section is followed by answers or by completions of the statement. Select the ONE lettered answer or completion that is BEST in each case.

1. Under normal conditions, the major mechanism of body heat loss is

   (A) radiation
   (B) evaporation
   (C) perspiration
   (D) insensible perspiration
   (E) conduction

2. The introduction of cold water into one ear may cause giddiness and nausea. The primary cause of this phenomenon is

   (A) temporary immobilization of otoliths
   (B) decreased movement of ampullar crests
   (C) increased discharge rate in vestibular afferents
   (D) decreased discharge rate in vestibular afferents
   (E) creation of convection currents in endolymph

3. Phosphorylation activates or inhibits all of the following enzymes EXCEPT

   (A) glycogen phosphorylase
   (B) lipoprotein lipase
   (C) triacylglycerol lipase
   (D) glycogen synthase
   (E) phosphorylase kinase

4. Which virus is most resistant to chemical and physical agents?

(A) mumps
(B) measles
(C) influenza
(D) serum hepatitis
(E) polio

5. The development of which tumor is associated with the ingestion of aflatoxin?

(A) hepatocellular carcinoma
(B) pulmonary sarcomas
(C) chordomas of the lower spine
(D) uterine leiomyomas
(E) sebaceous carcinoma of the eyelid

6. All the following sedatives have pharmacologically active metabolites EXCEPT

(A) prazepam
(B) chlordiazepoxide
(C) diazepam
(D) lorazepam
(E) clorazepate

7. All the following statements concerning neurons are correct EXCEPT

(A) neurons lack the ability to store glycogen
(B) neurons are the basic unit of the nervous system
(C) neurons contain Nissl bodies
(D) neurons contain neurotubules
(E) neurons are capable of reproducing themselves

8. Secretion of renin by the juxtaglomerular apparatus directly results in

(A) conversion of angiotensinogen to angioten-sin I
(B) secretion of ACTH
(C) secretion of aldosterone
(D) vasodilation
(E) increased renal potassium retention

9. The key regulatory enzyme of fatty acid synthesis is

(A) citrate cleavage enzyme
(B) ATP citrate lyase
(C) acetyl-CoA carboxylase
(D) malonyl-CoA decarboxylase
(E) malonyl transacylase

10. Which of the following is a bactericidal chemotherapeutic agent?

(A) sulfonamides
(B) erythromycin
(C) ampicillin
(D) chloramphenicol
(E) tetracyclines

11. Which of the following findings is considered diagnostic of Hirschsprung's disease on histologic examination of a rectal biopsy specimen?

(A) hypertrophy of the muscle coat of the wall of the rectum
(B) atrophy of the mucosal lining of the wall of the rectum
(C) absence of the nerve fibers that innervate the wall of the rectum
(D) absence of parasympathetic ganglion cells in the submucosal and myenteric plexus
(E) presence of multiple small polyps along the mucosal surface of the rectal wall

12. Which of the following antineoplastic agents acts by competitive inhibition of hormonal action?

(A) vincristine
(B) bleomycin
(C) busulfan
(D) tamoxifen
(E) melphalan

13. The functions of the ego include all of the following EXCEPT

(A) psychologic defense mechanisms
(B) reality testing

(C) thinking

(D) perception

(E) instinctual drives

14. Which of the following cranial nerves emerge from the sulcus between the olive and pyramid?

 (A) the abducens

 (B) the hypoglossal

 (C) the vagus

 (D) the glossopharyngeal

 (E) the spinal accessory

15. The principal form in which iron is stored within cells of the intestinal mucosa is

 (A) free ferrous ions

 (B) free ferric ions

 (C) apoferritin

 (D) ferritin

 (E) hemoglobin

16. The major carrier of cholesterol in the bloodstream is

 (A) chylomicrons

 (B) high-density lipoprotein (HDL)

 (C) low-density lipoprotein (LDL)

 (D) a sulfate ester

 (E) albumin-cholesterol complex

17. Penicillin would be LEAST effective in treating

 (A) syphilis

 (B) gonorrhea

 (C) pneumococcal pneumonia

 (D) mycoplasmal pneumonia

 (E) streptococcal pharyngitis

18. In the United States the most common etiology of an abdominal aortic aneurysm is

 (A) Marfan's syndrome

 (B) atherosclerosis

 (C) syphilitic infection

 (D) bacterial infection

 (E) acute rheumatic fever

19. All the following agents are useful in the treatment of rheumatoid arthritis EXCEPT

 (A) acetaminophen

 (B) gold

 (C) acetylsalicylic acid (aspirin)

 (D) glucocorticoids

 (E) penicillamine

20. All the following statements concerning homosexuality are correct EXCEPT

 (A) onset of same-sex erotic feelings usually occur in adolescence or before

 (B) genetic and biologic factors may play an important role in homosexuality

 (C) American Psychiatric Association's diagnostic manual defines homosexuality as a psychiatric disorder

 (D) female–female relationships tend to be more stable than male–male relationships

 (E) "coming out" may be an important milestone

21. First-order sensory neurons are located in all the following structures EXCEPT

 (A) the anterior gray column

 (B) the trigeminal ganglion

 (C) the geniculate ganglion

 (D) the dorsal root ganglion

 (E) the mesencephalic nucleus of the trigeminal

22. Glucagon's effects on hepatocytes include all the following EXCEPT

 (A) elevate intracellular cAMP

 (B) glycogenolysis

 (C) conversion of phorylase b to phosphorylase a

 (D) inactivation of phosphorylase b kinase

 (E) generation of glucose-1-phosphate

23. The pituitary prohormone proopiomlanocortin is the precursor of all the following hormones EXCEPT

    (A) thyroid-stimulating hormone (TSH)
    (B) melanocyte-stimulating hormone (MSH)
    (C) adrenocorticotropin (ACTH)
    (D) β-endorphin
    (E) γ-lipotropin

24. The antiphagocytic property of group A streptococci is associated with

    (A) M protein
    (B) hyaluronidase
    (C) streptolysin O
    (D) streptolysin S
    (E) DNAse

25. Which of the following forms of muscular dystrophy are inherited as an X-linked disorder and produce symptoms before the age of 4 years?

    (A) benign (Becker variety)
    (B) severe (Duchenne variety)
    (C) limb–girdle variety
    (D) myotonic dystrophy
    (E) facioscapulohumoral variety

26. Potassium supplementation is often necessary for patients taking

    (A) spironolactone
    (B) triamterene
    (C) furosemide
    (D) amiloride
    (E) captopril

27. Which of the following statements is true concerning sexual abuse in children?

    (A) the abuser is usually a stranger
    (B) sexual abuse in childhood usually does not result in long-lasting sequelae
    (C) sexually abused children seldom develop depression

    (D) about 2 to 8 % of allegations of sexual abuse are false
    (E) most perpetrators are eventually discovered and incarcerated

28. A 90° clockwise rotation of the intestinal loop usually results in which of the following?

    (A) an omphalocele
    (B) a retrocecal appendix
    (C) a retrocecal ureter
    (D) a transverse colon passing behind the duodenum
    (E) a vitelline cyst

29. Acetylcholine (ACh) is a critical link in the transmission of signals at the neuromuscular junction (NMJ). Its precise function at the NMJ is best summed up as

    (A) activating postsynaptic stimulatory G proteins that open potassium channels
    (B) directly opening postsynaptic voltage-gated sodium channels
    (C) opening postsynaptic ACh-gated cation channels
    (D) reducing the postsynaptic muscle cell's threshold for achieving an action potential
    (E) lowering the threshold for presynaptic transmitter release

30. The active form of the cofactor required for oxidative decarboxylation reactions is

    (A) thiamine
    (B) thiamine pyrophosphate
    (C) thiamine monophosphate
    (D) thiamine triphosphate
    (E) hydroxyethyl thiamine pyrophosphate

See color insert following page 270. (Photograph courtesy of Joseph M. Campos. From Jenson and Baltimore, *Pediatric Infectious Diseases*, Appleton & Lange, 1995, plate 1F.)

31. A 30-year-old man is diagnosed as having tuberculosis. He has been ill for about 7 months with symptoms that include a productive cough, intermittent fever, night sweats, and a weight loss of 27.3 kg (60 lb). Numerous acid-fast bacilli are seen in a sputum examination, and more than 50 colonies of organisms grow out in culture. Persons who have been in contact with this man and who have a positive skin test but show no other signs of disease should

    (A) receive prophylactic isoniazid (INH)
    (B) receive a full course of INH and ethambutol
    (C) be checked periodically by roentgenography
    (D) be immunized with bacille Calmette-Guérin (BCG) vaccine
    (E) be checked periodically by sputum culture

32. Hyponatremia resulting from the inappropriate secretion of ADH is most often associated with which one of the following lung tumors?

    (A) squamous cell carcinoma
    (B) adenocarcinoma
    (C) large-cell carcinoma
    (D) small cell carcinoma
    (E) bronchioloalveolar carcinoma

33. Which of the following antibiotics has a mechanism of action of binding to the 30 S ribosomal subunit and thus interfering with the initiation of protein synthesis?

    (A) chloramphenicol
    (B) vancomycin
    (C) nitrofurantoin
    (D) trimethoprim
    (E) gentamicin

34. Which of the following statements is true concerning substance abuse?

    (A) cocaine abuse causes mania but not depression
    (B) tobacco is habituating, but does not cause addiction
    (C) most cases of addiction to opioids are iatrogenic
    (D) tolerance does not develop to cannabis use
    (E) if a narcotic analgesic is to be given to an opioid-dependent person, the dose should be significantly increased

35. The primitive intestinal loop rotates around an axis formed by which of the following arteries?

    (A) the inferior epigastric
    (B) the superior epigastric
    (C) the obturator
    (D) the inferior mesenteric
    (E) the superior mesenteric

36. A lesion that produces partial or total blindness but spares the pupillary light response is most likely to be located in the

    (A) optic nerve
    (B) optic chiasm
    (C) optic tract
    (D) pretectal area
    (E) geniculocalcarine tract

37. In the presence of a poison that uncouples oxidative phosphorylation, what would be the net energy yield of the complete oxidation of one mole equivalent of glucose in muscle?

   (A) 1 mole equivalent ATP
   (B) 2 moles equivalent ATP
   (C) 3 moles equivalent ATP
   (D) 4 moles equivalent ATP
   (E) 5 moles equivalent ATP

38. A 7-month-old girl who has a history of pyogenic infections is hospitalized for a yeast infection that does not respond to therapy. On physical examination her spleen and lymph nodes are not palpable. A differential white blood cell count shows 95% neutrophils, 1% lymphocytes, and 4% monocytes. A bone marrow specimen contains no plasma cells or lymphocytes. Roentgenography reveals absence of a thymic shadow. Tonsils are absent. These findings are most compatible with

   (A) multiple myeloma
   (B) severe combined immunodeficiency disease
   (C) X-linked agammaglobulinemia
   (D) Wiskott–Aldrich syndrome
   (E) chronic granulomatous disease

39. The major scavenger cell involved in the inflammatory response is the

   (A) neutrophil
   (B) lymphocyte
   (C) plasma cell
   (D) eosinophil
   (E) macrophage

40. The sulfonylurea tolbutamide

   (A) will never cause severe hypoglycemia
   (B) is best used in insulin-dependent diabetes
   (C) needs to be injected subcutaneously

   (D) acutely stimulates the pancreas to secrete insulin
   (E) appears to prevent cardiovascular complications from diabetes

41. A patient who believes that he cannot eat as all his guts have rotted may be said to be

   (A) hallucinating
   (B) delusional
   (C) depressed
   (D) neurotic
   (E) phobic

42. The third aortic arch forms which of the following structures?

   (A) the maxillary artery
   (B) the hyoid and stapedial arteries
   (C) the common carotid artery
   (D) the pulmonary arch
   (E) the brachiocephalic artery

43. The foramen rotundum opens into which of the following areas?

   (A) the infratemporal fossa
   (B) the pterygopalatine fossa
   (C) the posterior cranial fossa
   (D) the orbital cavity
   (E) the oral cavity

44. Which of the following steps is common to both gluconeogenesis and glycolysis?

   (A) fructose 6-phosphate to glucose 6-phosphate
   (B) pyruvate to oxaloacetate
   (C) glucose 6-phosphate to glucose
   (D) fructose 1,6-bisphosphate to fructose 6-phosphate
   (E) oxaloacetate to phosphoenolpyruvate

45. Interferon causes antiviral resistance by inducing intracellular formation of antiviral proteins that

(A) interfere with adsorption of viruses to other cells
(B) prevent penetration of viruses
(C) inhibit viral uncoating
(D) block transcription of viral nucleic acid
(E) block translation of viral nucleic acid

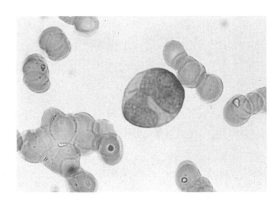

See color insert following page 270. (Photograph courtesy of Chi V. Dang, MD, PhD. From Stobo et al; *The Principles and Practice of Medicine 23/E*, Appleton & Lange, 1996, plate 8D.)

46. Auer rods are most characteristic of

(A) chronic lymphocytic leukemia
(B) acute lymphoblastic leukemia
(C) chronic myelocytic leukemia
(D) acute myeloblastic leukemia
(E) erythroleukemia (Di Guglielmo's syndrome)

47. The most common problem associated with use of nonsteroidal antiinflammatory agents, such as ibuprofen and naproxen, is

(A) toxic amblyopia
(B) fluid retention
(C) gastrointestinal complaints
(D) renal failure
(E) drowsiness

48. A 35-year-old man is admitted to the hospital for an elective operation. After 3 days in the hospital, during which various examinations are performed, he receives general anesthesia for an abdominal operation. Two days after the operation he becomes agitated and accusatory, is visibly tremulous, and seems to be hallucinating. In relation to this man's agitation and possible hallucinations, a history of which of the following would have the most immediate relevance in management plans?

(A) schizophrenia in the family
(B) alcoholism
(C) LSD use
(D) depression
(E) traumatic early childhood

49. The tensor veli palatini muscle is innervated by which of the following nerves?

(A) the facial
(B) the trigeminal
(C) the glossopharyngeal
(D) the vagus
(E) the ansa cervicalis

DIRECTIONS (Questions 50 through 60): Each group of items in this section consists of a list of lettered headings followed by a set of numbered words or phrases. For each numbered word or phrase, select the ONE lettered heading that is most closely associated with it. Each lettered heading may be selected once, more than once, or not at all.

Questions 50 through 52

For each description below, choose the organ with which it is associated.

(A) muscle
(B) liver
(C) red blood cell
(D) brain
(E) adipose tissue

50. Uses only glucose for energy but can adapt to use ketone bodies after long periods of starvation

51. Releases free fatty acids to the bloodstream

52. Produces ketone bodies

Questions 53

For the statement below, choose the most appropriate virus.

    (A) influenza virus
    (B) rubeola virus
    (C) human immunodeficiency virus
    (D) poliomyelitis virus
    (E) herpes virus

53. Antibodies to viral core protein p24 or the viral envelope glycoprotein gp46 are of diagnostic value

Questions 54

    (A) rifampin
    (B) erythromycin
    (C) puromycin
    (D) chloramphenicol
    (E) gentamicin

54. Blocks translation by mimicking a charged transfer RNA in the ribosome acceptor site

Questions 55

    (A) Yellow fever virus
    (B) Smallpox virus
    (C) Corona virus
    (D) Polyoma virus
    (E) Influenza virus

55. Hemagglutination mediated by what is called H (or HA) glycoprotein

Questions 56 and 57

For each statement below choose the MOST appropriate condition listed.

    (A) chondroma
    (B) osteogenic sarcoma
    (C) osteoid osteoma
    (D) chondrosarcoma
    (E) multiple endochondromatosis

56. A benign tumor composed of bone and osteoid

57. A malignant tumor composed of cartilage

Questions 58 through 60

For each of the following agents, select the pharmacologic effect with which it is associated.

    (A) blockade of muscarinic receptors
    (B) selective blockade of β_1-adrenergic receptors
    (C) inhibition of breakdown of cholinergic neurotransmitters
    (D) stimulation of α_1-adrenergic receptors
    (E) blockade of nicotinic receptors

58. *d*-Tubocurarine

59. Physostigmine

60. Atropine

DIRECTIONS (Questions 60 through 111): Each of the numbered items or incomplete statements in this section is followed by answers or by completions of the statement. Select the ONE lettered answer or completion that is BEST in each case.

61. At her child's 2-month "well baby" visit, a mother says she is quite distressed that her baby vomits after every feeding. The baby, who weighed 3.4 kg (7 lb, 8 oz) at birth, now weighs 6.0 kg (13 lb, 2 oz). The most likely cause of the baby's vomiting is

 (A) pyloric stenosis
 (B) overfeeding
 (C) adrenogenital syndrome
 (D) child abuse
 (E) inborn error in metabolism

62. During a routine physical examination, a child is observed to do the following: assume a sitting position without assistance; transfer objects from one hand to the other; stand, but only briefly, by holding someone's hand; and say "ma ma," "ba ba," and "da da." Assuming that the child has had normal growth and development to date, the age of this child is most likely to be

 (A) 5 months
 (B) 6 months
 (C) 8 months
 (D) 10 months
 (E) 12 months

63. An infant with hyaline membrane disease is being treated with supplemental oxygen. The most accurate way of monitoring this infant's oxygen requirements would be by which of the following tests?

 (A) serial chest roentgenography
 (B) pulmonary function tests
 (C) transcutaneous monitoring
 (D) capillary blood pH and oxygen content
 (E) arterial blood pH and oxygen content

64. A 9-year-old girl has had recurrent pulmonary infections. Chest roentgenography reveals an anterior mediastinal mass. All the following conditions could result in an anterior mediastinal mass EXCEPT

 (A) teratoma
 (B) thymoma
 (C) lymphoma
 (D) thymic cyst
 (E) bronchogenic cyst

65. Pubertal changes in adolescent girls typically progress in which of the following sequences?

 (A) sparse pubic hair, breast buds, darker pubic hair, axillary hair
 (B) sparse pubic hair, breast buds, axillary hair, darker pubic hair
 (C) breast buds, axillary hair, sparse pubic hair, darker pubic hair
 (D) breast buds, sparse pubic hair, axillary hair, darker pubic hair
 (E) breast buds, sparse pubic hair, darker pubic hair, axillary hair

66. A 57-year-old man complains of severe crushing chest pain while at work; he then collapses. A fellow worker rushes to his aid, notes absence of carotid pulses and spontaneous breathing efforts, and initiates cardiopulmonary resuscitation. The victim is brought to the hospital and, despite continued resuscitative efforts, dies in the emergency room. Which of the following statements is true concerning this type of death?

 (A) the vast majority of victims have no underlying cardiac disease
 (B) the precipitating rhythm disturbance is most commonly complete heart block
 (C) survivors are at increased risk for future infarcts
 (D) premature ventricular contractions on routine ECG are not associated with increased risk
 (E) it is a relatively rare type of death

See color insert following page 270. (Photograph courtesy of A. Brian West. From Jenson & Baltimore, *Pediatric Infectious Diseases,* Appleton & Lange, 1995, plate 2H.)

67. An 83-year-old widow has severe left-lower-quadrant abdominal pain, nausea, and vomiting. Her abdomen is distended but compressible, and frequent bowel sounds are heard. Her abdominal roentgenogram is shown below. The next step in management would be

   (A) colonoscopy
   (B) gastric lavage
   (C) abdominal ultrasonography
   (D) hemicolectomy
   (E) percutaneous drainage

68. A 29-year-old man has had malaise, myalgias, and chills for 4 weeks. On examination he is slightly jaundiced and has mild right-upper-quadrant tenderness. His SGOT, SGPT, and serum bilirubin levels are all twice normal. Serum serologies are as follows:

   hepatitis B surface antigen—negative
   hepatitis B e antigen—negative
   antibody to hepatitis B surface antigen—
     negative
   antibody to hepatitis B core antigen—
     positive

   These results support the conclusion that the man described

   (A) is in the incubation phase of hepatitis B infection
   (B) is a chronic carrier of hepatitis B virus
   (C) has had a recent hepatitis B infection
   (D) has never been exposed to hepatitis B virus
   (E) has just been exposed to hepatitis B virus

69. Calcium channel blockers are effective for all of the following EXCEPT

   (A) slowing the ventricular response to atrial fibrillation
   (B) termination of paroxysmal atrial tachycardia
   (C) treatment of vasospastic and fixed coronary artery disease
   (D) treatment of ventricular tachycardia
   (E) treatment of hypertension

See color insert following page 270. (Photographs courtesy of Bruce Benjamin. From Benjamin B: *A Colour Atlas of Pediatric Otorhinolaryngology*. Martin Dunitz Publishers/JB Lippincott. 1995: 291, 292.)

70. A 4-year-old boy has inspiratory stridor. All the following disorders cause inspiratory stridor EXCEPT

(A) epiglottitis

(B) acute bronchospasm

(C) infectious laryngotracheitis

(D) aspiration of a foreign body

(E) angioneurotic edema

71. Which of the following diagnostic tests is most likely to reveal osteomyelitis in a child who stepped on a nail 4 days ago?

(A) roentgenogram of the foot

(B) technetium bone scan

(C) gallium bone scan

(D) CT scan of the foot

(E) blood count and sedimentation rate

72. Turner's syndrome is associated with all the following abnormalities EXCEPT

(A) aortic stenosis

(B) coarctation of the aorta

(C) lack of sexual maturation

(D) cubitus valgus

(E) short stature

73. In the initial psychiatric interview, it is most important to

(A) establish a working alliance

(B) examine cognitive mental status

(C) recognize transference

(D) obtain a patient history

(E) assess motivation for change

74. All the following statements are true concerning chloramphenicol EXCEPT

(A) it may cause gray baby syndrome

(B) it is readily absorbed from the gastrointestinal tract

(C) it is effective for treating severe *Salmonella* infection

(D) it may cause brown discoloration of teeth in newborns

(E) it may cause idiosyncratic aplastic anemia

75. A 67-year-old man has a long history of constipation and recurrent, brief episodes of gripping lower-abdominal pain. He is currently asymptomatic. A recent barium enema roentgenogram is shown on page 262. Which of the following treatments would be most appropriate?

(A) surgical resection

(B) colonoscopy with biopsy

(C) administration of a histamine receptor antagonist

(D) administration of a corticosteroid rectal enema

(E) administration of bulk-producing colloids

76. In psychiatry, the term *psychosis* best refers to a disorder in

(A) cognition

(B) perception

(C) mood

(D) reality testing

(E) impulse control

77. The most commonly used chemical preservative in the food industry is

(A) sugar

(B) salt

(C) sulfur dioxide

(D) carbon dioxide

(E) benzoic acid

Figure for use with question 75.

78. Which of the following statements regarding human breast-feeding or breast milk is NOT correct?

(A) human breast milk contains IgA

(B) human breast milk contains maternal macrophages

(C) infants being exclusively breast-fed should receive supplemental iron

(D) infants being exclusively breast-fed should receive supplemental fluoride after 6 months of age

(E) infants being exclusively breast-fed should receive supplemental vitamin C

See color insert following page 270. (Photograph courtesy of Andrew P. Schachat, MD. From Stobo, T*he Principles and Practice of Medicine, 23/E*, Appleton & Lange, 1996, plate 7B.)

79. A slightly drowsy 42-year-old man is admitted with severe diabetic ketoacidosis, nausea, serum potassium of 6.1 mEq/L, and a BUN of 46 mg/dL. Which of the following statements is correct regarding this patient?

(A) despite the high serum potassium, his total body potassium is depleted and potassium replacement should be started at once

(B) the need to initiate potassium replacement is determined primarily by repeated measurements of serum potassium

(C) initial replacement should consist of 120 mEq of potassium given orally over a 4-hour period

(D) administration of bicarbonate to treat the acidosis may hasten the development of hypokalemia and magnify its intensity

(E) intravenous administration of potassium should not exceed 15 mEq/hour

80. The most common cause of a lower gastrointestinal bleed is

(A) colon cancer
(B) upper GI bleed
(C) colonic diverticuli
(D) colonic arteriovenous malformation
(E) colonic at adenomatas polyp

81. All the following phrases correctly characterize delusions EXCEPT

(A) false beliefs incongruent with an individual's experience
(B) common in schizophrenic disorders
(C) common in mania
(D) common in personality disorders
(E) resistant to empathic and logical argument

82. Bacterial contamination is LEAST likely to occur with which of the following commercial methods of food storage?

(A) pasteurization
(B) canning
(C) refrigeration
(D) freezing
(E) drying

83. Which of the following statements regarding brain tumors in children is NOT correct?

(A) seizures are the most common presenting complaint
(B) short stature is occasionally the presenting sign
(C) sexual precocity is occasionally the presenting sign
(D) half or more of the tumors arise in the posterior fossa
(E) half or more of the tumors occur in the midline

84. A 39-year-old woman has the sudden onset of weakness and "fluttering" in her chest. She is pale; her pulse is 160/min and irregularly irregular; and her blood pressure is 82/64 mm Hg. Her ECG is shown below. Immediate treatment of choice is

(A) digitalis
(B) verapamil
(C) quinidine
(D) coumarin
(E) cardioversion

85. Seminoma of the testicle is correctly described by all of the following statements EXCEPT

(A) it is the most common germinal testicular tumor
(B) it is more prevalent in cryptorchidism
(C) it is highly radioresistant
(D) it spreads through the lymphatics
(E) prognosis is excellent

Figure for use with question 84.

86. Antidepressant medications would be least effective in the treatment of which of the following psychiatric disorders?

   (A) bulimia
   (B) obsessive–compulsive disorder
   (C) delusional (paranoid) disorder
   (D) panic disorder
   (E) atypical depression

87. Under Social Security Administration (SSA) rules, a disabled worker is described as one who

   (A) can no longer perform the same type of work as previously
   (B) can no longer perform the same amount of work as previously
   (C) can no longer work at all
   (D) can no longer engage in gainful activity
   (E) has not been able to work for 6 months or more

88. A drug of choice for treating children who have petit mal or absence seizure is

   (A) ethosuximide
   (B) phenytoin
   (C) diazepam
   (D) diphenhydramine
   (E) phenobarbital

89. A 28-year-old man has the acute onset of gross hematuria and colicky pain in the left costovertebral angle radiating into the groin. Abdominal roentgenography discloses a stone in the left ureter. The man spontaneously passes the stone. The most likely cause of this stone is

   (A) chronic urinary tract infections
   (B) vitamin D excess
   (C) primary hyperparathyroidism
   (D) idiopathic hypercalciuria
   (E) gout

90. All the following statements concerning pericardial tamponade are correct EXCEPT

   (A) central venous pressure is elevated
   (B) pulse pressure is elevated
   (C) left atrial pressure measurement is not helpful in the diagnosis
   (D) normal cardiac shadow on chest roentgenogram does not rule out the diagnosis
   (E) pericardiocentesis is helpful in the diagnosis

91. A 30-year-old man is brought unconscious to the local emergency room. Supportive measures are initiated. Physical examination is remarkable for hyperactive deep-tendon reflexes and abdominal scars that suggest numerous surgical procedures. The man is admitted for intensive care observation. A few hours later he becomes responsive but screams that he is blind. Neurologic work-up is unremarkable; a CT scan of the head is negative, although he refuses the contrast-dye study because of allergy. Upon entering the man's room the next morning, his physician finds him reading. When confronted, the man becomes angry and storms out of the hospital. The most likely diagnosis is

   (A) chronic factitious disorder
   (B) conversion disorder
   (C) antisocial personality disorder
   (D) schizophrenia
   (E) drug abuse

92. Nosocomial infections lead to excess health care cost. In terms of the proportion of excess direct cost in US hospitals, the most costly are infections of the

   (A) urinary tract
   (B) surgical wound
   (C) respiratory tract
   (D) bloodstream
   (E) other nosocomial infections

93. A 22-year-old primigravid woman is in premature labor at 30 weeks' gestation. Despite administration of tocolytics to stop labor, it appears that she is likely to deliver soon. Pulmonary maturity in the fetus might be enhanced by the administration of

(A) magnesium sulfate
(B) betamethasone
(C) hydroxyprogesterone
(D) chloroprocaine
(E) bupivacaine

94. Which of the following statements regarding basal skull fractures in children is NOT correct?

(A) can result in ecchymosis around the eyes (raccoon eyes sign)
(B) can result in ecchymosis overlying the mastoid bone (Battle's sign)
(C) may be associated with nasal discharge of cerebrospinal fluid
(D) associated with increased risk of bacterial meningitis
(E) generally are easily recognized on skull roentgenographic films

95. A 74-year-old woman complains of progressive weakness, anorexia, and weight loss. She appears dehydrated and lethargic; her temperature is 38.9°C (102°F); pulse is 100/min; respirations are 20/min; and blood pressure is 90/70 mm Hg. She is cachectic, and her skin has increased pigmentation. Serum sodium level is 129 mEq/L, potassium is 5.7 mEq/L, BUN is 59 mg/dL, and glucose is 88 mg/dL. Immediate management would consist of intravenous administration of

(A) antibiotics
(B) hypertonic sodium chloride solution
(C) sodium bicarbonate
(D) arginine vasopressin
(E) hydrocortisone

96. A patient receiving prophylactic oral ampicillin develops colicky abdominal pain, diarrhea, fever, abdominal distention, and leukocytosis. Sigmoidoscopic examination reveals yellowish-white, raised mucosal plaques separated by edematous hyperemic mucosa. The antibiotic of choice for treating this condition is

(A) clindamycin
(B) penicillin
(C) metromidazole
(D) sulfa preparations
(E) erythromycin

97. Central dopamine receptor blockade is the mechanism of action of which of the following classes of psychotropic drugs?

(A) antipsychotics
(B) antidepressants
(C) anxiolytics
(D) hypnotics
(E) antiparkinsonian drugs

98. All the following statements about the chi-square test are true EXCEPT

(A) it is designed to compare two proportions in paired or independent samples
(B) it can be expanded to the comparison of several proportions
(C) it can compare measured quantities, ranks, or percentages
(D) it involves the concept of degrees of freedom
(E) it is a relatively simple formula to understand and apply

99. A pregnant insulin-requiring diabetic woman is receiving weekly nonstress tests. Her nonstress test at 32 weeks is somewhat equivocal. It is repeated the next day and still found to be equivocal. An oxytocin challenge test is performed, which is read as showing no distress. The proper procedure at this point would be to

(A) repeat the nonstress test in 5 to 7 days
(B) perform an emergency cesarean section
(C) order daily estriol determinations
(D) perform amniocentesis to determine the lecithin/sphingomyelin (L/S) ratio
(E) order daily human placental lactogen determinations

100. A previously well 8-month-old child is brought to the hospital because of the onset of cyanosis. Except for the presence of cyanosis, which is not relieved by oxygen, physical examination is entirely within normal limits. Arterial blood gas obtained while the child is breathing room air reveals a pH of 7.35 and a Po_2 of 90 torr. The most appropriate drug to administer for this child would be

(A) furosemide

(B) physostigmine

(C) atropine

(D) methylene blue

(E) amyl nitrite

101. A 52-year-old man presents with widespread psoriasis. Disorders associated with this condition include all of the following EXCEPT

(A) Koebner's phenomenon

(B) arthritis

(C) pleurisy

(D) hyperuricemia

(E) pitted nails

See color insert following page 270. (Photograph courtesy of Antoinette F. Hood, MD. From Stobo, *The Principles and Practice of Medicine, 23/E,* Appleton & Lange, 1996, plate 5A.)

102. A 75-year-old man comes to the emergency room because of pain in the abdomen and back. He is found to be hypotensive, with a pulsatile, tender abdominal mass. The correct management of this man consists of

(A) immediate transfer to the operating room

(B) immediate sonography

(C) immediate CT scan

(D) immediate administration of intravenous fluids

(E) work-up in the emergency room to rule out myocardial infarction

103. In the work-up of which of the following individuals would a CT scan of the brain be LEAST indicated?

(A) a 51-year-old woman with confusion of unknown etiology

(B) a 68-year-old man with dementia of unknown etiology

(C) a 19-year-old man with a newly discovered psychosis

(D) a 38-year-old woman with a newly discovered major depression

(E) a 60-year-old woman with a dramatic change in personality

104. An 18-year-old male student comes to you for a precollege physical examination. He states that he drinks alcoholic beverages at least twice each week, and when he does he normally consumes a six-pack. On this evidence, you should advise him that

(A) any consumption of alcoholic beverage above this limit will be dangerous to his health

(B) men should not drink more than six "units" of alcohol a day

(C) he is at no greater risk for illness than his peers

(D) women are at the same risk as men in relation to alcohol consumption

105. All of the following would be considered acceptable therapy for carcinoma in situ of the cervix EXCEPT

(A) cryosurgery
(B) cold-knife conization of the cervix
(C) laser conization of the cervix
(D) total hysterectomy
(E) radical hysterectomy

See color insert following page 270. (Photograph courtesy of Henry M. Feder, Jr. From Jenson & Baltimore, *Pediatric Infectious Diseases,* Appleton & Lange, 1995, plate 3F.)

106. A 7-year-old boy has red cheeks that have a slapped appearance. He also has a generalized rash in a lacy, reticular pattern. The most likely diagnosis is

(A) rubeola
(B) rubella
(C) popsicle panniculitis
(D) Kawasaki's disease
(E) erythema infectiosum

107. A 49-year-old woman has had progressive, generalized pruritus for the past 6 weeks. Systemic diseases commonly known to present in this fashion include all of the following EXCEPT

(A) chronic renal failure
(B) systemic lupus erythematosus
(C) primary biliary cirrhosis

(D) polycythemia vera
(E) hyperthyroidism

108. Concerning insulinoma, all the following statements are true EXCEPT

(A) the tumor is frequent during the fourth to seventh decades of life
(B) the diagnostic feature is the association of low blood sugar with a high insulin level
(C) approximately 10% of the tumors are malignant
(D) angiography localizes the majority of the tumors
(E) streptozocin is useful in treating malignant tumors

109. The insanity defense in American jurisprudence is correctly described by which of the following statements?

(A) the insanity defense is invoked often in US court cases
(B) the insanity defense often is successful in US court cases
(C) laws toughening the criminal justice system would likely lead to decreased use of the insanity defense
(D) "insanity" is a medical term, not a legal term
(E) none of the above

110. Which organism is discovered to be most responsible as a pathogen for diseases of the lower respiratory tract (pneumonia) in acute care hospitals in the United States?

(A) *Pseudomonas*
(B) *Staphylococcus*
(C) *Klebsiella*
(D) *Enterobacter*
(E) *Escherichia coli*

See color insert following page 270. (Photograph courtesy of Joseph M. Campos. From Jenson & Baltimore, *Pediatric Infectious Diseases,* Appleton & Lange, 1995, plate 1B.)

111. Glomerulonephritis is recognized as a complication of β-hemolytic streptococcal infections. Which of the following statements regarding this condition is true?

  (A) it most frequently occurs in children between the ages of 10 and 14 years
  (B) males are affected twice as often as females
  (C) all strains of streptococci are equally associated
  (D) it frequently recurs
  (E) the prevalence is similar in most population groups

DIRECTIONS (Questions 112 through 120): Each group of items in this section consists of lettered headings followed by a set of numbered words or phrases. For each numbered word or phrase, select the ONE lettered heading that is most closely associated with it. Each lettered heading may be selected once, more than once, or not at all.

Questions 112 and 113

For each congenital condition listed below, select the genetic screening test most commonly employed for its detection.

  (A) fetal blood sampling
  (B) amniotic fluid cell culture
  (C) amniotic fluid analysis
  (D) maternal urinalysis
  (E) ultrasonography

112. Achondroplasia

113. Open meningomyelocele

Questions 114 through 117

For each class of psychoactive drug, select the specific agent that is a member of that class.

  (A) phenelzine
  (B) amitriptyline
  (C) benztropine
  (D) clonazepam
  (E) haloperidol

114. Tricyclic antidepressant

115. Neuroleptic (antipsychotic)

116. MAO inhibitor

117. Benzodiazepine

Questions 118 through 120

For each of the organizations listed below, choose the type of health care planning with which it is usually associated.

  (A) population-based planning
  (B) institution-based planning
  (C) financial planning
  (D) program planning
  (E) morbidity planning

118. Local health department or health systems agency

119. Prepaid health plan or health maintenance organization (HMO)

120. Maternal and child health care system

SETTING I: UNSCHEDULED PATIENTS

Unscheduled patients seeking both urgent and routine care are encountered in both office and clinic settings. The following case studies reflect those types you might encounter in this setting.

DIRECTIONS (Questions 121 through 180): Each of the numbered items or incomplete statements in this section is followed by answers or by completions of the statement. Select the ONE lettered answer or completion that is BEST in each case.

Questions 121 through 124

An 83-year-old woman has her blood pressure checked in the shopping mall. During the test, the nurse asks her if she has had any headaches during the past few months and the woman says yes. The nurse advises her to see her doctor. She calls her doctor's office, and he is out of town. She becomes nervous and decides not to wait for his return. She comes to you because you are the doctor covering for hers. She presents with a blood pressure of 185/85 mm Hg. Blood pressure assessments are repeated during the next three visits scheduled over the next 3 months, and persistently elevated systolic pressures are noted.

121. What is the most appropriate step in this patient's care?

   (A) follow-up for repeat blood pressure visit in 1 month
   (B) initiation of nonpharmacologic approach to blood pressure management
   (C) initiation of diuretic therapy
   (D) initiation of diuretic therapy and ACE inhibitor therapy
   (E) 24-hour blood pressure monitoring

122. This patient numerous cardiovascular changes that accompany normal aging. In comparing resting heart rate and exercise heart rate between this 83-year-old patient and a 33-year-old patient, the older patient has

   (A) a lower resting heart rate and a higher heart rate with exercise
   (B) a higher resting heart rate and a lower heart rate with exercise
   (C) similar resting heart rate and similar heart rate with exercise
   (D) similar resting heart rate and a lower heart rate with exercise
   (E) a lower resting heart rate and a lower heart rate with exercise

123. The average life expectancy of this patient is

   (A) 1 to 2 years
   (B) 2 to 4 years
   (C) 5 to 9 years
   (D) 10 years or greater
   (E) difficult to determine since the patient is already over the expected national average of life expectancy

124. The fastest growing group in America is patients 80 years and older. Which of the following most likely represents the relation between longevity and disability?

   (A) people are living longer than ever and increasingly are in good health up to the last few weeks of life
   (B) while the average life expectancy is not changing, we are seeing less and less chronic illness
   (C) people are living longer than ever before, but more and more people are doing so with increased burdens of disability for increasing years before death
   (D) the maximum achievable human lifespan is likely to increase 10 years by the year 2030
   (E) there is no clear relationship between longevity and disability noted

Questions 125 through 127

An 86-year-old man gets lost while trying to go to the grocery store he has been shopping in for the past 15 years. His daughter is upset by this because she is leaving town for a couple of days and concerned for her father's welfare while she is gone. She decides to bring him to the office for a checkup. She reports that family members are concerned about her father, as they have noted increasing memory impairment over the past year.

125. The most common cause of memory impairment (dementia) like the patient's is

   (A) Alzheimer's disease
   (B) cerebrovascular accidents
   (C) old age
   (D) excessive medication use
   (E) carotid artery stenosis

126. The management of memory impairment (dementia) in this patient should include

   (A) use of multiple psychoactive agents
   (B) environmental cues and reorientation
   (C) acute hospitalization in the supervised setting
   (D) vitamin therapy
   (E) attention to the patient's advanced directives

127. The best office assessment test for dementia concerns evaluation of

   (A) orientation
   (B) registration
   (C) attention and calculation
   (D) recall
   (E) language

Questions 128 through 130

An active 75-year-old woman relocates to your town for a warmer climate. She has hypertension, arthritis, and diabetes and decides to visit the office upon moving in. Her medication regimen includes hydrochlorothiazide, potassium elixir, diltiazem, acetaminophen, ibuprofen, and glipizide.

128. The factor most related to compliance with the medication regimen is

   (A) age
   (B) number of drugs in the regimen
   (C) gender
   (D) number of comorbid diseases
   (E) use of tablets versus use of elixirs

129. Changes with age in the ability to handle drugs is noted for all of the following processes EXCEPT

   (A) absorption
   (B) distribution into fat
   (C) distribution into water
   (D) excretion
   (E) metabolism

130. Six weeks after the initial clinic visit, the patient is seen again for complaints of urinary incontinence. Causal factors related to this incontinence include all of the following EXCEPT

   (A) calcium channel blockers
   (B) restricted mobility
   (C) impaired mentation
   (D) loss of functioning nephrons
   (E) diabetes

Question 31. *(Photograph courtesy of Joseph M. Campos)*

Question 46. *(Photograph courtesy of Chi V. Dang, MD, PhD)*

Question 68. *(Photograph courtesy of A. Brian West)*

Question 70. *(Photographs courtesy of Bruce Benjamin. From Benjamin B: A Colour Atlas of Pediatric Otorhinolaryngology. Martin Dunitz Publishers/JB Lippincott. 1995. 291, 292)*

Question 79. *(Photograph courtesy of Andrew P. Schachat, MD)*

Question 101. *(Photograph courtesy of Antoinette F. Hood, MD)*

Question 106. *(Photograph courtesy of Henry M. Feder, Jr.)*

Question 111. *(Photograph courtesy of Joseph M. Campos)*

Question 141. *(Photograph courtesy of Joseph M. Campos)*

Question 169–171. *(Photograph courtesy of Antoinette F. Hood, MD)*

SETTING II: SCHEDULED APPOINTMENTS

This is an office setting where most patients seen are by appointment. Most of the patients would be known to you; however, you sometimes see patients of your associates. The following case studies reflect those types you might encounter in this setting.

Questions 131 through 136

An 84-year-old hypertensive white male is brought into the office by his daughter. He is a heavy smoker and for the past 4 months has been known to have carcinoma of the lung, for which he has refused treatment. The daughter reports that her father has shown increasing confusion and lethargy over the previous 3 weeks. The daughter requests that you determine the source of his confusion. Physical examination is normal except for a blood pressure of 156/94, early hypertensive retinopathy, a palpable bladder, scattered pulmonary rhonchi, and a very enlarged prostate.

131. Which of the following tests would be LEAST appropriate in the initial work-up?

   (A) serum BUN and creatinine
   (B) urinalysis
   (C) urine electrolytes
   (D) thyroid functions
   (E) CT scan of the chest

132. Laboratory studies demonstrate a hemoglobin of 11.6, white blood cell count of 12.5, blood urea nitrogen of 87, serum creatinine of 4.8, and mildly abnormal liver function tests. Of the following studies, which would be LEAST likely to confirm the tentative diagnosis?

   (A) CT scan of the abdomen
   (B) intravenous pyelogram
   (C) plain film of the kidneys, ureter, and bladder
   (D) ultrasound of the abdomen
   (E) retrograde ureterography

133. The most appropriate additional diagnostic procedure at this time is

   (A) suprapubic aspiration
   (B) repeat rectal examination
   (C) cystoscopy
   (D) insertion of a Foley catheter
   (E) pelvic ultrasound

134. Outlet obstruction may be ruled out if

   (A) suprapubic aspiration reveals pyuria
   (B) less than 30 mL urine are obtained by catheterization
   (C) KUB films are negative
   (D) physician is unable to pass Foley catheter
   (E) renal arteriography is normal

135. While appropriate diagnosis is made and initial treatment begun, the patient is noted to be increasingly lethargic and confused. Repeat BUN is found to be 98, with a creatinine of 5, potassium of 6, and blood pressure of 88/60. He refuses to be admitted to the hospital. Of the following options, which should NOT be considered?

   (A) increased ingestion of magnesium compounds
   (B) restriction of protein intake
   (C) expansion of volume
   (D) adjustment of total caloric intake to 35 to 50 kcal/kg/day
   (E) correction of acidosis

136. Despite conservative measures, the patient becomes progressively lethargic and expires. The greatest fear of the dying patient is

   (A) pain and loss of control
   (B) how the survivors will manage
   (C) suffering alone and being deserted
   (D) financial

Questions 137 through 146

A 34-year-old white male presents to the office with a 2-month history of low-grade fever, weight loss, easy fatigability, and anorexia. He admits to a history of IV drug abuse. Physical examination is positive for subungual splinter hemorrhages. Cardiac auscultation is unremarkable. Laboratory studies include a negative HIV test, normochromic, normocytic anemia with a normal white blood cell count. Rheumatoid factor is positive.

137. The most likely diagnosis at this stage of evaluation would be

   (A) false negative HIV infection
   (B) rheumatoid arthritis
   (C) infective endocarditis
   (D) pyelonephritis
   (E) tuberculosis

138. Appropriate additional studies confirm a diagnosis of infective endocarditis. Which of the following statements is NOT correct?

   (A) up to 10% of patients have no murmur
   (B) clubbing and splenomegaly are common
   (C) retinal infarcts may be noted
   (D) Osler's nodes are tender nodules in fingers and toes
   (E) a single positive blood culture is inadequate to make the diagnosis of infective endocarditis

139. The pathogenesis of infective endocarditis involves all of the following EXCEPT

   (A) endothelial damage secondary to turbulent flow across a valve lesion
   (B) vegetations secondary to platelet-fibrin thrombus
   (C) transient bacteremia seeding from the sinuses, gums, or other locations
   (D) multiplication of the bacteria outside the thrombus
   (E) extension of infection to supporting valve structures

140. Of the following, which condition is MOST likely to be associated with infective endocarditis?

   (A) chronic CHF
   (B) chronic atrial fibrillation
   (C) atrial septal defect
   (D) mitral valve prolapse
   (E) purely stenotic valvular lesions

See color insert following page 270. (Photograph courtesy of Joseph M. Campos. From Jenson & Baltimore, *Pediatric Infectious Diseases*, Appleton & Lange, 1995, plate 1A.)

141. In the case presented, the most common infecting organism would be

   (A) group D streptococci
   (B) *Streptococcus viridans*
   (C) gram-negative bacilli
   (D) *Staphylococcus aureus*
   (E) fungi

142. In the case presented, the most common valve affected would be

   (A) tricuspid
   (B) mitral
   (C) aortic
   (D) pulmonary

143. Treatment of infective endocarditis should include high-enough antimicrobial concentration to eradicate all microorganisms from the vegetation. For enterococcal endocarditis, which of the following is MOST effective?

(A) cephalosporins

(B) penicillin G

(C) penicillin plus an aminoglycoside

(D) vancomycin

(E) nafcillin

144. The most common cause of recurrent fever during treatment of infective endocarditis is

(A) drug reaction

(B) drug resistance

(C) noncompliance

(D) factitious

(E) emboli

145. Complications of infective endocarditis include all of the following EXCEPT

(A) glomerulonephritis

(B) arthritis

(C) myocarditis

(D) meningitis

(E) urethritis

146. Prophylaxis of endocarditis in patients with valvular heart disease undergoing dental work may include all of the following EXCEPT

(A) ampicillin plus gentamicin IV or IM

(B) penicillin V orally

(C) cephalosporins IM or IV

(D) vancomycin IV

(E) erythromycin orally

Questions 147 through 150

A 16-year-old female presents to the office with a 2-week history of lethargy, low-grade fever, sore throat, and swollen glands. She has been absent from school during this time and has not yet sought medical care. She reports being exposed to a friend with mononucleosis 50 days previously. Examination is remarkable only for a temperature of 100.2°F and epitrochlear adenopathy.

147. Which of the following additional studies would be of LEAST importance in the initial evaluation of this case?

(A) heterophil titer

(B) complete blood count

(C) bone marrow examination

(D) HIV

(E) rapid strep screen

148. Which of the following is incorrect regarding infectious mononucleosis?

(A) the incubation period is 30 to 50 days

(B) most patients will complain of headache and malaise

(C) abdominal pain and hepatomegaly are usually noted

(D) complications may include encephalitis and seizures

(E) absolute lymphocytosis is present in about 75% of cases

149. Of the following, which is the correct statement regarding the potential complications of infectious mononucleosis?

(A) hepatitis is common

(B) neurologic complications never present as the sole symptom

(C) no hematologic complications have been observed

(D) electrocardiogram abnormalities and coronary artery spasm are not observed complications of mononucleosis

(E) splenic rupture may occur in 52% of cases

150. Parents of adolescents with mononucleosis should be advised of all of the following EXCEPT

(A) the disorder is self-limiting

(B) contact sports should be avoided for 6 to 8 weeks after the onset of the illness

(C) recovery may be gradual

(D) return to school or work is determined solely by symptoms

(E) fever is infrequently present during the course of the disease

Questions 151 through 154

A teenage first-time mother brings her newborn into the office. The infant is 2 weeks old. There is a family history of autism in several cousins on the father's side and cerebral palsy in one of the mother's cousins. The parent has numerous concerns regarding the infant's normal expected motor and social development and behavior patterns.

151. Which of the following is correct regarding the expected social behavior during the first year of life?

    (A) during the newborn period, there is a visual preference for the human face

    (B) social smile is noted at 20 weeks

    (C) response to sound of the child's name takes place at 5 months

    (D) playing peekaboo is noted at about 3 to 4 months

    (E) waves bye-bye at 18 weeks

152. Which of the following is INCORRECT regarding motor behavior during the first year of life?

    (A) walks with one hand held at 52 weeks

    (B) creeps or crawls at 12 weeks

    (C) sits up alone and indefinitely without support, back straight at 40 weeks

    (D) when prone, turns head side to side at 4 weeks

    (E) head lags on pull to sitting at 8 weeks

153. Of the following reflexes, which reflex would NOT be expected to be noted upon newborn examination?

    (A) Moro's

    (B) stepping

    (C) sucking and rooting

    (D) placing

    (E) Landau's

154. Persistence of tonic neck reflexes beyond 9 months may indicate which of the following?

    (A) hypothyroidism

    (B) usually normal finding

    (C) central motor lesions

    (D) possible nutritional disorder

    (E) meningitis

SETTING III: HOSPITAL ROUNDS

Hospital Rounds can include general medical service, critical care units, pediatric, geriatric, or obstetric services. The following case studies reflect those types you might encounter in this setting.

Questions 155 through 158

A 79-year-old woman falls in a grocery store and is taken to a local community hospital. A diagnosis of hip fracture is made in the hospital emergency room and the patient is subsequently hospitalized.

155. All of the following statements regarding hip fractures in the elderly are true EXCEPT

    (A) most hip fractures occur in patients 65 and older

    (B) hip fractures accompany 50% of falls in this age group

    (C) risk factors attributable to hip fracture include cognitive impairment, psychoactive medications, and poor vision or balance

    (D) subcapital hip fractures result in a distribution of blood flow to the femoral head

    (E) intertrochanteric hip fractures result in no disruption of blood flow to the femoral head

156. After repair of the hip fracture, the patient is considered for anticoagulation therapy during her hospital stay. Which of the following therapeutic strategies represents the best management of anticoagulation in this elderly patient?

    (A) no anticoagulation is needed, as the risks of bleeding far outweigh the benefits in respect to deep-vein thrombosis

    (B) anticoagulation should be initiated, and a target prothrombin time of 15 should be the gold standard of therapy

(C) anticoagulation should be initiated, and a target prothrombin time of 24 should be the gold standard of therapy

(D) anticoagulation should be initiated, and a target INR level of 2.0 should be the gold standard of therapy

(E) anticoagulation should be initiated, and a combination of heparin and dextran therapy is indicated

157. During the patient's hospital stay, the patient develops a pneumonia with fever, treated with antibiotics. In addition, as a result of the patient's lack of access to water and immobile state, the patient becomes dehydrated and is treated with intravenous fluids. On approximately the third hospital day, the patient is known to be confused and asking to see the hairdresser for her three o'clock appointment. The diagnosis of delirium is suggested by this presentation. The best test for delirium in this patient is

(A) serum ammonia level
(B) attention and calculation
(C) delayed recall
(D) confrontational naming
(E) generative naming

158. Contributing factors to the patient's delirium include all the following EXCEPT

(A) medications
(B) electrolyte imbalance
(C) nutritional deficiency
(D) Alzheimer's disease
(E) immobility

Questions 159 through 161

An 89-year-old male is admitted to the hospital with a diagnosis of acute myocardial infarction.

159. Which of the following statements is true regarding the acute management of myocardial infarction (MI) in the elderly?

(A) thrombolysis is contraindicated because of the increased risk of bleeding in the elderly

(B) beta-blockers are contraindicated because of the risk of central nervous system side effects

(C) aggressive use of anticoagulation is inappropriate because of the risk of bleeding

(D) 20% of all MI deaths occur in patients 65 and older

(E) inpatient mortality rates reach 33% in patients 75 and older

160. After a prolonged stay in the intensive care unit, the patient was transferred to the stepdown unit on the medical service. A decubitus ulcer was noted by the nursing staff. Factors contributing to the pathogenesis of decubitus ulcer include all of the following EXCEPT

(A) pressure
(B) shear
(C) immobility
(D) friction
(E) moisture

161. The following are true concerning the management of decubitus ulcers EXCEPT

(A) the hospital prevalence for the disease approaches 10%

(B) about two-thirds of ulcers occur in patients over the age of 70

(C) this disorder is not associated with mortality and morbidity but represents a minor complication in many older patients

(D) common areas for ulcers include the sacral ischial tuberosity and calcaneus

(E) the most common complication of decubitus ulcers is infection

Questions 162 and 163

An energetic alert 80-year-old male is admitted to the hospital for elective treatment of abdominal aortic aneurysm. The patient has congestive heart failure that is well controlled with a combination of digoxin, angiotensin-converting enzyme inhibitor, and diuretic therapies. The blood pressure is 160/90 without postural changes, heart sounds are normal, and no jugular venus distention is present. Roentgenographic films and routine laboratory and urine testings are unremarkable.

162. All the following characteristics increase the risk of cardiac complications of surgery EXCEPT

    (A) age over 70
    (B) emergent operation
    (C) intra-abdominal procedure
    (D) echocardiogram ejection fraction less than 30%
    (E) $PO_2 < 60$

163. Using the Goldman Cardiac Risk Index, this patient's risks of cardiac death or life-threatening complications are:

    (A) 2% death, 5% life-threatening
    (B) 2% death, 11% life-threatening
    (C) 10% death, 30% life-threatening
    (D) 22% death, 56% life-threatening
    (E) unable to calculate

Questions 164 through 168

A 77-year-old female smoker with a history of chronic obstructive lung disease is maintained on theophylline and albuterol. The patient has an acute exacerbation of bronchospasm requiring hospitalization on the medical service.

164. All the following medications are useful for the treatment of acute exacerbation of chronic obstructive lung disease EXCEPT

    (A) ipratropium
    (B) beta-adrenergic drugs
    (C) oxygen

    (D) inhaled corticosteroids
    (E) intravenous corticosteroids

165. Changes that accompany normal aging with reference to the pulmonary system include all of the following EXCEPT

    (A) increased chest compliance
    (B) decreased resting PO_2
    (C) increased residual volume
    (D) decreased lung elasticity
    (E) decreased respiratory muscle strength

166. Results of admission laboratory tests are now available in the medical record. Routine laboratory screening that was done is remarkable for the urine culture with 100 000 colonies/cc per milliliter. The patient has no complaints of urinary burning, urinary frequency, or urinary urgency. The most common organism associated with infection is

    (A) *Escherichia coli*
    (B) *Pseudomonas aeruginosa*
    (C) *Klebsiella pneumoniae*
    (D) *Proteus mirabilis*
    (E) normal urinary flora

167. Which of the following statements is true concerning the management of this patient's clinical condition?

    (A) discharge should be delayed until the infection is treated
    (B) treatment eradicates bacteria in almost all cases without sequelae
    (C) ciprofloxacin is more effective than ampicillin in the treatment of this disorder
    (D) asymptomatic bacteriuria is a common finding in the older patient and does not require treatment
    (E) descending routes of infection are the most common cause of bacteriuria, and a diagnostic work-up should be initiated

168. The patient has been managed with a variety of medications for COPD and appears ready for discharge. The patient is now complaining of gastritis and symptoms consistent with duodenal ulcer. A decision is made to start the patient on cimetidine therapy, and post-discharge plans are made. One week later the patient presents to your office with tachycardia and vomiting and a serum theophylline level of 25 mg/deciliter (therapeutic range, 10 to 20 mg/dL). What is the most likely explanation for these findings?

(A) noncompliance with theophylline

(B) noncompliance with beta-adrenergic blockers

(C) noncompliance with corticosteroid therapy

(D) interaction between cimetidine and theophylline

(E) interaction between corticosteroids and theophylline

SETTING IV: EMERGENCY DEPARTMENT

In an emergency room, most patients you will see will be new to you. Generally, patients seen here are seeking urgent care. The following case studies reflect those types you might encounter in this setting.

Questions 169 through 171

A 30-year-old woman with a history of intravenous drug abuse presents to the Emergency Department with a chief complaint of a nonproductive cough and shortness of breath for 2 days. Physical examination reveals a cachectic woman in moderate respiratory distress with a blood pressure of 100/60 mm Hg, pulse of 110/min, respiratory rate of 24/min, and temperature of 38.3°C (101°F). Head and neck examinations show temporal wasting, white plaques in the posterior pharynx and on the soft palate, and cervical lymphadenopathy. On auscultation of the chest there are diffuse rhonchi. Room air pulse oximetry reveals a saturation of 91%.

See color insert following page 270. (Photograph courtesy of Antoinette F. Hood, MD. From Stobo et al., *The Principles and Practice of Medicine 23/E*, Appleton & Lange, 1996, plate 2A.)

169. The most likely finding on chest roentgenogram is

(A) none (normal chest radiograph)

(B) lobar infiltrate

(C) diffuse interstitial infiltrates

(D) nodular infiltrates

(E) pleural effusion

170. Laboratory findings to confirm the diagnosis would be an elevation of the

(A) peripheral leukocyte count

(B) serum lactate dehydrogenase

(C) serum glucose

(D) serum sodium

(E) none of the above

171. The most appropriate initial therapy would be

(A) erythromycin, intravenously

(B) trimethoprin-sulfamethoxazole, intravenously

(C) isoniazid, rifampin, and ethambutol, orally

(D) cefuroxime, intravenously

Questions 172 through 174

A 14-year-old boy is brought to the Emergency Department with lower abdominal pain, nausea, and vomiting that occurred shortly after gym class. Physical examination reveals normal vital signs and a nontender abdomen with normal bowel sounds.

172. Which of the following findings on physical examination would suggest torsion of the spermatic cord?

    (A) relief of pain on elevation of the scrotum
    (B) painless, unilateral scrotal swelling
    (C) a visible "blue dot" on the upper pole of the testis
    (D) absent cremasteric reflex
    (E) penile discharge

173. Once the diagnosis of testicular torsion is suspected, the most appropriate next step is to obtain

    (A) radionuclide testicular scan
    (B) emergent urologic consultation
    (C) urine for urinalysis
    (D) Doppler ultrasound
    (E) CT scan

174. The most appropriate next step in management is

    (A) administer intravenous diazepam and place patient in Trendelenburg
    (B) attempt manual detorsion in the Emergency Department
    (C) discharge the patient with scrotal support and urologic follow up
    (D) Foley catheterization
    (E) scrotal elevation and observation in the Emergency Department

Questions 175 through 177

A 70-year-old man presents to the Emergency Department complaining of chest pain. Shortly after arrival, the patient collapses. He has no palpable pulse. A "quick look" with the cardiac monitor reveals ventricular fibrillation.

175. The most important first step is to

    (A) verify the rhythm by checking another lead
    (B) defibrillate with 200 joules
    (C) administer epinephrine 1:10 000 IV
    (D) administer lidocaine 100 mg IV
    (E) administer 100% oxygen by mask

176. In the event that intravenous access is lost, all of the following can be administered via the endotracheal tube EXCEPT

    (A) lidocaine
    (B) epinephrine
    (C) naloxone
    (D) sodium bicarbonate
    (E) atropine

177. All of the following are true concerning ventricular fibrillation EXCEPT

    (A) it is the initial monitored rhythm in approximately two thirds of prehospital cardiac arrests
    (B) it is almost always initiated by a run of ventricular tachycardia
    (C) it is never accompanied by a pulse or blood pressure
    (D) 5% of patients with ventricular fibrillation will survive to discharge
    (E) bretylium is indicated in the treatment of refractory ventricular fibrillation

Questions 178 through 180

A 65-year-old woman comes to the Emergency Department because of epigastric abdominal pain and vomiting for 1 day. She has a past medical history significant for hypertension and diabetes mellitus. On examination she has a blood pressure of 120/70 mm Hg, her pulse is 100/min, and her respirations are 22/min. Examination of her abdomen reveals normal bowel sounds and right-upper-quadrant tenderness. Her electrocardiogram is normal.

178. Other expected physical findings include all of the following EXCEPT

    (A) a palpable gallbladder
    (B) stool positive for occult blood
    (C) fever
    (D) mild icterus
    (E) a positive Murphy's sign

179. The best test to confirm the diagnosis is

    (A) upper GI series
    (B) abdominal sonogram
    (C) radionuclide scanning of the biliary tree
    (D) CT scan of abdomen
    (E) abdominal roentgenogram

180. Laboratory examination reveals an elevated peripheral leukocyte with a left shift, a serum glucose of 455 with trace acetone, and a venous pH of 7.30. The most important immediate therapeutic step is administration of

    (A) fluids, intravenously
    (B) insulin, intravenously
    (C) sodium bicarbonate, by intravenous injection
    (D) cefoxitin, intravenously
    (E) potassium, intravenously

ANSWERS AND EXPLANATIONS

1. **(A)** A wide variety of environmental conditions provoke several mechanisms to come into play to maintain body temperature by balancing heat production and heat loss. The loss of heat by infrared rays (radiation) accounts for more than 60% of normal heat loss. Conduction of heat to objects or to air (ie, convection) accounts for 15%, and evaporation about 25%. Sweating is an important form of heat loss and is regulated by various body mechanisms. Insensible perspiration through the skin and lungs, although important, remains relatively constant despite environmental changes and thus does not provide a major mechanism to regulate body temperature. *(Guyton, pp 911–914)*

2. **(E)** When water that is either higher or lower than body temperature is introduced into the external auditory meatus, convection currents can occur within the endolymph of the inner ear. These currents may result in the stimulation of the semicircular canals by causing movements of the ampullar crests, and vertigo and nausea may ensue. Decreased movement or immobilization of the otoliths is not caused by such changes in temperature. Furthermore, changes in the discharge rate of vestibular afferents, which must occur with caloric stimulation, are most likely to be caused by the changes in the activity of the receptors rather than being a direct response to changes in temperature. *(Ganong, p 166)*

3. **(B)** Except for lipoprotein lipase, which is a blood lipoprotein delipidation enzyme activated by interaction with C-II apolipoproteins, all the enzymes listed in the question are part of cyclic AMP-dependent cascades that are either activated or deactivated by phosphorylation. During stimulation of glycogenolysis (and concurrent inhibition of glycogen synthesis), hormone-stimulated increases in cyclic AMP levels activate protein kinase, which activates phosphorylase kinase by catalyzing its phosphorylation. The protein kinase also inhibits glycogen synthase by catalyzing its phosphorylation. The activated phosphorylase kinase activates glycogen phosphorylase by accelerating its phosphorylation. Triacylglycerol lipase is also activated by phosphorylation after cyclic AMP-medi-

ated stimulation of protein kinases. *(Stryer, pp 590–597,605–606)*

4. **(D)** Hepatitis B virus is practically indestructible. Disposable syringes, needles, and other equipment that may carry the pathogen must be carefully used and discarded. The increased use of drugs in the United States has greatly increased the occurrence of hepatitis B in the population and hence has also increased the danger of transmission by any procedures that involve skin puncture or bleeding. The characteristic incubation period for hepatitis B is 60 to 160 days. Hepatitis A has a much shorter incubation period, 15 to 40 days, and the incubation period of non-A, non-B hepatitis varies widely, with reported incubations from 14 to 77 days. These differences probably reflect variations in the viral growth rate. It is important to note that the longer the incubation period, the longer the individual will be able to spread the agent, either in the feces (in hepatitis A) or via blood transfusions or other means (in hepatitis B and the non-A, non-B form). *(Joklik et al, pp 1039–1047)*

5. **(A)** Aflatoxin is a known potent chemical carcinogen which can produce hepatocellular carcinoma in humans. It is a fungal-derived contaminant of improperly stored foods. An increased incidence of liver cell carcinoma parallels those geographic areas, such as Africa and the Far East, in which aflatoxin-tainted foodstuffs arise. *(Rubin and Farber, p 772)*

6. **(D)** Most benzodiazepines, with the exception of oxazepam, lorazepam, temazepam, triazolam, and midazolam are metabolized to active intermediates, which can significantly prolong the duration of action. This is because the active metabolites undergo a much slower biotransformation than the parent compound. For example, the half-life of flurazepam is 2 to 3 hours, but the half-life of one of its active metabolites is 50 hours. Therefore, the selection of a particular benzodiazepine for its duration of action, must factor in the duration of action of active metabolites as well. *(Hardman et al, pp 368–370)*

7. **(E)** Neurons are so specialized that most are incapable of reproducing themselves. The neuron is the basic unit of the nervous system. The Nissl bodies are basophilic aggregates located in the cell body and dendrites of each neuron. Neurons, unlike most cells, lack the ability to store glycogen. Each neuron contains numerous fibrillar organelles called neurotubules. *(Moore, pp 15–22)*

8. **(A)** Renin secretion directly results in the conversion of angiotensinogen into angiotensin I, which is subsequently converted in the lungs to angiotensin II, a potent vasoconstrictor. Angiotensin induces aldosterone secretion, whose effects on the kidney include increased sodium and water resorption as well as increased potassium secretion. *(Guyton, pp 227–230,363–364)*

9. **(C)** The formation of the three-carbon CoA thioester malonyl CoA from acetyl CoA is the regulatory step of fatty acid synthesis. Acetyl-CoA carboxylase catalyzes this reaction:

$$\text{Acetyl CoA} + \text{HCO}_3 + \text{ATP} \rightleftharpoons$$
$$\text{malonyl CoA} + \text{ADP} + \text{P}_i$$

Citrate, which serves as the means of transport of acetyl CoA from the mitochondria to the cytosolic site of fatty acid synthesis, is the key allosteric regulator of acetyl-CoA carboxylase. It shifts the enzyme from an inactive protomer to an active filamentous polymer. The end product of the cytosolic fatty acid synthetase complex, palmitoyl CoA, inhibits the carboxylase. Although acetyl-CoA carboxylase is the prime regulatory enzyme of fatty acid synthesis, it is not a part of the fatty acid synthetase complex, the site where most of the reactions of fatty acid synthesis take place. *(Stryer, pp 614–617)*

10. **(C)** Ampicillin is a bactericidal antibiotic because it inhibits cell wall synthesis, which leads to lysis and death of the ampicillin-susceptible bacterial cells. Erythromycin, chloramphenicol, and tetracycline inhibit bacterial protein synthesis that is not associated

with the lysis or death of the bacterial cell. Bacteria remain viable but cannot multiply. Therefore, these antibiotics, as well as sulfonamides, which are competitive inhibitors of *p*-aminobenzoic acid, are bacteriostatic antibiotics. *(Joklik, pp 154–160,173–175)*

11. **(D)** Hirschsprung's disease (idiopathic megacolon) usually appears soon after birth, with abdominal distention, failure to pass stool, and, occasionally, acute intestinal obstruction. The pathogenesis involves abnormal functioning and coordination of the propulsive forces in the distal segment of the large bowel. This motility disorder occurs because of an absence of parasympathetic ganglion cells in the submucosal and myenteric plexus, the diagnostic histologic feature of Hirschsprung's disease. Hypertrophied, disorganized nonmyelinated nerve fibers are often identified in place of ganglion cells. The length of large bowel involved varies. Proximal to the involved segment, however, the colon may be dilated and hypertrophied. The mucosa often appears normal or inflamed. A full-thickness rectal biopsy is the standard procedure employed in diagnosis. Mucosal polyps are not associated with Hirschsprung's disease. *(Rubin & Farber, pp 671–672)*

12. **(D)** Tamoxifen is a nonsteroidal compound used in the treatment of breast carcinoma in postmenopausal women. It acts by competing with estrogen for the estrogen receptor, thus blocking the growth-promoting effects of the hormone on estrogen-dependent tumors. Vincristine is a vinca alkaloid that disrupts the mitotic spindle. Bleomycin causes DNA strand breakage. Busulfan and melphalan are alkylating agents. *(Hardman, pp 1275–1276)*

13. **(E)** The ego functions include emotions, defense mechanisms, and cognitive and perceptual functions. The ego is the agent of the personality system that mediates between the demands of the id, which is the reservoir of instinctual drives, and the demands of the superego, which represents parental and societal values. The ego also mediates between the personality system and external reality. *(Kaplan and Sadock, pp 247–248)*

14. **(B)** The hypoglossal nerve emerges from the sulcus between the olive and pyramid. The third, sixth, and twelfth cranial nerves emerge from the anterior brainstem in a longitudinal line just lateral to the midsagittal plane. The fifth, seventh, ninth, tenth, and eleventh cranial nerves emerge from the lateral aspect of the brainstem. *(Noback, pp 8–9)*

15. **(D)** Iron is readily absorbed by mucosal cells in the intestine, primarily in the duodenum and the jejunum. The major form in which iron is absorbed is as ferrous ions. After the ions have entered the cells, a complex of ferric hydroxyphosphate, surrounded by the 24-subunit protein apoferritin, may form. This complex, known as ferritin, is the principal storage form of iron within cells, accounting for approximately 30% of the iron within the body. *(Ganong, pp 440–441)*

16. **(C)** Cholesterol is required by all eukaryotic cells. It is a major component of the plasma membranes of these cells. Cholesterol is transported in the bloodstream to peripheral tissues largely in the form of low-density lipoprotein. LDL can be taken up by those tissues that require cholesterol. The uptake of LDL is mediated by LDL receptors on the cell surface. *(Stryer, pp 697–701)*

17. **(D)** *Mycoplasma* organisms do not have a cell wall and are therefore resistant to penicillin. Other forms of bacteria that have lost parts or all of their cell wall are spheroplasts and protoplasts, which are formed from gram-negative and gram-positive bacteria, respectively, through the action of penicillin or by other procedures that remove the cell wall or interfere with its formation. The other organisms listed in the question are all susceptible to the action of penicillin, although certain strains of *Gonococcus* have acquired a β-lactamase-producing plasmid. Tetracyclines, erythromycin, and the aminoglycosides are effective antibiotics for the treatment of mycoplasmal infections. *(Joklik et al, pp 730–737)*

18. **(B)** Atheroclerosis is he most common cause of aortic abdominal aneurysms in the United States. These aneurysms are rare before age 50 and are more common in males than in females. Hemodynamic and genetic factors may potentiate the development of the aneurysms. Small asymptomatic aneurysms may be inconsequential. Larger aneurysms, particularly those that are symptomatic, may be treated surgically. (*Cotran, pp 500–501*)

19. **(A)** The mainstay therapy of many forms of rheumatoid arthritis is nonsteroidal anti-inflammatory drugs (NSAIDs). Aspirin is the prototype and is used to reduce symptoms of swelling, fever, or pain associated with arthritis. It does not affect tissue proliferation or alter the course of the disease. Numerous other NSAIDs are available including indomethacin, phenylbutazone, ibuprofen, sulindac, and piroxicam. The selection of these agents for use in arthritis remains somewhat arbitrary. Acetaminophen is a useful antipyretic and analgesic that is without significant anti-inflammatory action and is less useful than aspirin for arthritis. When physical rehabilitation and NSAIDs fail to control synovitis or when erosive disease becomes apparent, several disease modifying antirheumatic drugs (DMARDs) are available including gold compounds and penicillamine (as well as chloroquine, methotrexate, sulfasalazine, and azathioprine). These diverse groups of drugs decrease rheumatoid factor and may inhibit the disease process itself. They are usually used in conjunction with NSAIDs and great caution is required, as toxic effects are significant. Glucocorticoids are a last-choice therapy for rheumatoid arthritis and inhibit all phases of inflammation including vascular, cellular, and connective tissue repair processes. They are most commonly used while waiting for remittive agents to work or when significant systemic features (weight loss, anemia, fatigue) accompany rheumatoid arthritis. In general, they are more useful for systemic lupus erythematosus, systemic vasculitis, and various hypersensitivity states, and their prolonged use should be avoided. (*Craig and Stitzel, pp 485–500*)

20. **(C)** In 1973, homosexuality was eliminated as a diagnostic category by the American Psychiatric Association and removed from the Diagnostic and Statistical Manual of Mental Disorders. (*Kaplan and Sadock, pp 658–661*)

21. **(A)** The anterior gray column contains alpha, gamma, and preganglionic autonomic neurons. First-order sensory neurons are located in the dorsal root ganglia and cranial nerve equivalent. (*Noback, pp 107–108,109–111*)

22. **(D)** The binding of glucagon to the hepatocyte cell membrane initiates a complex chain reaction. Intracellular cAMP rises, which in turn activates a protein kinase that *activates* phosphorylase b kinase. The activated form of this enzyme converts phorylase b to phosphorylase a, which proceeds to degrade glycogen to glucose-1-phosphate. Glucose-1-phosphate is subsequently dephosphorylated. (*Guyton, pp 978–979*)

23. **(A)** Proopiomelanocortin can give rise to five peptide hormones of the anterior pituitary. ACTH and β-lipotropin, a prohormone, are formed by cleavage of proopiomelanocortin. Alpha-melanocyte-stimulating hormone (α-MSH) is a cleavage product of ACTH, whereas β-endorphin and γ-lipotropin are cleavage products of β-lipotropin; β-MSH is a cleavage fragment of β-endorphin. This sequence is summarized below:

Thyroid-stimulating hormone (TSH), a hormone of the anterior pituitary gland, is not derived from proopiomelanocortin. (*Stryer 3rd ed., pp 993–994*)

24. **(A)** Group A streptococci produce two antiphagocytic surface components, hyaluronic

acid and M protein, which interfere with ingestion. The streptolysins are able to kill phagocytic cells by membrane disruption (streptolysin O) or by leukotoxicity, but are exhibited only after phagocytosis. Other streptococcal extracellular products that may have a deleterious effect on leukocytes include DNAse, proteinase, and RNAse. Hyaluronidase and streptokinase are virulence factors that may play a role in the organism's spread through the body. (*Joklik et al, pp 418–426*)

25. **(B)** Although there have been numerous ways of attempting to classify the various forms of muscular dystrophy, the present one is based on the mode of inheritance. There are types that are sex-linked inheritances: the Becker variety and the Duchenne variety. The Duchenne variety differs from the Becker variety by being more severe and producing its effects earlier in life, usually before the age of 4 years, whereas in the Becker variety, the disease produces its effects somewhere between the age of 5 and 25. The limb–girdle variety is inherited by autosomal recessive inheritance and the facioscapulo and myotonic dystrophies by autosomal dominant inheritance. (*Chandrasoma and Taylor, pp 941–943*)

26. **(C)** Spironolactone is a competitive antagonist of aldosterone and therefore may cause hyperkalemia if administered concomitantly with potassium supplements. Likewise, the potassium-sparing diuretics triamterene and amiloride cause potassium retention. Captopril inhibits production of angiotensin II and therefore inhibits aldosterone production. Furosemide promotes renal potassium excretion and often requires concomitant supplemental potassium administration. (*Hardman, pp 706–709*)

27. **(D)** The majority of child sexual abuse is committed by adults within the immediate or extended family and thus are known to the child. The psychological and physical effects of sexual abuse in children are often long-lasting and serious, including symptoms of post-traumatic stress disorder as well as,

commonly, depression. Most cases of sexual abuse of children are never discovered because of the victim's feelings of guilt, shame, and fear. (*Kaplan and Sadock, pp 787–790*)

28. **(D)** In some cases, there is reversed rotation of the intestinal loop where the primitive loop then rotates 90° in a clockwise direction. In such an abnormality, the transverse colon passes behind the duodenum. Remnants of the vitelline duct may appear as a vitelline ligament, cyst, fistula, or Meckel's diverticulum. Frequently the appendix develops posterior to the cecum and is called a retrocecal appendix. (*Sadler, pp 245–271*)

29. **(C)** Acetylcholine (ACh) released from motor neurons in the neuromuscular junction (NMJ) binds to nicotinic ACh receptors on the postsynaptic muscle cells. These receptors are ligand-gated cation channels. Binding of ACh results in their opening, allowing the passage of sodium into the cell. The resulting depolarization can initiate a muscle action potential. (*Guyton, pp 87–90*)

30. **(B)** Vitamin B_1 is obtained as thiamine from pork, yeast, whole grains, and nuts. Its active form in enzymatic reactions is thiamine pyrophosphate (TPP), a form to which it is converted in the body. During decarboxylation, substrates form a hydroxyethyl-TPP intermediate, which is then oxidized to an acetyl group before being transferred off of TPP. A deficiency of thiamine leads to beriberi, a wasting disease with nervous system damage and edema. (*Stryer, pp 514–518*)

31. **(A)** Exposure to the tuberculosis bacillus does not *ensure* disease, but a positive skin test makes the diagnosis more likely. Chemoprophylaxis with isoniazid (INH) would be the treatment of choice for contacts of actively infected persons. Ethambutol is very effective against most mycobacteria and is used in the treatment, not prophylaxis, of tuberculosis. The skin test is the most sensitive index of infection, and, for individuals who have already shown a positive response, roentgenography would not add much infor-

mation. Sequential roentgenograms months apart might indicate if the lesion were increasing in size, but that is most certainly not a high-priority procedure for contacts of infected persons. Immunization with the live attenuated TB strain bacille Calmette–Guérin (BCG) would be pointless, because the contacts have already developed an infection if the skin test is positive. Individuals receiving INH should periodically be checked by sputum culture and by roentgenography to be sure that the therapy is effective. *(Joklik et al, pp 498–510)*

32. **(D)** Ectopic hormone production is sometimes seen in association with pulmonary neoplasms. Some tumor types may produce two or more different hormones. This phenomenon has been associated in particular with small cell carcinoma. Small cell carcinoma may produce hyponatremia by the ectopic production and inappropriate secretion of ADH. It, along with bronchial carcinoid tumors, has also been associated with Cushing's syndrome and the carcinoid syndrome. Squamous cell carcinoma is associated with hyperparathyroidism, and all types of lung tumors, including adenocarcinoma and large-cell carcinoma, have been linked to gynecomastia resulting from the secretion of ectopic gonadotropin. In addition to endocrine abnormalities, oat cell carcinoma may also produce confusional psychosis, encephalomyelitis, sensory neuropathy, and muscular dysfunction. *(Chandrasoma and Taylor, pp 290–291)*

33. **(E)** Gentamicin is a member of the aminoglycoside family of antibiotics, which are rapidly bactericidal. Aside from interfering with the initiation of protein synthesis, aminoglycosides can also induce the incorporation of incorrect amino acids during protein synthesis and cause premature termination of translation of messenger RNA. Chloramphenicol binds to the 50 S ribosomal subunit, nitrofurantoin forms a highly reactive intermediate which selectively damages bacterial DNA. Vancomycin inhibits cell wall synthesis by binding to particular cell wall

precursor units. Trimethoprim selectively inhibits the reduction of bacterial dihydrofolate to tetrahydrofolate, thereby inhibiting DNA synthesis. *(Hardman et al, pp 1105–1106)*

34. **(E)** Cocaine abuse and withdrawal is often associated with depression, protracted dysphoria and anhedonia. Tobacco addiction is the most common type of drug dependency in the United States. Opioids administered to treat pain seldom results in addiction. Repeated use of cannabis results in tolerance. If indicated for pain, narcotic analgesics should be increased by 25 to 50% in an opioid-dependent individual because of tolerance to the analgesic action. *(Leigh and Reiser, pp 245–266)*

35. **(E)** The primitive intestinal loop rotates around an axis formed by the superior mesenteric artery. The superior and inferior epigastric vessels anastomose within the rectus sheath. The inferior mesenteric artery supplies the transverse, descending, and sigmoid colon. *(Sadler, pp 260)*

36. **(E)** The constriction of the pupil of the eye in response to light is mediated by a pathway that travels from the retina through the optic nerves, the optic chiasm, and the optic tracts. Lesions in these areas are therefore likely to impair this reflex. The pathway leaves the optic tracts anterior to the lateral geniculate to enter the pretectal area. Lesions in this area would, therefore, also prevent normal functioning of the reflex. A lesion of the geniculocalcarine tracts, which convey visual information from the lateral geniculate bodies to the occipital cortex, would cause partial or total blindness in humans but would not affect the pupillary reflex. *(Ganong, pp 135–136)*

37. **(D)** Under normal aerobic conditions, 30 net ATP are formed from the complete oxidation of glucose. Glycolysis yields 2 net ATP from substrate-level phosphorylation, the citric acid cycle yields 2 ATP (as guanosine triphosphate [GTP]) from substrate-level phosphorylation, and oxidative phosphorylation yields 26 ATP. In the presence of an uncoupling

agent, such as dinitrophenol, substrate-level phosphorylation still proceeds. Thus, 4 net ATP would be produced. *(Stryer, pp 551–552)*

38. **(B)** The girl described in the question has a profound deficiency of both the B-cell and T-cell components of the immune response (ie, severe combined immunodeficiency disease). The dramatic absence of lymphocytes and lymphoid tissue would not be found in any of the other conditions listed. Patients with acquired immunodeficiency syndrome (AIDS) may have a similar immune function deficit (absence of effective B-cell and T-cell responses); however, they have adequate lymphoid tissues. The cells are present, perhaps in diminished numbers, but are not mature and functional. *(Joklik et al, pp 333–335)*

39. **(E)** Macrophages are derived from monocytes and are the major scavenger cells in the inflammatory process, especially in late stages of inflammation. They gather up and digest debris, dead cells, proteins, and foreign material, as well as release degradative enzymes. They also release chemotactic and permeability factors, induce leukocytosis and fever, secrete proteins important in defense, release factors to aid healing, and have a function in the immune-mediated response. Macrophages are large, long-lived cells with an eccentric nucleus and abundant cytoplasm. They belong to the reticuloendothelial system (mononuclear phagocyte system) of cells, which are specialized for pinocytosis and phagocytosis. Neutrophils are the most important cells in the acute inflammatory response and are important in the initial engulfment and destruction of microorganisms and foreign material. Lymphocytes are inflammatory cells involved in chronic inflammation in immune reactions and delayed hypersensitivity responses. Plasma cells are modified lymphocytes involved in antibody production and secretion in immune-mediated inflammatory responses. Eosinophils are inflammatory cells whose true function is unknown. They are involved in hypersensitivity

and allergic reactions as well as parasitic infections. *(Chandrasoma and Taylor, p 59)*

40. **(D)** Tolbutamide is one of several oral hypoglycemic agents that is used for diabetes of the non–insulin-dependent type in individuals who cannot be treated by diet alone or are unwilling to take insulin. If tolbutamide is used alone in insulin-dependent diabetes, therapy is certain to fail and the patient is at great risk. Although results from University Group Diabetes Program are controversial, most endocrinologists and investigators have interpreted data to be consistent with a lack of effect of oral hypoglycemics in reducing cardiovascular complications associated with diabetes. All oral hypoglycemics are capable of producing profound hypoglycemia. This may occur after even one dosage and may require days of glucose therapy. Incontrovertible is that the mechanism underlying the effect of these drugs is to cause the pancreas to secrete insulin. *(Hardman, pp 1507–1509)*

41. **(B)** An hallucination is a perception without a stimulus, whereas an illusion is a distorted perception in the presence of a stimulus. For example, a patient seeing a dragon perching on the bed is experiencing a hallucination, but a patient who mistakes an intravenous pole for a gallows is experiencing an illusion. Delusion is a fixed idea or belief that does not correspond to reality. In this case, the patient has the fixed idea that his guts have rotted. As the delusion is of a depressive nature, the patient may also be depressed, but the phenomenon that is described is best described as delusional. *(Leigh and Reiser, pp 145–155)*

42. **(C)** The first arch persists to form the maxillary artery. The second arch persists as the hyoid and stapedial arteries. The third arch persists as the common carotid artery. The fourth arch persists as the pulmonary arch. The aortic sac forms right and left horns, which give rise to the brachiocephalic artery. *(Sadler, pp 212–215)*

43. **(B)** The foramen rotundum leads to the pterygopalatine fossa. The pterygopalatine fossa leads to the orbital cavity via the superior orbital fissure, to the oral cavity via the palatine canals, to the infratemporal fossa via the pterygomaxillary fissure. It does not lead to the posterior cranial fossa. *(Woodburne, pp 319–322)*

44. **(A)** Phosphoglucose isomerase catalyzes the reversible conversion of fructose 6-phosphate to glucose 6-phosphate in both glycolysis and gluconeogenesis. In fact, most of the steps of glycolysis are simply reversed in gluconeogenesis. However, the three regulatory steps in the conversion of glucose to pyruvate are not reversible. These steps are (1) glucose → glucose 6-phosphate, which is catalyzed by hexokinase; (2) fructose 6-phosphate → fructose 1,6-bisphosphate, which is catalyzed by phosphofructokinase; and (3) phosphoenolpyruvate → pyruvate, which is catalyzed by pyruvate kinase. The reversal of these steps in gluconeogenesis requires the enzymes glucose 6-phosphatase and fructose 1,6-bisphosphatase for the formation of glucose and fructose 6-phosphate, respectively. The formation of phosphoenolopyruvate from pyruvate is more complicated in that the four following steps are involved: (1) Pyruvate carboxylase catalyzes the conversion of pyruvate to oxaloacetate; (2) oxaloacetate is reduced to malate by mitochondrial malate dehydrogenase; (3) malate is reconverted to oxaloacetate by extramitochondrial malate dehydrogenase; and (4) oxaloacetate is transformed to phosphoenolpyruvate by GTP-dependent phosphoenolpyruvate carboxykinase. *(Stryer, pp 485–487,570–572)*

45. **(E)** Interferon activates cellular genes that code for antiviral proteins. The main target is the translational step in viral replication, which is blocked by two mechanisms. A protein kinase that is activated by double-stranded RNA (dsRNA) inactivates initiation factor EF-2 by phosphorylation. In the other mechanism, a nuclease, also activated by dsRNA, destroys messenger RNA. *(Joklik et al, pp 863–865)*

46. **(D)** Auer rods are round, rodlike, or elongate cytoplasmic inclusions in the cytoplasm of immature, abnormal granulocytes or myeloblasts. They represent aberrant forms of the cytoplasmic azurophilic granules produced by abnormal cytoplasmic maturation in the leukemic blast cells. Although they may occasionally be seen in chronic myelocytic leukemia in blast crisis, they are most characteristic of acute myeloblastic leukemia. Erythroleukemia (Di Guglielmo's syndrome) is an acute myeloid leukemia that is predominantly a disorder of erythroid precursors. At some stage of the disease, myeloid precursors may also be abnormal. In these instances, Auer rods may be seen when myeloblasts are present. Acute lymphoblastic leukemia and chronic lymphocytic leukemia are leukemias of the lymphocyte cells and do not demonstrate Auer rod formation. *(Rubin and Farber, pp 1058–1062)*

47. **(C)** The most common and distressing side effect of nonsteroidal anti-inflammatory agents is gastrointestinal complaints. Of those persons taking ibuprofen, 5% to 15% have symptoms referable to the digestive system. A similar incidence has been observed for naproxen. Toxic amblyopia is an unusual complication of ibuprofen therapy. Edema formation and renal failure have uncommonly been associated with both drugs. Drowsiness is an extremely rare side effect. *(Hardman, pp 639–640)*

48. **(B)** Agitation, tremulousness, and hallucinations indicate the likely presence of delirium tremens. If the hallucinations are primarily visual and frightening, and if there is other evidence of sympathetic activation, the diagnosis would be more likely. Physicians should be aware that alcoholic patients often drink in the hospital and fail to disclose the extent of their alcohol use. Following an operation, patients may develop an alcoholic withdrawal state as a result of their restricted oral intake. *(Leigh and Reiser, pp 305–323)*

49. **(B)** The mandibular division of the trigeminal nerve provides the nerve to the tensor veli palatini and tensor tympani muscles. The

levator veli palatini is innervated by the vagus. Muscles of facial expression are innervated by the facial nerve. The glossopharyngeal innervates the stylopharyngeus. The ansa cervicalis innervates the infrahyoid muscles. (*Woodburne, pp 195–197,252–254,278*)

50–52. (50-D, 51-E, 52-B) Brain does not store any sources of energy. Rather it depends on a continuous supply of glucose for its energy needs. During starvation the available sources of glucose are scarce. To provide sufficient energy to the brain, the liver begins to synthesize significant levels of the ketone bodies, acetoacetate and 3-hydroxybutyrate. These are formed in a pathway that begins with the condensation of two molecules of acetyl CoA to yield acetoacetyl CoA. Ketone body production occurs only in the liver. The acetyl CoA is derived by oxidation of fatty acids released by adipose tissue. Fatty acids are stored in adipose tissue in the form of triacylglycerols. Free fatty acids are derived from the stored triacylglycerols by the action of lipases and transported to the liver as complexes with albumin. (*Stryer, pp 612–613,770–777*)

53. (C) Influenza, rubeola, poliomyelitis, or the herpes virus do not contain enzymes that synthesize DNA from RNA (reverse transcriptase), or p24 and gp46 viral proteins that are of diagnostic value. Also, destruction of OKT4 lymphocytes is not a known attribute of these viruses. All of the above-indicated attributes are found in the human immunodeficiency virus. (*Joklik, pp 896–900,1051–1054*)

54. (C) Puromycin is an effective inhibitor of protein synthesis in animal and other cells. It is structurally similar to a portion of transfer RNA, a structural analog, and inhibits synthesis by terminating the growth of polypeptide chains, thus preventing cell growth. Chloramphenicol inhibits protein synthesis by blocking bond formation. Erythromycin blocks the translocation step by interfering with the release of the charged transfer RNA bound to the donor site (p site) of the ribosome after peptide bond formation. (*Joklik et al, p 176*)

55. (E) The ability of certain viruses, such as the orthomyxoviruses and paramyxoviruses, to agglutinate chicken red blood cells or human type O red blood cells is called hemagglutination. Hemagglutination is mediated by what is called the H(or HA) glycoprotein, which is a proteinaceous spike located on the envelope of the orthomyoviruses and paramyxoviruses. The H glycoprotein is an important antigen that is involved in the antigenic variation of influenza viruses. Since hemagglutination is a common feature of orthomyxoviruses and paramyxoviruses, this test is used for the presumptive identification of these viruses. (*Joklik et al, pp 766–767*)

56–57. (56-C, 57-D) Osteoid osteoma is a variant of a benign tumor that produces primitive bones and some denser bone in a very characteristic fashion, which can be recognized radiologically and pathologically but which does not metastasize. It may reoccur locally if not entirely and properly excised.

Chondrosarcoma is a highly malignant tumor of cartilage that is distinguished from its benign counterpart, chondroma, by pleomorphism, appearance of the cells, and invasive capacity. It also metastasizes through the bloodstream and may become widespread.

Osteogenic sarcoma is the bone, or osteoid, equivalent of chondrosarcoma and is also highly malignant and distinguishable from the osteoid osteoma.

Multiple endochondromatosis, a series of benign cartilaginous tumors that occur in the central portions of the shafts of bones both large and small, may occur throughout the body, producing gross deformities. They are benign and do not metastasize.

The distinction among these various types of benign and malignant tumors of both osteoblastic and chondroblastic origins is very important and requires a combination of clinical history and age, radiologic, and pathologic assessment. It is dangerous to rely on any one of these parameters alone to make a very clear distinction, which is of fundamental importance in the management and treatment of a patient. (*Rubin and Farber, pp 1316–1321*)

58–60. **(58-E, 59-C, 60-A)** Neurohumoral transmission may be classified into two basic types—cholinergic and adrenergic transmission. Cholinergic transmission involves the stimulation of either nicotinic or muscarinic receptors by acetylcholine. Postsynaptic nicotinic receptors may be blocked by *d*-tubocurarine; blockade of these receptors at motor end plates results in muscle paralysis. Muscarinic receptors of postganglionic parasympathetic fibers are also stimulated by acetylcholine; however, these receptors are blocked by atropine and not by *d*-tubocurarine. The activity of cholinergic neurotransmitters (eg, acetylcholine) is rapidly terminated by acetylcholinesterase. This enzyme may be inhibited reversibly by anticholinesterases, such as physostigmine. *(Hardman, pp 150,161–163,177–182)*

61. **(B)** Most infants gain an average of an ounce of weight a day during the first 4 months of life. Infants who gain more than this amount of weight and are spitting up usually are being overfed. Overfeeding often affects infants of primigravida mothers. Pyloric stenosis first becomes manifest at about 3 weeks of age, and affected infants gain weight poorly. Adrenogenital syndrome and inborn errors in metabolism also present in the first weeks of life and result in poor weight gain. Neglected infants would not be expected to be overfed. *(Rudolph et al, pp 136–137,1001)*

62. **(C)** Infants begin to sit by 5 months of age, but they usually do not attain the sitting position without assistance until they are 8 months old. At 8 months of age, children typically begin to stand with someone holding their hand. Children at this age also typically start to verbalize (eg, "ma ma" and "da da"). *(Rudolph et al, pp 18–20)*

63. **(E)** Hyaline membrane disease is a major cause of morbidity and mortality in newborn infants. Because both hyperoxemia and hypoxemia can lead to serious sequelae, it is of utmost importance to maintain normal blood oxygen levels in affected infants. Measuring arterial P_{O_2} is the most accurate way of monitoring oxygenation. Transcutaneous and capillary measurements frequently are used to monitor blood oxygen levels, but they aren't as precise as arterial samplings. Serial chest roentgenograms and pulmonary function tests are of no help in following the oxygen requirements of infants who have hyaline membrane disease. *(Rudolph et al, pp 1485–1492)*

64. **(E)** Anterior mediastinal masses are not uncommon in children. Teratomas, thymomas, lymphomas, and thymic cysts can all arise in the anterior mediastinal space. On the other hand, bronchogenic cysts arise in the middle mediastinal region. *(Rudolph et al, p 1474)*

65. **(E)** Tanner developed a scale (I to V) to describe the pubertal changes of girls and boys. Stage I is the prepubertal stage. Breast buds are the first signs of female pubertal development, and their appearance corresponds to Tanner stage II. Sparse pubic hair, the second sign, also corresponds to Tanner stage II, whereas dark pubic hair occurs during Tanner stage III. Axillary hair begins to form during the beginning of Tanner stage IV. Stage V represents full pubertal development. *(Oski et al, pp 766–769)*

66. **(C)** In the United States, sudden cardiac death (SCD) accounts for as many as 500 000 deaths yearly, almost half of all deaths caused by heart disease. Current research aims at identifying populations at risk in order to prevent SCD. In addition to the known risk factors for cardiovascular disease (eg, smoking and hypertension), the following factors are associated with increased risk for SCD: ventricular ectopic beats and arrhythmias; myocardial infarction, whether complicated or not; angina pectoris; prolonged QT interval on ECG; previous attack of SCD; and admission to intensive care with coronary artery disease and chest pain but without acute infarction. The vast majority of victims have underlying coronary artery disease, although not all have had prior symptoms. The most common precipitating arrhythmia is ventricular fibrillation, frequently preceded

by ventricular tachycardia. *(Isselbacher, pp 193–198)*

67. **(A)** The roentgenogram that accompanies the question demonstrates a dilated loop of large bowel with the ascending, transverse, and descending colon dilated proximally. This pattern is highly suggestive of a sigmoid volvulus. Immediate decompression by rectal tube or colonoscopy may be curative. In rare cases, if bowel infarction is suspected, surgical intervention is indicated. Gastric lavage would not be helpful. Abdominal ultrasonography might yield additional information but would not alter the need for immediate treatment. Percutaneous drainage would not relieve the obstruction and would be dangerous. Colonic volvuli recur in 55% of cases and may be complicated by colonic perforation. *(Hazzard, p 1270)*

68. **(C)** Serologic markers are extremely useful in the diagnosis of hepatitis B infections. In the typical case, titers of surface antigen (HBsAg) and e antigen (HBeAg) rise either before or simultaneously with clinical symptoms then fall to unmeasurable levels. Shortly thereafter, antibodies to surface antigen (anti-HBsAg) appear. The short interval between the disappearance of HBsAg and the appearance of anti-HBsAg is the so-called window period, when hepatitis is present despite negative serologic results. Another antibody is present during this period—antibody to hepatitis B core antigen (anti-HBcAG). This antibody persists for years after the infection has resolved. In the case presented in the question, the serologic findings show either that the man is in the window period of acute hepatitis B infection, in which case anti-HBsAg will appear on retesting, or that anti-HBcAg is persisting from a previous hepatitis B infection and the current hepatitis is due to another agent (eg, hepatitis C) or a toxin. Anti-HBcAg usually does not indicate either a chronic carrier state or immunity. *(Isselbacher, pp 1459–1478)*

69. **(D)** Calcium channel blockers are not effective in the treatment of ventricular tachycardia. They do slow conduction through the AV node and may, therefore, slow the ventricular response to atrial fibrillation or terminate reentry rhythms such as paroxysmal atrial tachycardia. All calcium blocking drugs have been shown to be effective for relief of angina in vasospastic and fixed coronary artery disease. Because of their vasodilatory action, these drugs can be used to treat hypertension and some patients with congestive heart failure. *(Isselbacher, pp 1024,1081–1082, 1127–1129)*

70. **(B)** Inspiratory stridor is the hallmark of upper airway obstruction. Among the disorders that can involve the upper airway and cause stridor are epiglottitis, infectious laryngotracheitis, angioneurotic edema, and foreign-body aspiration. In contrast, acute bronchospasm prolongs the expiratory phase of respiration and causes predominantly expiratory wheezing rather than inspiratory stridor. *(Rudolph et al, pp 959–960)*

71. **(B)** Osteomyelitis can be diagnosed in its earliest stage by technetium bone scanning. Plain roentgenographic films typically take at least 10 days to reveal the early changes of osteomyelitis. Gallium scans are helpful in proving the effectiveness of therapy at the end of treatment. Blood counts and sedimentation rates are helpful in monitoring the progression and response to treatment of osteomyelitis but do not prove or disprove the existence of disease. *(Rudolph et al, pp 1945–1946)*

72. **(A)** Turner's syndrome children are phenotypically female with an XO-chromosome pattern. The diagnosis, if missed at birth, becomes obvious during the pubertal years, when affected girls do not mature sexually and have short stature and cubitus valgus (deviation of the forearm to the radial side when extended). Coarctation of the aorta, but not aortic stenosis, has been reported in association with Turner's syndrome. *(Rudolph et al, pp 1658–1659)*

73. **(D)** Regardless of the clinical setting or the type of treatment being contemplated, it is of primary importance in the initial psychiatric

interview to obtain a careful patient history. Evaluation of mental status is next in importance, because it sheds light on the patient's orientation, cognition, and reality testing and may disclose the presence of organic disturbances. Establishing a working alliance is critical but should occur as a concomitant of careful and empathic introductory interviews. (*Kaplan and Sadock, vol 1, pp 522–526*)

74. **(D)** The antibiotic chloramphenicol is effective against a variety of organisms, including *Salmonella*. However, the side effects from the use of this drug are significant, and some are potentially lethal. Gray baby syndrome (peripheral vascular collapse) can occur in newborns receiving large doses of chloramphenicol. Aplastic anemia can develop as an idiosyncratic response (not dose-related) to treatment, and a reversible anemia also can occur. Discoloration of teeth is a side effect in newborns of maternal tetracycline therapy. Chloramphenicol is absorbed readily from the gastrointestinal tract. (*Rudolph et al, p 534*)

75. **(E)** The barium enema roentgenogram shown in the question reveals multiple sigmoid diverticuli. Most cases of colonic diverticular disease do not require surgery, even for active gastrointestinal bleeding. Colonoscopy is not necessary unless the barium enema reveals additional lesions or the diagnosis is in doubt. Histamine H_2-receptor antagonists such as cimetidine and ranitidine are useful for treating peptic ulcer disease but not for diverticulosis. Rectal corticosteroid enemas have a role in inflammatory bowel disease but not in diverticular disease. Appropriate management of the acute attack consists of bed rest, liquid diet, and perhaps anticholinergics. Thereafter, a high-fiber diet should be prescribed to help prevent further recurrences. Bran, raw vegetables, legumes, and hydrophilic colloids such as psyllium seed derivatives are all useful. (*Isselbacher, pp 1418–1420*)

76. **(D)** Psychosis is best defined as a state of gross impairment in reality testing. This condition may be demonstrated by imagined perceptions (hallucinations), belief in irrational thoughts (delusions), or marked inability to integrate and respond to important aspects of the environment. Psychosis may indicate underlying functional psychiatric illness or organic disease. (*APA, pp 404–405*)

77. **(A)** In the food industry, sugar is the most commonly used chemical preservative. At concentrations of 65% or greater, sugar prevents the growth of bacteria, yeasts, and molds. Bacteria rarely survive in concentrations greater than 25%. Salt is also an effective preservative, but because of its taste is not as readily acceptable as sugar. From a health standpoint, both substances have disadvantages. Benzoic acid, prohibited in some countries, is permitted in concentrations of as much as 0.1 percent for certain foods in the United States. Carbon dioxide is rarely used, except in carbonated beverages. Sulfur dioxide is used in some food-drying processes. (*Last, pp 605–607*)

78. **(E)** Human breast milk constitutes an optimal and almost perfect diet for young infants. It contains IgA and maternal macrophages, both of which presumably offer some immunologic protection to the newborn. Although the amount of iron in human milk is very small, it is very well absorbed, much better than in cow's milk. It is generally recommended, however, that breast-fed infants receive supplemental iron. Human milk generally contains little fluoride, regardless of the mother's dietary fluoride intake, and for this reason, it is recommended that supplementation with fluoride begin after 6 months of age. Normal infants fed breast milk exclusively probably require no vitamin supplementation. Supplementation with vitamin D, however, is deemed advisable and is most important in dark skinned infants or infants receiving minimal exposure to sunlight. (*Rudolph et al, pp 236–244*)

79. **(D)** Hypokalemia is magnified by bicarbonate treatment of acidosis, which causes potassium to enter cells. Patients with severe diabetic ketoacidosis always have a depletion of

their total body potassium even though the serum potassium may be elevated. This patient's hyperkalemia, however, still represents a risk because of its potential to produce cardiac arrest, a risk that may be greatly accentuated if potassium replacement is begun too early. Patients should be monitored very carefully to obtain unequivocal evidence that serum potassium has begun to fall before potassium therapy is started. Oral potassium is unwise in a drowsy, nauseated patient. The electrocardiogram is more reliable than serum potassium levels to assess the need for potassium replacement. Potassium can be administered at 30 mEq/hour with caution if potassium deficiency becomes severe. *(Isselbacher, pp 1990–1993)*

80. **(B)** Lower GI bleeding is a common presentation of a variety of colonic and non-colonic pathology. Due to the significantly more common occurrence of upper GI bleeding, it is by far the most common cause of "lower" GI bleeding. If only considering true colonic pathology as the cause diverticuli of the colon are the most common disease state leading to lower GI blood loss. Artenovenous malformations and colon cancer are less frequently the cause of lower GI bleeding. Benign polyps of the colon usually present with heme-positive stools and not frank GI bleeding. *(Greenfield, pp 1041–1053)*

81. **(D)** Delusions are fixed false beliefs of which a person cannot be dissuaded by empathic or logical argument. They may be present whenever reality testing is obstructed by a psychotic process; thus, they may occur in association not only with schizophrenia but also with mania, depression, or organic disturbances. Commonly encountered delusions include those of persecution, grandiosity, and physical disease. *(Kaplan and Sadock, pp 563–564)*

82. **(B)** Commercially canned foods are less likely to be contaminated by bacteria than foods stored by the other methods listed in the question. Temperatures of 120°C (250°F) or higher have to be used in the canning process. This temperature is obtained by steam under pressure and continues for a stipulated period of time that varies inversely with the amount of heat used. The desired effect be-gins when the temperatures achieved are 105°C (220°F) or higher. By this method, at least 90% of all organisms are killed. Pasteurization is also a form of heat treatment, in which lower temperatures are used for longer time periods. This method is adequate to prevent bacterial growth, but it may not be bactericidal. Refrigeration and freezing prevent bacterial multiplication, but food stored by these methods needs to be adequately cooked unless, like ice cream, it is to be eaten shortly after removal from the cold environment. Drying is a relatively safe method of storage, as pathogenic bacteria tend to die in the absence of water in foods that have been dried to 10 to 20% of their original weight. *(Last, pp 604–607)*

83. **(A)** Seizures actually are one of the less common initial manifestations of brain tumors in children. This is easily understood when one realizes that 50 to 60% of pediatric brain tumors are infratentorial and 75% or more occur in the midline, third and fourth ventricles, optic chiasm, and brainstem. Ataxia, cranial nerve involvement, and heat tilt are common presentations of brain tumors in children. Hypothalamic and endocrine dysfunctions occasionally are the presenting complaints. These can include growth failure and either sexual infantilism or sexual precocity. The most common tumors presenting in this manner are the craniopharyngioma and the chiasmal glioma. Occasionally pineal tumors and teratomas also may involve hypothalamicstructures. *(Rudolph et al, pp 1731–1747)*

84. **(E)** The ECG that accompanies the question shows atrial fibrillation with a rapid ventricular response. When atrial fibrillation is of recent onset and associated with hemodynamic compromise resulting from a rapid ventricular rate, treatment of choice is emergency cardioversion. In the absence of hypotension and severe symptoms, or if the atrial fibrilla-

tion is paroxysmal, digitalis, calcium channel blockers, or beta-adrenergic blockers may be given to slow the ventricular rate. If atrial fibrillation has been present for several days, elective cardioversion may be performed with concurrent anticoagulation to prevent embolism of any thrombus that may have formed. Quinidine, procainamide, and disopyramide are sometimes given at the time of cardioversion in hope of maintaining sinus rhythm. (*Isselbacher, pp 1022–1023*)

85. **(C)** Seminoma is the most common germinal tumor of the testes. The incidence of seminoma is higher in men with cryptorchidism. The tumor is highly radiosensitive, and the overall survival rate is approximately 85%. The tumor spreads by the lymphaticstoretroperitonealnodules. Hematogenous spread occurs late in the course of the disease and is not common. (*Lieskovsky, pp 508– 514*)

86. **(C)** Antidepressant drugs have long been effectively used in the pharmacologic management of major affective disorder (primarily recurrent depression), the depressive phases of bipolar illness, and atypical depression. Over the past several years clinical research has revealed that the major symptoms of a number of other psychiatric syndromes can be ameliorated pharmacologically with these same agents. The binge eating of certain bulimic individuals diminishes in frequency and intensity when these individuals are treated with certain antidepressant medications. Ruminative thinking and compulsive behaviors characteristic of obsessive–compulsive disorder diminish in severity when antidepressant medications are administered. Similarly, persons who experience panic attacks or phobias (specific anxiety disorders) often achieve symptomatic relief when given an antidepressant. It is not clear that the same serum levels necessary to effectively treat major depressive episodes must be established in treating these other syndromes. Antidepressant drugs are not effective in the treatment of delusional (paranoid) disorders. (*Dunner, pp 717–776*)

87. **(D)** A worker who can no longer do the type of work or amount of work that was previously performed is generally described as partially disabled. However, the Social Security Administration (SSA) system defines disability as the "inability to engage in any substantial gainful activity by reason of a medically determinable physical or mental impairment that can be expected to result in death, or has lasted or can be expected to last for a continuous period of not less than 12 months." The important phrases are "any substantial gainful activity," which begins to give some indication of how much activity can be undertaken by someone who is disabled; "by reason of a medically determinable physical or mental impairment," which implies that there must be some ability to define the condition in medical terminology and on the basis of a definable condition; and an estimated outcome that either will result in death or has resulted or will result in continuous disability for more than 12 months. In addition, the SSA has listed "severe impairments" that automatically qualify for medical disability. Some of these descriptions are very detailed. (*Last, pp 583–584*)

88. **(A)** Ethosuximide and valproic acid are the drugs of choice in the treatment of petit mal absence seizures, which cause transient loss of consciousness. Phenobarbital and phenytoin are excellent anticonvulsants but are not first-line medications for treating this disorder. Diphenhydramine is an antihistamine of no benefit in treating this disorder, and diazepam, which is useful in treating status epilepticus, also is not a drug used in the treatment of petit mal seizures. (*Rudolph et al, pp 1774–1775*)

89. **(D)** Nearly 90% of renal stones are visible on a plain abdominal roentgenography, and the majority contain calcium oxalate. The most common cause of calcium stone disease is idiopathic hypercalciuria. Almost half of affected persons daily excrete > 4 mg of calcium/kg body weight in the absence of hypercalcemia. Causes of hypercalciuria are sarcoidosis, hyperthyroidism, and Paget's

disease of bone. Idiopathic hypercalciuria is believed to result from either increased gastrointestinal absorption of calcium, increased calcium resorption from bone, or excessive renal calcium leakage into the urine. *(Isselbacher, pp 1329–1333)*

90. **(B)** Cardiac tamponade is the most frequent sign of intrapericardial injury. Elevation of central venous pressure is the most reliable sign for making the diagnosis. Left atrial pressure measurement through a Swan–Ganz catheter is of little value, because it may be normal or low. Decreased pulse pressure, when present, is diagnostic of cardiac tamponade. Normal cardiac shadow does not rule out cardiac tamponade; because of the suddenness with which cardiac tamponade occurs, the pericardium does not have sufficient time to expand; as little as 20 to 30 mL of accumulated fluid can produce the condition. Pericardiocentesis is helpful in the diagnosis. Aspiration of 10 to 20 mL may dramatically improve the patient's condition. However, it is important to remember that the pericardial tap may be falsely negative in 19% and falsely positive in 6% of cases. *(Greenfield, p 289)*

91. **(A)** Diagnostic criteria for chronic factitious disorder (Munchausen syndrome) include the presentation of physical symptoms that are consistent with genuine illness but are under the person's voluntary control. The disorder reflects a need to become a patient and receive care. Physical condition can deteriorate as a result of the multiple invasive procedures affected persons typically undergo. Unlike chronic factitious disorder, malingering reflects the simple desire to avoid unpleasant circumstances or to obtain undue compensation. *(APA, pp 316–318)*

92. **(B)** Although urinary tract infections are the most common nosocomial infections in US hospitals, responsible for 42% of such infections, they are responsible only for 9.9% of excess direct cost. Surgical wound infections, 23.7% of total nosocomial infections, are responsible for 48.4% of excess direct cost.

Thus, they are the most costly type of nosocomial infection. *(Kelley, p 1823)*

93. **(B)** The only agents currently recognized to enhance production of fetal pulmonary surfactant are glucocorticoids, and their use is controversial. These substances were first used by Liggins and Howie in fetal lambs. Some subsequent studies have shown them to be successful in enhancing pulmonary maturation; follow-up studies show no long-term consequences in the offspring. However, some data compiled from studies on animals show limitation of growth of certain organs. Of the agents listed in the question, magnesium sulfate will block eclamptic seizures and stop uterine contractions; hydroxyprogesterone is used experimentally on a chronic basis to decrease premature labor; and chloroprocaine and bupivacaine are anesthetics. *(Cunningham, pp 864–865)*

94. **(E)** Basal skull fractures are notoriously difficult to visualize on skull roentgenographic films, at least in part because of the complicated features of the base of the skull. Usually, the diagnosis is made on the basis of clinical findings. These include the seepage of blood over the mastoid area (Battle's sign), about the eyes (raccoon eyes sign), and into the middle ear (hemotympanum), as well as nasal bleeding or discharge of cerebrospinal fluid. As basal skull fractures may involve the middle ear or sinuses, bacterial meningitis is a concern. *(Rudolph et al, pp 1758–1760)*

95. **(E)** The history, examination, and laboratory findings of the patient described in the question all suggest acute adrenal insufficiency (addisonian crisis). The most common cause is exogenous steroid therapy causing suppression of adrenocorticosteroid production. Discontinuing or rapid tapering of the exogenous hormone often precipitates the crisis. Less common causes of adrenal insufficiency are hypopituitarism or primary adrenal lesions (eg, autoimmune destruction or tumor). In these settings, crisis is often precipitated by infection or stress. Once the diagnosis is suspected, a plasma cortisol level

should be drawn, but treatment should not be delayed to await definitive testing. Intravenous administration of hydrocortisone sodium succinate is the treatment of choice, along with fluids to replenish extracellular volume. Antibiotics, hypertonic saline, or sodium bicarbonate may be needed but are not essential to immediate management. Arginine vasopressin is used to treat diabetes insipidus. (*Isselbacher, pp 1970–1973*)

96. **(C)** Antibiotic-related colitis is the result of enterotoxin produced by *Clostridium difficile.* It has been reported with the use of practically every antibiotic except vancomycin. When diarrhea is the only manifestation, discontinuing the antibiotic is all that is necessary. In more severe cases, treatment requires administering metromidazole. Vancomycin by mouth is also adequate in treating *C. difficile* but due to its expense is not the first line drug. Rarely, total colectomy and ileostomy are required to treat toxic megacolon and perforation. (*Schwartz, pp 1226–1228*)

97. **(A)** Antipsychotic (neuroleptic) medications exert their pharmacologic effects by a central dopamine receptor blockade. Decreased dopaminergic activity accounts for the parkinsonian side effects commonly produced by these drugs. Other drugs, like amphetamines, that promote increased dopaminergic activity in the brain can lead to psychosis or exacerbate an existing schizophrenic illness. (*Hales and Frances, pp 178–179*)

98. **(C)** The general formula of chi-square is

$$\chi^2 \,(df) = \Sigma \frac{(O - E)^2}{E}$$

where O is the observed count in the category and E is the expected count in the category if the null hypothesis is true. The formulation applies only to counts of the number of observations and not to measured quantities, ranks, percentages, or proportions. It is designed to make comparisons or proportions, but the data must be presented in raw numerical form. The concept of degrees of freedom (df) is involved.

The test is designed for the comparison of paired or independent samples—for example, the proportion of persons exposed to a certain level of radiation developing leukemia compared with the number of those who also develop the disease but who have not been exposed. (*Kramer, pp 168–171*)

99. **(A)** Antepartum fetal monitoring in the form of nonstress testing, stress testing, or biophysical profile evaluation is commonly used to help ensure fetal well-being. There is no general agreement as to which type of test is best or when it is best initiated. Therefore, centers will generally use one or more of these tests and begin evaluation between 25 to 36 weeks, depending on high-risk indications. The tests would generally be performed at weekly intervals unless a higher risk (such as previously nonreactive nonstress tests) indicates the need for more frequent testing. (*Cunningham, pp 1031–1044*)

100. **(D)** This child, who is cyanotic despite the administration of oxygen and despite an arterial PO_2 of 90 torr, probably has methemoglobinemia. If the cyanosis were due to cardiac or pulmonary disease, one would expect hypoxemia as well as corresponding findings on physical examination. There are a variety of causes of methemoglobinemia, but the sudden onset in this previously well child suggests the ingestion of a toxin. Nitrites from well water is one notorious cause of methemoglobinemia. It also has been suggested that home-prepared infant vegetable purees may be very rich in nitrates, which if improperly stored are reduced to nitrites, causing methemoglobinemia. A simple test is to place a drop of the patient's blood on filter paper. If the blood appears brown, the level of methemoglobin is greater than 15%. The treatment of nitrite poisoning and methemoglobinemia is methylene blue administered intravenously. Physostigmine is useful in counteracting the symptoms of tricyclic ingestion; atropine is the drug of choice for organic phosphate poisoning; and amyl nitrite is used for cyanide poisoning. (*Rudolph et al, pp 808–809*)

101. **(C)** Psoriasis is a chronic skin disease characterized by well-demarcated, erythematous papules and plaques covered by flakes or scales. Common sites of involvement are the scalp, back, extensor surfaces of the knees and elbows, perianal region, and genitalia. Psoriasis is associated with nail dystrophy (pits, grooves, or crumbling), arthritis (usually involving the digits), involvement of traumatized areas (Koebner's phenomenon), and hyperuricemia (caused by rapid nucleic acid turnover). Pleurisy is not an associated feature of psoriasis. *(Isselbacher, p 276)*

102. **(A)** Ruptured abdominal aortic aneurysm is characterized by the diagnostic triad of abdominal or back pain, hypotension, and a tender, pulsatile abdominal mass. Treatment consists of control of hemorrhage, restoration of blood volume, and replacement of the aneurysm with a graft. Survival of affected individuals depends on how soon the bleeding is controlled. Control over continued hemorrhage is best achieved in the operating room. Delay can prove fatal, because blood pressure may fall precipitously at any moment. All painful procedures, which may increase blood pressure and thereby aggravate bleeding, should be deferred until the patient is in the operating room and the surgical team is ready to open the abdomen at a moment's notice. *(Greenfield, pp 1711–1722)*

103. **(D)** Organic causes of psychiatric illness must always be considered, but some clinical presentations warrant special attention. By definition, delirium is organic, not functional, in nature and therefore must be fully investigated. Confusion, dementia, and sudden personality change all can arise from such "nonpsychiatric" causes as neoplastic, metabolic, cardiovascular, and infectious disease. Similarly, first psychotic episodes must not be attributed to a schizophreniform disorder without first performing an organic work-up. Although major depression can be simulated by organic causes, such as thyroid disease, a CT scan of the brain is less indicated in the workup of depression than the other clinical situations mentioned above. *(Hales and Frances, pp 287–289)*

104. **(A)** In Australia, the National Health and Medical Research Council has recommended "safe" levels for drinking. Their recommendations are based on a "unit" of alcohol being 8 to 10 g of alcohol as opposed to the Canadian and American standard of 13.6 g. Men should not drink more than the equivalent of 40 g of absolute alcohol per day on a regular basis. Women are generally more susceptible to the effect of alcohol and should drink no more than half the consumption of men. In essence, no level of consumption of alcohol will always be safe for all individuals under all conditions. *(Last, pp 743–744)*

105. **(E)** Many factors contribute to the decision regarding what type of therapy a woman should receive for carcinoma in situ of the cervix. Extended or radical hysterectomy is usually not considered because, by definition, carcinoma in situ is not invasive and does not involve pelvic lymph nodes. If an affected woman has completed her childbearing, hysterectomy is usually the treatment of choice. Either conization or cautery is possible for women who wish to maintain fertility. The major advantage of cryosurgery is that it can be performed on an outpatient basis, whereas conization requires some form of anesthesia. However, the recurrence rates after cryosurgery are higher than those of conization. The success rate with all of the methods is quite good. All women should, however, be followed up for recurrence of disease, including women who have had a hysterectomy. *(Gant, pp 221–230)*

106. **(E)** Slapped red cheeks and a generalized lacy reticular rash are classic signs of erythema infectiosum, which is caused by human parvovirus. (This disease is also known as "fifth disease," because it was the fifth disease, after rubella, measles, scarlet fever, and Filatov–Dukes disease, described with this type of rash.) Sucking on a Popsicle also can lead to reddish discoloration of the

cheeks, a condition called Popsicle panniculitis. Kawasaki's disease, rubeola, and rubella are associated with a variety of skin manifestations, but the "slapped cheeks" sign is not a characteristic finding. *(Feigin and Cherry, p 1647)*

107. **(B)** As many as 50% of patients presenting with a principal complaint of persistent, generalized pruritus have an occult systemic disease. Chronic renal failure is a common cause of itching; postulated mechanisms include elevated serum histamine or kinin levels and mast cell hyperplasia. Pruritus is the initial symptom in almost half of all patients with primary biliary cirrhosis and eventually affects almost all. Other hepatic disorders to rule out are hepatitis and extrahepatic biliary obstruction (accumulation of bile salts is thought to cause the pruritus). Half of all patients with polycythemia vera suffer from itching that is characteristically worsened by hot baths. Pruritus is associated with a poorer prognosis in Hodgkin's disease and mycosis fungoides. Pruritus associated with thyrotoxicosis, occurring in as many as 10% of cases, is also thought to be caused by increased kinin activity. Numerous other causes, including occult malignancy and parasitic infections, should be carefully considered. However, lupus is not especially associated with generalized pruritus as a presenting complaint. *(Wyngaarden, pp 2283–2284)*

108. **(D)** Localization of insulinoma is not always easy. Angiography and splenic venous sampling localizes the tumor in only 30% of the patients. At operation the pancreas has to be mobilized and tumor carefully looked for. If no tumor is found, distal pancreatectomy is done and blood sugar determined after 30 minutes. Elevation of blood sugar is an indicator of tumor removal. *(Schwartz, pp 1426–1427)*

109. **(E)** Insanity is defined by law, not by psychiatry, and definition of insanity varies from state to state. The insanity defense is employed infrequently in US courts for several reasons, including relative lack of success

and the prospect that harsh institutional life awaits those persons found not guilty by reason of insanity. As laws are passed to toughen the US criminal justice system and thus make the possibility of imprisonment even more intimidating, defendants may well opt more often for the insanity defense. At present, there is a movement to consider restricting the use of the insanity defense to sentencing and not to determination of guilt or innocence. *(Halleck, pp 207–224)*

110. **(A)** In fact, the data produced by the Centers for Disease Control in 1984 reveals that the organisms listed in the question occur in descending order of frequency as listed. *Pseudomonas* was then reported to be the pathogen in 16.9% of cases of lower respiratory tract infection reported in acute-care hospitals. The patterns are constantly changing, but these changes are noted only over a period of years. *(Kelley, p 1827)*

111. **(B)** The peak incidence of poststreptococcal glomerulonephritis occurs between the ages of 3 and 7 years. Not all strains of streptococci are equally associated with glomerulonephritis—particular association has been noted with type 12, and also with types 1, 4, 25, and 29. Because these strains are not evenly spread throughout the communities, the prevalence of poststreptococcal glomerulonephritis can vary widely between different population groups. There is little tendency for the condition to recur, and therefore there is little indication for secondary preventive measures. *(Clark and Mac-Mahon, pp 228–229)*

112–113. **(112-E, 113-C)** A variety of congenital disorders can be diagnosed in utero. Achondroplasia, a form of dwarfism, is readily noted on ultrasonography, which discloses shortened fetal limbs. A fetus with an open meningomyelocele secretes measurable quantities of alpha-fetoprotein (AFP) into the amniotic fluid, which can be obtained by amniocentesis. Sickle cell anemia will be detectable on a fetal blood sample obtained during fetoscopy. Hunter's syndrome, a disorder of mucopolysaccharide storage, can be detected in cells grown in culture from amniotic fluid. *(DeCherney, pp 344–349)*

114–117 (114-B, 115-E, 116-A, 117-D) Both phenelzine and amitriptyline are used in the treatment of major depression. Phenelzine, an MAO inhibitor, augments available catecholamine neurotransmitters for release into the synaptic cleft by inhibiting the intraneuronal breakdown of norepinephrine, serotonin, and dopamine. The degree of enzyme inhibition appears to be directly related to the antidepressant effect. Persons treated with phenelzine or any other MAO inhibitor must eliminate tyramine-containing foods from their diet or risk the possibility of a hypertensive crisis.

Amitriptyline, a tricyclic antidepressant, exerts its therapeutic effect by means of inhibition of serotonin reuptake into the presynaptic neuron, thus enhancing the availability of neurotransmitter for action on the postsynaptic neuron. The structurally related compounds nortriptyline and protriptyline also are effective antidepressants.

Clonazepam is a benzodiazepine used originally as an anticonvulsant in the treatment of akinetic and myoclonic seizures. In recent years it has also been prescribed for its antianxiety effects as well. Haloperidol is a high-potency antipsychotic agent with minimal anticholinergic properties and maximal dopamine-blocking properties; it is used in the treatment of schizophrenia, manic-depressive disorder, and other psychotic states. Benztropine is an anticholinergic used to manage the pseudoparkinsonian and extrapyramidal side effects of the higher-potency antipsychotic agents like haloperidol. *(Tupin et al, pp 3–5,54–59,62–64)*

118–120. (118-A, 119-B, 120-D) Local health departments or health systems agencies are concerned with making plans for the entire population of an area and with developing a comprehensive population-based plan. This involves estimating health requirements, matching them with existing resources, and outlining the strategy based on the deficit or surplus that has been demonstrated. A distinction is frequently made between what the patient wants (which would be used if available and free), what the patient needs (services determined by professionals to be appropriate), and what the patient demands (services that are actually used in the current market situation).

Planning for an HMO is based on that segment of the population that is "the market" for the organization. The population may or may not live in a contiguous area. The planning is designed to identify goals and objectives in institutional terms: eg, to determine the market for the services the organization provides, and to estimate future demands. The population need (as opposed to the population demand) is not necessarily a concern of institutional planners.

Program planning concerns itself with neither the need for a particular service nor its marketability. By definition, "the program" is the focus (eg, maternal and child health care will be provided). Planning is directed toward the way in which the already established goals will be carried out. This type of planning is frequently necessary to implement government-sponsored prgrams. *(Last, pp 1080–1081)*

UNSCHEDULED PATIENTS

121. (B) The patient has documented isolated systolic hypertension (ISH), which is the most common type of hypertension observed in the elderly. Given the results of the major study, the Systolic Hypertension in the Elderly Program, management of this disorder leads to decreased cerebrovascular mortality and morbidity. The most appropriate next step in this patient's management is initiation of a nonpharmacologic approach to control blood pressure. If the blood pressure is not controlled after a 3-month interval, initiation of therapy with a diuretic or beta-blocker should follow. There is no indication for starting two pharmacologic therapies at the same time. No further diagnostic evaluation for blood pressure measurement should be attempted at this time without a specific intervention planned, and 24-hour ambulatory blood pressure monitoring is not indicated in this setting. *(SHEP; Applegate and Rutan)*

122. **(D)** With normal aging, there is a down-regulation of the beta-adrenergic receptors in normal cardiac muscle. At rest, this finding is not clinically important, as older patients have the same heart rate as younger patients. However, with exercise and challenge to the sympathetic nervous system, there is an expected increase in catecholamine discharge but a less-than-expected increase in heart rate as a result of the down-regulation of the beta-receptors as described above. *(Geokas et al; Wei)*

123. **(C)** While the average life expectancy of a person born in the United States is currently 75 years for a man and 79 years for a woman, these figures represent a 50%:50% chance of reaching a specific chronologic age. Given the fact that the patient is currently 83 years old, there is still an expected average life expectancy of approximately 7 years, suggesting that there is a 50% chance that the patient will live 7 years or longer. This advanced age is a reflection of the survivorship in this patient. Even at age 83, this patient will continue to experience additional life and additional health care needs. *(Avorn, 1986; Soldo and Manton, pp 12–22)*

124. **(C)** Fries described three important terms in measuring human health in advancing years: disease, morbidity, and mortality. There is a period of time when the *disease* is present in the individual, but no symptoms are clinically apparent. Screening is helpful at this time to provide information on asymptomatic conditions which, if detected and treated early, may lead to improved life expectancy. Once a disease is clinically manifest, the disease is responsible for *morbidity* in the given individual, and with advancing age, there is an increasing frequency of co-morbid conditions. The third step as described by Fries is *mortality*, and although there have been great increases in average

life expectancy throughout the 20th century, the maximum life expectancy has remained the same at approximately 110 years. No foreseeable extension in the maximum lifespan can be predicted at this time. *(Avorn, 1984; Fries)*

125. **(A)** Dementia, defined as significant memory impairment, is relatively uncommon in all patients over the age of 65 but may be present in as many as 50% of patients over the age of 80. The most frequent etiology of memory impairment in the older individual is dementia of the Alzheimer's type (DAT), also known as Alzheimer's disease. This entity is responsible for approximately 60% of all memory impairment. Memory impairment resulting from cerebrovascular accidents is seen in approximately 20% of individuals. Reversible causes of memory impairment, such as drug-induced illness, are seen in approximately 20% of individuals. The remaining 5% of memory loss can be explained by a variety of illnesses, including Parkinson's disease, Pick's disease, and other neurodegenerative conditions. Old age in and of itself is not related to memory loss: when a patient presents to the office with memory impairment, a diagnostic search should begin to rule out common clinical and pathophysiologic conditions that may be responsible for memory loss. *(Katzman; Odenheimer)*

126. **(B)** Given the patient's deficits in memory, efforts should be made by the clinician to educate the patient around the activities of daily living and structural support in his or her home environment. This education should extend not only to the patient but also to the family and should include information on the activities of daily living. In addition, the physician should use other strategies such as simplification of the medication regimen, written information to supplement oral information, and home visitation to enhance therapeutic outcomes in these patients. Psychoactive agents are not indicated in the management of dementia unless psychotic features are noted. Acute hospitalization may

be necessary for other illnesses that occur in the later stages of dementia, such as pressure ulcers caused by decreased mobility in these patients, but are not indicated early in the management of this disorder. There is no role for vitamin therapy in the management of dementia. While a discussion with the patient and family is recommended concerning advance directives and the appointment of a health care proxy, this step, again, should not be foremost in the clinician's mind in prioritizing the treatment strategies for this patient. (*Winograd and Jarvik; Wasson et al*)

127. **(D)** The magnitude of the memory impairment can be evaluated using the Folstein Mini-Mental State Examination, a low-tech standardized test. A deficit in delayed recall, the inability to learn new information, is the typical finding in patients with dementia of the Alzheimer's type and several other dementing illnesses. Testing can be done dynamically by reciting three words, asking the patient to immediately repeat the words back to the examiner and remember them for later testing, and asking the patient to recall the words after a five-minute interval. The ability to recall distant information is relatively preserved in dementia. Deficits in orientation and language may be noted as well but are not pathognomonic of dementia. Both registration and attention and calculation deficits are not consistent with dementia but rather are more consistent with delirium or acute confusional state, which represents another important mental disorder in the elderly. If deficits are noted in any of these two spheres, a diagnostic work-up separate from that for management of dementia should be commenced. (*Folstein et al; Lachs et al*)

128. **(B)** Compliance can be defined as the ability of the patient to adhere to the treatment regimen, in this situation the medication regimen. While a number of studies have been performed relating factors such as patient demographics to compliance, there is no clear relationship between age or gender and the magnitude of compliance. The one factor that has consistently been noted as related to medication compliance is the number of medications in the patient's regimen: the level of compliance is inversely related to the number of medications, with the poorest compliance noted with increasing number of medications. The number of comorbid diseases is not in itself related to compliance, and there is no evidence of a difference in compliance between tablets versus elixirs. (*Darnell et al; Monane et al*)

129. **(A)** Pharmacokinetics is the area dealing with "what the body does to the drug." Four specific processes are identified—absorption, distribution, excretion, and metabolism. With normal aging, there is an increased amount of body fat and a decreased amount of body water, which directly affects the volume of distribution of medications. Medications that are renally excreted have markedly prolonged half-lives, as a result of a decreasing number of function nephrons with normal aging. Phase I metabolism, which includes oxidative reactions of the P450 systems, is markedly impaired in the older individual, while Phase II processes such as conjugation are relatively well preserved. Absorption is essentially unchanged in the older versus the younger individual. (*Montamat et al; Avorn and Gurwitz, pp 66–77*)

130. **(D)** Urinary incontinence is one of the most common conditions in the older individual, affecting 10% to 15% of patients in the community setting. The etiology of urinary incontinence in many individuals is related to factors outside of the genitourinary tract, and many of these factors are potentially reversible or amenable to therapy. Calcium channel blockers lead to overflow incontinence by decreasing the action of smooth muscle responsible for bladder emptying. Restricted mobility is responsible for lack of access to the bathroom and may result in incontinence, and impaired mentation may lead to inappropriate central nervous system response to bladder contractions. Diabetes may be responsible for urinary incontinence as a result of increasing osmolarity of the urine. Although the number of functioning nephrons

decreases with normal aging, the relationship between this physiologic change in older individuals and the onset of urinary incontinence is not clinically important. *(Resnick and Yalla; Ouslander et al)*

SCHEDULED APPOINTMENTS

131. (E) With a known history of pulmonary carcinoma, evaluation of the chest by CT scan is unlikely to yield additional information concerning the recent problem of confusion. Considering the palpable bladder and enlarged prostate, serum blood urea nitrogen (BUN) and creatinine, urinalysis, and urinary electrolytes are reasonable tests to rule out renal failure or obstructive uropathy. Thyroid function tests may be performed in this elderly individual with confusion to rule out hypothyroidism. *(Kursh, pp 135–137)*

132. (B) Since there is suspicion of acute renal failure, one must determine the etiology. The classic distinction is among prerenal, renal, and postrenal. Radiologic examination is essential in the evaluation. In view of the elevated BUN and creatinine, combined with the history of enlarged prostate and palpable bladder, CT scan of the abdomen (may detect uric acid stones not visible on KUB), ultrasound of the abdomen (rules out hydronephrosis), KUB film (rule out stones), and retrograde ureterography are all appropriate. With the creatinine above 2.5, an intravenous pyelogram is of minimal value. *(Kursh, p 137)*

133. (D) The most vital office procedure performed in acute renal failure is insertion of a Foley catheter. It is both diagnostic and therapeutic. Foley insertion should be performed whether one can palpate the bladder or even if the bladder is nonpalpable. With outlet obstruction resulting from benign prostatic hypertrophy or tumor, the Foley insertion will be both diagnostic and therapeutic. *(Kursh, p 137)*

134. (B) Renal failure involves the inability of the kidneys to maintain metabolic homeostasis. This will result in multiple metabolic, acid–base, and volume disorders. If output is less than 500 mL/d, it may be termed oliguric renal failure. Renal failure is not due to outlet obstruction when residual is less than 30 mL. Some findings on history and physical examination that *are* consistent with anatomic lesions and outlet obstruction include flank pain, history of ureterolithiasis, and difficult voiding. On examination, palpable kidneys may indicate polycystic kidney disease or lymphoma. *(Kursh, p 137)*

135. (A) While it is reasonable to restrict protein, correct volume depletion, and control caloric intake and acidosis, one should refrain from the use of magnesium-containing compounds. Conservative management may include daily weight, serial laboratory studies, and monitoring of fluid intake and output. While protein intake should be limited to 0.5 g/kg/d, highly catabolic patients (burns, postoperative) may require higher amounts. Hypertension also needs to be aggressively treated. *(Woodley, p 221)*

136. (C) Of more concern than a painful death is the fear of suffering alone. Patients may fear being abandoned by their physician, which leads to despair. Reduced conversation and the tendency to withdraw will aggravate the patient's sense of loneliness. A touch, examination, or even the taking of the pulse serves to support patient– physician bonding and reduce patient anxiety. *(Rakel, p 184)*

137. (C) While TB and collagen vascular disease need to be considered in any individual with prolonged fever and malaise, the history of IV drug use and physical findings should prompt a search for infective endocarditis. Other possible disorders in the setting of prolonged fever and malaise may include neoplasia and viral infection. Rheumatic fever also needs to be considered in the differential. The history, cardiac examination, and blood cultures, along with an index of suspicion, will confirm the diagnosis. Remember also that the clinical picture will depend on the specific infecting organism. *(Rakel, p 443)*

138. **(B)** Clubbing and splenomegaly are seen only in neglected cases of over 6 weeks' duration. Patients with infective endocarditis may be noted to have fatigue, petechiae, and embolic infarcts in the spleen, retina, or cerebral circulation. Retinal infarcts (Roth's spots) may be also noted in other vascular disorders, such as systemic lupus erythematosis (SLE). Immune complex disease may present as nephritis, Osler's nodes, and arthralgias. Patients with acute bacterial endocarditis may be critically ill, whereas those with subacute bacterial endocarditis may appear chronically ill, presenting with weight loss and anorexia. Up to 10% of patients may have no murmur, and this is especially noted in patients with tricuspid valve involvement. Abnormal laboratory findings include normochromic, normocytic anemia in up to 90% to cases. *(Rakel, p 440)*

139. **(D)** When increased turbulence is present along a valve, as a result of pre-existing disease, endothelial damage occurs. Sterile platelet-fibrin thrombi are formed. Bacteremia that involves an organism with the ability to adhere to either the endothelium or the platelet-fibrin thrombi could result in infection. Phagocytosis does not occur on valve leaflets, so bacteria multiply within the thrombus. The infection may extend to supporting structures, resulting in additional damage. Vascular occlusion may result from the embolization of the vegetations. Suppurative metastatic lesions may also then occur. *(Rakel, p 440)*

140. **(D)** Low turbulence found in low-pressure-gradient conditions is unlikely to result in infective endocarditis. Conditions such as chronic congestive failure, atrial septal defect, and purely stenotic valvular lesions most often have low pressure gradients. Other low-flow conditions include chronic atrial fibrillation and atrial septal defects. The low pressure gradients result in less turbulence. Such lesions are at a low risk for infective endo-

carditis. A greater risk is noted in insufficient valvular lesions, which are associated with a high pressure gradient and increased turbulence. *(Rakel, p 440)*

141. **(D)** Eighty percent of endocarditis cases are due to streptococci and staphylococci. *Streptococcus viridans* is the most frequent organism in natural valve endocarditis. The increased frequency of streptococci in endocarditis is related to the bacteria's ability to adhere to valve tissue. Although the majority of natural valve and late prosthetic valve infective endocarditis cases are due to *S viridans*, in the IV drug user, the most common isolate is *Staphylococcus aureus*. The skin is the most common source of microorganisms that result in the IV drug abuser's infection. *S bovis*, when noted as a cause of endocarditis, is associated with colonic neoplasia in greater than 50% of cases. *(Rakel, p 441)*

142. **(A)** Tricuspid valve is affected in over 50% of infective endocarditis cases in IV drug abusers. Infections with multiple organisms are common, and the onset is often acute. Most addicts with initial endocarditis infection do not have previously damaged heart valves. Pulmonary emboli are common in tricuspid valve endocarditis. Murmurs are often absent in these cases. Some of these infections involve fungal endocarditis. Fungal endocarditis is more common in the settings of open heart surgery, prolonged intravenous therapy, and IV drug abuse. *(Wilson, p 521)*

143. **(C)** Bactericidal effect against enterococci is not obtained with the single antimicrobials listed. Enterococcal organisms are very resistant to the cephalosporins. As penicillin, vancomycin, and ampicillin are not bactericidal for the enterococci, combination therapy including an aminoglycoside is necessary. The addition of an aminoglycoside creates a synergistic bactericidal effect. Antibiotics should be administered by the parenteral route. The concentration should be sufficient to destroy all microorganisms in the vegetation. The duration of antibiotic treatment is usually 4 to 6 weeks. *(Wilson, p 524)*

144. (A) Drug reaction is the most common cause of fever during treatment, with emboli and metastatic abscess formation as less common causes. Within one week of initiation of antimicrobial therapy, fever will most often subside. Continued fever and bacteremia may also be noted with myocardial abscess formation. If a rash develops during treatment, antihistamines may be given. If the rash is progressive and severe, the treatment program should be changed. The main cause of death during or after therapy is heart failure. *(Wilson, p 523)*

145. (E) Manifestations of infective endocarditis include embolic episodes, neurologic symptoms, cardiac and renal failure. Also noted are fever and murmurs. With early endocarditis and in tricuspid valve endocarditis, a murmur may not be appreciated. With chronic disease, clubbing may be noted. Neurologic manifestations may also be noted. Circulating immune complexes secondary to high antibody titers against the infecting organism contribute to glomerulonephritis and arthritis. These manifestations will usually have their onset within 2 weeks of the initial bacteremia. The onset may be slow (as with *S viridans*) or acute (as with *S aureus*). *(Wilson, p 522)*

146. (C) Prophylaxis is necessary for prevention of endocarditis in those patients at increased risk. This includes patients with rheumatic heart disease, patients with previous infective endocarditis, calcific aortic stenosis, most forms of congenital heart disease, mitral valve prolapse with mitral insufficiency, and those individuals with prosthetic valves. Oral procedures do not require parenteral medication, even in those individuals at high risk. Parenteral antibiotics are advised for high-risk patients who undergo gastrointestinal or genitourinary procedures. Cephalosporins should not be used for prevention of endocarditis. *(Woodley, p 261)*

147. (C) The diagnosis of mononucleosis needs to be considered in this scenario. With an incubation of 30 to 50 days, infectious mononucleosis presents with an insidious onset of fever and sore throat. The virus is spread by oral transmission and also by respiratory spread of saliva. Lymphadenopathy and hepatosplenomegaly may be noted. Edema of the eyelids and maculopapular rashes may be evident on examination. HIV seroconversion may present as a "flulike" illness, with fever and lethargy. A complete blood count will assist in screening for mononucleosis (atypical lymphocytosis). While the differential diagnosis also includes toxoplasmosis, cytomegalovirus, and hepatitis A, these may be evaluated by serologic testing. Bone marrow study is unnecessary in the initial evaluation. *(Behrman, p 671)*

148. (C) Abdominal pain is infrequent, except where the spleen has ruptured. Rapid enlargement of the spleen may occasionally cause left-upper-quadrant discomfort. This pain may be the presenting complaint. Hepatomegaly is uncommon and noted in less than one third of patients. Mild hepatic tenderness may be noted in up to 50% of cases. Splenomegaly is noted in about 50% of patients. *(Behrman, p 671)*

149. (A) Hepatitis is common, with over 90% of patients demonstrating abnormal liver function tests. Other complications include splenic rupture, airway obstruction, and interstitial pneumonia. Hemolytic anemia, thrombocytopenia, pancreatitis, and Reye's syndrome may also be noted. The most common neurologic complications include cranial nerve palsies and encephalitis. Cardiac complications are uncommon but include myocarditis, coronary artery spasm, and pericarditis. *(Wilson, p 791)*

150. (E) Recovery from mononucleosis is gradual, and the disorder is self-limiting. Avoiding contact sports for 6 to 8 weeks may prevent splenic rupture. Timing of return to school or work is determined by the degree of symptoms. Fever is present in over 90% of patients and may reach 40°C (104°F). The fever most often continues for 1 to 2 weeks. Lymphadenopathy often persists for 3 weeks.

Malaise is noted to be the most persistent symptom. Pharyngitis reaches a peak at about 1 week, then resolves over the next 7 to 10 days. 80% of patients with mononucleosis who are given penicillin will develop a generalized rash. Treatment with glucocorticoids is reserved for the symptoms of airway obstruction and perhaps in those cases where hemolytic anemia is present. *(Wilson, p 793)*

151. **(A)** While newborns have a visual preference for the human face, a social smile, cooing, and listening to voice occur at about 8 weeks. At about 12 weeks, the infant is noted to demonstrate sustained social contact. At 16 weeks, the baby will laugh out loud and is excited at the sight of food. At 28 weeks, the baby babbles and enjoys a mirror. Response to his or her name, waving bye-bye, and peekaboo games take place at approximately 10 months. *(Behrman, p 33)*

152. **(B)** At 16 weeks, the infant will not display head lag upon being pulled to a sitting position. At 28 weeks, the infant will sit briefly and lean forward on the hands. Motor activity of creeping or crawling occurs at approximately 40 weeks. At 40 weeks, sitting up alone is accomplished, without support and with the back straight. At 1 year, motor activity includes walking with one hand held and walking while holding onto furniture. *(Behrman, p 33)*

153. **(E)** Only subcortical (brainstem and spinal cord) reflexes may be tested for at birth. At this stage, major cerebral defects may not be detected. Reflexes that are present at birth include Moro's, stepping, placing, sucking, rooting palmar grasp, and plantar grasp. Landau's reflex appears at approximately 3 months and persists to about 2 years of age. It consists of extension of the head, trunk, and hips while the infant is supported in a prone position. If the examiner flexes the head, the trunk and hips will flex. At 2 months, tonic neck reflexes will be noted, while at 9 months the parachute reaction is noted. *(Behrman, p 1279)*

154. **(C)** The tonic neck reflex consists of extension of the arm and leg on the same side. This occurs when the infant's head is turned quickly to one side. Also noted is flexion of the extremities on the opposite side, similar to the pose of a fencer. This reflex is noted in infants between the ages of 2 to 4 months. Persistence of tonic neck reflexes is noted in infants with central motor lesions (eg, spastic cerebral palsy). *(Behrman, p 1279)*

HOSPITAL ROUNDS

155. **(B)** While falls increase in prevalence with age, fractures are seen in only 5 to 10% of subjects who fall. Another 30 to 40% of persons who fall will sustain soft-tissue injury. In 1990, there were over 250 000 hip fractures, and patients over the age of 65 accounted for 87% of these cases. These hip fractures are generally classified into two groups: subcapital (femoral neck) fractures and intertrochanteric or subtrochanteric fractures. Of note, a major differentiation between the two groups is the disruption of the blood supply to the femoral head. Subcapital fractures are associated with disruption of blood flow to the femoral neck and lead to a higher incidence of nonunion and necrosis of the femoral head. Intertrochanteric fractures, which do not disturb the blood flow to the femoral neck, have a lower incidence of nonunion and necrosis but are more commonly associated with acute complications associated with fracture (eg, major bleeding and instability). Factors correlated with hip-fracture risk in the elderly include advancing age, dementia of the Alzheimer's type, psychotropic medications including long-acting benzodiazepines, female gender, and osteopenia. *(Pierron et al; Tinetti et al)*

156. **(D)** Venous thromboembolism represents a major cause of complications after hip fracture. Before the advent of thromboembolic prophylaxis, deep-vein thrombosis developed in about 50% of patients with hip fractures, pulmonary emboli in about 10% of pa-

tients, and death in 2 to 5% of patients. Therefore treatment for prophylaxis of deep-vein thrombosis should be initiated preoperatively if possible and continued throughout the hospital stay. In choosing antithrombotic agents, the use of dextran is generally not considered for the older patient because of the opportunities for fluid overflow and increased bleeding associated with its use. Warfarin has been used and shown effective in the prevention of thromboembolic disease. Formerly, the prothrombin time was useful in the management of anticoagulation in patients on warfarin therapy; however, a change in thromboplastin agents used by the various hospitals resulted in marked variation in values of prothrombin levels. Therefore, the International Normalized Ratio (INR) is now considered the standard of care for the management of anticoagulation. An INR level of 2.0 to 2.5 is acceptable for the management of thromboembolic disease in this patient. (*Amstutz et al; Hirsh and Poller*)

157. **(B)** The patient has an acute confusional state or delirium, which occurs in approximately 10 to 25% of hospitalized patients. The hallmark of this disorder is decreased attention with disorganized thinking developing over hours or days, with fluctuations throughout the day. The best test for diagnosing this disorder is low-tech in nature and is provided through the Folstein Mini-Mental State Examination. A test for attention and calculation could include either a digit span examination, asking the patient to repeat five digits forward and three digits backwards, or asking the patient to spell the word *world* backwards. Errors in these parameters suggests a diagnosis of delirium. Serum ammonia levels have been shown to increase in many diseases associated with confusion, especially those associated with hepatic degeneration, but these represent a poor correlation for either the diagnosis or management of confusion. Tests of delayed recall are especially helpful in judging the patient's short-term memory and could be a useful diagnostic test for Alzheimer's disease. Disturbance in naming, either confrontational or genera-

tive, are more often seen with severe dementias associated with white matter disease. (*Gustafson et al; Schor et al*)

158. **(D)** Delirium affects possibly 30 to 40% of all older persons admitted to the hospital. The new onset of confusion should be regarded as a medical emergency unless proven otherwise. Causes of acute confusional state can be described by the mnemonic DELIRIUM, and include drugs, such as anticholinergic agents and narcotics, as well as sedative-hypnotics; electrolyte imbalance, such as hypo- or hypernatremia and hypo- or hyperglycemia; lack of sleep; infection; reduced sensation; fecal impaction; urinary retention; and myocardium, including heart failure, cardiac arrhythmia, and myocardial infarction. While Alzheimer's disease is a predisposing factor for delirium, and delirium is often seen in patients with Alzheimer's disease, this acute confusional state cannot be attributed to the presence of Alzheimer's disease, and an investigative search should be commenced, examining the possible etiologies of the patient's current signs and symptoms and not attributing the condition to Alzheimer's disease. (*Francis et al; Johnson et al*)

159. **(E)** Despite an overall decline in cardiovascular disease mortality, heart disease remains a common and serious medical problem for the elderly. While adults 65 and older make up only 12% of the population, 80% of all deaths from acute myocardial infarction occur in patients 65 years and older. The inpatient case fatality rate for initial acute myocardial infarction reaches 33% in those 75 years and older. Given the dramatically poor outcomes of older patients as compared to younger patients, therapy with modern agents is exceedingly beneficial in this older age group. Despite the rationale for the use of beta-blockers for acute myocardial infarction and numerous studies suggesting efficacy even in the very old, many clinicians still resist prescribing these drugs for elderly MI patients. The same is true for chemical thrombolysis, although several placebo-

controlled mortality trials of thrombolytic therapy have shown decreased mortality and greater benefit for patients 70 years or older, with mortality decreased by 16.9% with lytic therapy in the higher age groups. In the Warfarin Reinfarction Study, mortality was reduced by 24% and reinfarction by 34% in patients who received anticoagulation therapy versus those who did not. (*Forman et al; Krumholz and Wei, pp 101–109*)

160. **(C)** Decubitus ulcers are common complications of hospital stay. The prevalence of decubitus ulcers reaches 10%. Causative factors for decubitus ulcers include pressure, as up to 200 mm Hg for 11 hours can cause a full-thickness ulcer. Shearing forces cause ulcers by tearing subcutaneous capillaries, such as the fragile subcutaneous capillaries over the sacrum. Friction produced by transferring or pulling patients across a bed surface can lead to abrasion. Moisture from perspiration or incontinence, both fecal and urinary, dramatically increases the likelihood of developing a pressure ulcer. While immobility in and of itself is not a risk factor for pressure ulcer, the relief of pressure through a number of devices or frequent turning of the patient every 2 hours from a left-lateral to right-lateral 30 to 60 degree oblique position is helpful in preventing decubitus ulcers. (*Allman; Brandeis et al*)

161. **(C)** Decubitus ulcers remain a difficult problem because of their propensity to occur among the frailest patients with multiple medical problems. The hospital prevalence of this disease is approximately 10%. The national cost for care of this disorder can reach seven billion dollars, and 70% of cases occur in patients over 70. A colonization is common with all hospital-acquired wounds, and sepsis may result from localized infection in the pressure ulcer, with mortality as high as 50%. Given the increased costs and complications associated with this disease in the older patient, prevention of decubitus ulcers represents an important approach for the hospitalized patient. The bony sacrum, ischial tuberoses, trochanter, heels, and lateral malleoli

account for 80% of all decubitus ulcers. (*Goode and Allman; Panel*)

162. **(D)** In a prospective study of patients undergoing surgery at the Massachusetts General Hospital, Goldman et al evaluated the risk of surgical morbidity of cardiac complications associated with noncardiac operations. Independent risk factors included age under 70; presence of jugular venus distention or third heart sound; myocardial infarction in the previous 6 months; less than five premature ventricular contractions per minute; cardiac rhythm other than sinus; emergency operation; intrathoracic, intraabdominal, or aortic surgery; significant aortic valvular stenosis; and general poor medical condition. This index provides a low-tech evaluation of a patient's risk for surgery. Another standardized index available to categorize elderly patients and their risk for surgical complications is the American Society of Anesthesiology (ASA) Physical Status Classification, which has been validated for individuals over 80. This classification system divides risk according to mild systemic disease, severe systemic disease, morbid condition, and emergency operation. (*Gilbert and Minaker; Goldman et al*)

163. **(A)** Using the Goldman Cardiac Risk Index, the patient could be classified according to the schema described above. In this patient, the age over 70 and the intra-abdominal nature of the procedure classify a total of 8 points out of a possible 53. The risk of a cardiac death associated with this procedure is 2%, and the risk of life-threatening complications is 5%. Alternatively, there are minor or no complications in 93% of surgical cases. Using the American Society of Anesthesiology Physical Status Classification, the patient is ASA II, associated with a mortality of approximately 1%. Geriatric patients commonly are candidates for elective as well as for emergency surgical intervention. The quality of their perioperative care often determines whether their outcome is successful. Surgery can be performed successfully on very old patients, and questions on the initial preoper-

ative assessment of the older patient should include: is the proposed surgery reasonable; is the operation consistent with the patient's values and wishes; and has the posthospital care been considered? *(Lubin; Minaker and Rowe, pp 415–424)*

164. (D) Chronic obstructive pulmonary disease (COPD) encompasses a group of diseases characterized by obstruction of expired air flow. Therapy for elderly patients with COPD is limited and directed toward controlling symptoms, increasing physical activity, promoting independent self-care, and reducing hospitalization. These important objectives can greatly benefit the lives of older patients with COPD. Bronchodilators such as theophylline remain useful in the care of the COPD patient despite controversy surrounding their role. Beta-adrenergic drugs are especially helpful as inhaled preparations and can provide effective bronchodilation with few if any side effects. Anticholinergic drugs such as ipratropium are helpful in the management and improving ventilatory functions in patients with COPD. Corticosteroids can benefit those with reactive airway disease, while inhaled corticosteroids represent a major therapeutic advance through the avoidance of systemic side effects as a result of chronic oral use. However, inhaled corticosteroids are not beneficial in the acute management of COPD but represent a major therapeutic strategy for long-term care. *(Ferguson and Cherniack; Skorodin)*

165. (A) With normal aging, growth and development of the human lung continues to about age 20. Following the variable period of stability, many parameters of function decline steadily with advancing age. With advancing age, loss of elastic recall causes closure of small airways in the lower regions of the lung during normal respiration and decreases gas exchange, resulting in an increased residual volume and a lower resting serum oxygen tension. Decreased lung elasticity is a result of changes in collagen. Respiratory muscle strength and endurance decreases with age. There is decreased chest

compliance with normal aging, not increased chest compliance. *(Tockman, pp 499–508; Williams and Evans)*

166. (A) *Escherichia coli* is the most common organism associated with urinary tract infection in women. While the prevalence of *E coli* as a causative organism reaches 80 to 90% in young women, there is a change in the epidemiology of urinary pathogens in the older individual. *E coli* remains the most likely organism in the older patient and is responsible for 50 to 60% of urinary tract infections, with an increasing frequency of gram-positive infections such as staphylococci and enterococci. *(Baldassarre and Kaye; Stamm and Hooton)*

167. (D) Asymptomatic bacteriuria represents a common condition in the older individual. Predisposing factors that lead to the development of colonization in the urinary tract include a short urethra, allowing access from the vagina and perianal area to the bladder, as well as atrophic vaginitis with a decrease in circulating serum estrogen and a loss of the normal mucosal barrier. There is no evidence that treatment of disorder is helpful in eradicating this colonization, and it can be detrimental because of the adverse side effects associated with treatment and in consideration of public health concerns about the emergence of resistant organisms. Ciprofloxacin and ampicillin are both useful antibiotics in the management of urinary tract pathogens; most urinary tract organisms can be treated with both agents with equal efficacy. The most common source of infection is the ascending route of infection from the vagina to the bladder, and descending routes are relatively less likely. There is no reason to delay hospital discharge for this patient. *(Boscia et al; Nicolle)*

168. (D) Toxicity is commonly associated with use of theophylline. The most frequent adverse effects are nausea, cardiac arrhythmias, confusion, and seizures and their incidence is only roughly correlated with serum drug levels. A number of factors affect the metabolism of theophylline and can raise normal serum levels to toxic levels; for example, the use of cimetidine can inhibit cytochrome P-450 metabolism of theophylline. Noncompliance with theophylline could also raise the patient's drug level to the toxic levels demonstrated in this case; however, underuse is generally more common than overuse in clinical practice. Noncompliance with the other medications listed is not a clinical factor associated with the case presented. There are no known pharmacokinetic or pharmacodynamic interactions between theophylline and corticosteroids. *(Vaz Fragoso and Miller; Vestal et al)*

EMERGENCY DEPARTMENT

169–171. (169-C, 170-B, 171-B) This case describes a woman with physical findings consistent with immune deficiency. The most likely diagnosis in a patient with acquired immune deficiency who presents with a shortness of breath and cough is *Pneumocystis carinii* pneumonia (PCP). PCP most commonly presents as diffuse interstitial infiltrates on chest radiograph. A lobar infiltrate is more suggestive of bacterial pneumonia.

The diagnosis of PCP is suggested by the absence of leukocytosis, hypoxia, and an elevation in serum LDH.

The drug of choice for treatment of *Pneumocystis carinii* is TMP–SMX (trimethoprim 20 mg/kg/d and sulfamethoxazole 100 mg/kg/d) intravenously for 2 to 3 weeks. Pentamidine (intravenously) is indicated as second-line therapy in the presence of TMP–SMX allergy or treatment failure after 4 to 5 days of TMP–SMX treatment. INH, rifampin, and ethambutol are indicated for the treatment of pulmonary tuberculosis. *(Rosen et al, 3rd ed, p 2316)*

172–174. (172-D, 173-B, 174-B) In several studies the cremasteric reflex could not be demonstrated in patients with proven torsion of the spermatic cord. The absence of this reflex strongly suggests the diagnosis of spermatic cord torsion. Prehn's sign, *worsening* of pain

caused by torsion by elevating the scrotal contents, is extremely unreliable in making the diagnosis. A "blue dot" sign is a classic sign of torsion of the testicular appendage.

Although testicular scans are useful, they should not be ordered before urologic consultation. Testicular scan and Doppler ultrasonography should be reserved for cases in which the diagnosis is questioned by an experienced examiner. Surgical exploration should not be delayed for the arrangement of diagnostic studies.

Surgery is the only definitive treatment for torsion of the spermatic cord. Manual distortion may be attempted in the emergency department while the patient is awaiting surgery. *(Fleisher and Ludwig, pp 237,239–240; Edelsberg and Surh)*

175. (B) Successful treatment of ventricular fibrillation depends on how rapidly defibrillation occurs. Immediate defibrillation should take precedence over all other interventions. Asystole needs to be verified by checking another lead, since ventricular fibrillation may appear as asystole if the fibrillatory vector is perpendicular to the recording lead. *(Rosen et al, 3rd ed, p 123)*

176. (D) Epinephrine, atropine, lidocaine, and naloxone can be administered via the endotracheal route. *(Rosen, 3rd ed, p 122)*

177. (D) Ten percent to 25% of patients with ventricular fibrillation will survive to discharge. *(Rosen et al, 3rd ed, p 123)*

178–179. (178-B, 179-C) Acute cholecystitis is more common in middle-aged to elderly women. Physical examination usually reveals right-upper-quadrant tenderness with rebound and guarding. In 30 to 70% of cases there is a palpable gallbladder. Mild to moderate jaundice is present, with severe jaundice suggesting obstruction of the common duct. Murphy's sign refers to pain on inspiration during palpation of the right-upper-quadrant as a result of diaphragm touching the inflamed gallbladder.

Ultrasound and CT scan can assess the

anatomy of the biliary tree and the presence of gallstones. However, confirmation of acute cholecystitis requires radionuclide scanning to demonstrate obstruction and is considered the test of choice. It is a noninvasive diagnostic test without the risk of intravenous contrast. *(Rosen et al, 2nd ed, p 1449; Rosen et al, 3rd ed, p 1617)*

180. (A) The most important step in the initial management of diabetic ketoacidosis (DKA) is fluid resuscitation. Patients may have a 5 to 6 liter fluid deficit. Fluid administration alone will considerably reduce both the acidosis and hyperglycemia. Sodium bicarbonate is indicated if the arterial pH falls below 7.1. *(Rosen et al, 3rd ed, p 2185)*

REFERENCES

Anatomy

Hollinshead WH, Rosse C. *Textbook of Anatomy.* 4th ed. Philadelphia: Harper & Row Publishers Inc; 1985.

Moore KL. *Clinically Oriented Anatomy.* 3rd ed. Baltimore: Williams & Wilkins; 1992.

Noback CR, Strominger NL, Demarest RJ. *The Human Nervous System.* 5th ed. Philadelphia: Lea & Febiger; 1996.

Sadler TW. *Langman's Medical Embryology.* 7th ed. Baltimore: Williams & Wilkins; 1995.

Woodburne RT, Burckel WE. *Essentials of Human Anatomy.* 9th ed. New York: Oxford University Press; 1994.

Behavioral Sciences

Leigh H, Reiser MF. *The Patient: Biological, Psychological, and Social Dimensions of Medical Practice.* 3rd ed. New York: Plenum Press; 1992.

Kaplan HI, Sadock BJ, Grebb JA. *Kaplan and Sadock's Synopsis of Psychiatry, Behavioral Sciences, Clinical Psychiatry.* 7th ed. Baltimore: Williams & Wilkins; 1994.

Scheiber SC, Doyle BB, eds. *The Impaired Physician.* New York: Plenum Publishing Corp; 1983.

Simons RC. *Understanding Human Behavior in Health and Illness.* 3rd ed. Baltimore, Md: Williams & Wilkins; 1985.

Tanner JM. *Growth at Adolescence.* 2nd ed. Oxford, England: Blackwell Scientific Publications; 1962.

Biochemistry

Stryer L. *Biochemistry.* 4th ed. New York: WH Freeman Co Publishers; 1995.

Emergency Medicine Case Studies

Edelsberg J, Surh Y. The acute scrotum. *Emerg Clin North Am.* 1988;6:521–546.

Fleisher G, Ludwig S. *Textbook of Pediatric Emergency Medicine.* 3rd ed. Baltimore, Md: Williams & Wilkins; 1993.

Rosen P, Baker F, Barkin R, et al. 2nd ed. *Emergency Medicine Concepts and Clinical Practice.* St. Louis, Mo: CV Mosby Co; 1988.

Rosen P, Barkin R, Braen R, et al. 3rd ed. *Emergency Medicine Concepts and Clinical Practice.* St. Louis, Mo: Mosby Year Book; 1992.

Hospital Rounds

Allman RM. Pressure ulcers among the elderly. *N Engl J Med.* 1989;320:850–853.

Amstutz HC, Friscia DA, Dorey F, et al. Warfarin prophylaxis to prevent mortality from pulmonary embolism after total hip replacement. *J Bone Joint Surg Am.* 1989;71:321–326.

Baldassarre JS, Kaye D. Special problems of urinary tract infection in the elderly. *Med Clin North Am.* 1991;75:375–390.

Boscia JA, Abrutyn E, Kaye D. Asymptomatic bacteriuria in elderly persons: treat or do not treat? *Ann Intern Med.* 1987;106:764–766.

Brandeis GH, Morris JN, Nash DJ, et al. The epidemiology and natural history of pressure ulcers in elderly nursing homes residents. *JAMA.* 1990;264:2905–2909.

Ferguson GT, Cherniack RM. Management of chronic obstructive pulmonary disease. *N Engl J Med.* 1993; 328:1017–1022.

Forman DE, Bernal J, Wei JY. Management of acute myocardial infarction in the very elderly. *Am J Med.* 1992;93:315–326.

Francis J, Martin D, Kapoor WN. A prospective study of delirium in hospitalized elderly. *JAMA.* 1990;263: 1097–1101.

Gilbert GH, Minaker KL. Principles of surgical risk assessment of the elderly patient. *J Oral Maxillofac Surg.* 1990;48:972–979.

Goldman L, Caldera DL, Nussbaum SR, et al. Multifactorial index of cardiac risk in noncardiac surgical patients. *N Engl J Med.* 1977;297:845.

Goode PS, Allman RM. The prevention and management of pressure ulcers. *Med Clin North Am.* 1989;73: 1511–1524.

Gustafson Y, Brannstrom B, Norberg A, et al. Underdiagnosis and poor documentation of acute confusional states in elderly hip fracture patients. *J Am Geriatr Soc.* 1991;39:760–765.

Hirsh J, Poller L. The International Normalized Ratio: a guide to understanding and correcting its problems. *Arch Intern Med.* 1994;154:282–288.

Johnson JC, Gottlieb GL, Sullivan E, et al. Using DSM-III criteria to diagnose delirium in elderly general medical patients. *J Gerontol.* 1990;45:M113–M119.

Krumholz HM, Wei JY. Acute myocardial infarction: clinical presentations and diagnosis. In: Gersh BH, Rahimtoola SH, eds. *Acute Myocardial Infarction.* New York, NY: Elsevier Press; 1991.

Lubin MF. Is age a risk factor for surgery? *Med Clin North Am.* 1993;77:327–333.

Minaker KL, Rowe JW. Anesthesia and surgery. In: Rowe JW, Besdine RW, eds. *Health and Disease in Old Age.* Boston, Mass: Little, Brown & Co Inc; 1982.

Nicolle LE. Urinary tract infection in the elderly. How to treat and when? *Infection.* 1992;(suppl 4):S261–S265.

Panel for the Prediction and Prevention of Pressure Ulcers in Adults. *Pressure Ulcers in Adults: Prediction and Prevention.* Rockville, Md: Agency for Health Care Policy and Research, Public Health Service, US Department of Health and Human Services; 1992. AHCPR Publication No. 92-0047. Clinical Practice Guideline, No. 3.

Pierron RL, Perry HM, Grossberg G, et al. The aging hip. *J Am Geriatr Soc.* 1990;38:1339–1352.

Schor J, Levkoff SE, Lipsitz LA, et al. Risk factors for delirium in hospitalized elderly. *JAMA.* 1992;267: 827–831.

Skorodin MS. Pharmacotherapy for asthma and chronic obstructive pulmonary disease: current thinking, practices, and controversies. *Arch Intern Med.* 1993; 153:814–828.

Stamm WE, Hooton TM. Management of urinary tract infections in adults. *N Engl J Med.* 1993;329: 1328–1334.

Tinetti ME, Speechley M, Greinter SF. Risk factors for falls among elderly persons living in the community. *N Engl J Med.* 1998;319:1701–1709.

Tockman MS. Aging of the respiratory system. In: Hazzard WR, Andres R, Bierman EL, et al, eds. *Principles of Geriatric Medicine and Gerontology.* 2nd ed. New York, NY: McGraw-Hill Book Co Inc; 1990.

Vaz Fragoso CA, Miller MA. Review of the clinical efficacy of theophylline in the treatment of chronic obstructive pulmonary disease. *Am Rev Resp Dis.* 1993; 147:540–547.

Vestal RE, Cusak BJ, Crowley JJ, et al. Aging and the response to inhibition and induction of theophylline metabolism. *Exp Gerontol.* 1993;28:421–433.

Williams JM, Evans TC. Acute pulmonary disease in the aged. *Clin Geriatr Med.* 1993;9:527–545.

Internal Medicine

Isselbacher KJ, Braunwald E, Wilson JD, et al, eds. *Harrison's Principles of Internal Medicine.* 13th ed. New York, NY: McGraw-Hill Book Co; 1994.

Hazzard WR, Bierman EL, Blass JP, et al., eds. *Principles of Geriatric Medicine and Gerontology.* 3rd ed. New York, NY: McGraw-Hill Book Co; 1994.

Wyngaarden JB, Smith LH Jr, eds. *Cecil's Textbook of Medicine.* 19th ed. Philadelphia, Pa: WB Saunders Co; 1992.

Microbiology

Joklik WK, Willett HP, Amos DB, et al. *Zinsser Microbiology.* 20th ed. Norwalk, Conn: Appleton & Lange; 1992.

Obstetrics and Gynecology

Cunningham FG, MacDonald PC, Gant NF. *Williams Obstetrics.* 19th ed. East Norwalk, Conn: Appleton & Lange; 1993.

Gant NF, Cunningham FG. *Basic Gynecology and Obstetrics.* East Norwalk, CT: Appleton & Lange; 1993.

DeCherney AM, Pernoll ML. Current Obstetric & Gynecologic Diagnosis & Treatment. 8th ed. East Norwalk, CT: Appleton & Lange; 1994.

Pathology

Chandrasoma P, Taylor CR. *Concise Pathology.* 2nd ed. Norwalk: Appleton and Lange; 1995.

Cotran RS, Kumar V, Robbins SL. *Robbins Pathologic Basis of Disease.* 5th ed. Philadelphia: WB Saunders Company; 1994.

Rubin E, Farber JL. *Pathology.* 2nd ed. Philadelphia, Pa: JB Lippincott; 1994.

Pediatrics

Berman SA, Balkany TJ, Simmons MA. Otitis media in infants less than 12 weeks of age: differing bacteriology among in-patients and out-patients. *J Pediatr.* 1978;93: 453.

Bland RD. Otitis media in the first six weeks of life: diagnosis, bacteriology and management. *Pediatrics.* 1972; 49:187.

Callaham ML. *Current Practice of Emergency Medicine.* 2nd ed. Philadelphia, Pa: BC Decker; 1991.

Dinarello CA, Cannon JG, Wolff SM. New concepts on the pathogenesis of fever. *Rev Infect Dis.* 1988;10:168.

Feigin RD, Cherry JD. *Textbook of Pediatric Infectious Diseases.* 2nd ed. Philadelphia, Pa: WB Saunders Co; 1987.

Gauthier B, Edelman CM, Barnett HL. *Nephrology and Urology for the Pediatrician.* Boston: Little, Brown & Co; 1982.

Ginsburg CM, Henle W, Henle G. Infectious mononucleosis in children: evaluation of Epstein-Barr virus-specific serologic data. *JAMA.* 1977;237:781.

Harlan WR, Cornoni-Huntley J, Leaverton PE. Blood pressure in childhood: *The National Health Examination Survey.* Hypertension 1979;1:559–565.

Kempe CH, Silver HK, O'Brien D, et al. *Current Pediatric Diagnosis and Treatment.* Norwalk, Conn: Appleton & Lange; 1987.

Lebenthal E. Recurrent abdominal pain in childhood. *Am J Dis Child.* 1980;134:347–348.

Levy JS. Total parenteral nutrition in pediatric patients. *Pediatr. Rev.* 1980;2:99.

Liebman WM. Recurrent abdominal pain in children: lactose and sucrose intolerance—a prospective study. *Pediatrics.* 1979;64:43–45.

Linshaw MA, Stapleton FB, Gruskin AB, et al. Blood pressure in childhood hypertension. *J Pediatr.* 1979; 95:994.

Lipson A, Beuhler B, Bartley J, Walsh D, et al. Maternal hyperphenylalaninemia fetal effects. *J. Pediatr.* 1984; 104:216–220.

Morb Mortal Wkly Rep. 1988;37:341.

Newth CJL. Recognition and management of respiratory failure. *Pediatr Clin North Am.* 1979;26: 617–618.

O'Donovan JC, Bradstock AS, Pharm BS. The failure of conventional drug therapy in the management of infantile colic. *Am J Dis Child.* 1979; 133:999.

Oski FA, DeAngelis CD, Feigin RD, et al. *Principles and Practice of Pediatrics.* Philadelphia, Pa: JB Lippincott; 1990.

Rogers MF. AIDS in children: a review of the clinical, epidemiologic and public health aspects. *Pediatr Infect Dis.* 1985;4:230–236.

Rudolph AM, Hoffman JIE, Rudolph CD. *Pediatrics.* 19th ed. Norwalk, Conn: Appleton & Lange; 1991.

Saenger P. Abnormal sex differentiation. *J Pediatr.* 1984; 104:1–17.

Schmitt BD. Nocturnal enuresis: an update on treatment. *Pediatr Clin North Am.* 1982;29:21–36.

Shurin PA, Howie VM, Pelton SI, et al. Bacterial etiology of otitis media during the first six weeks of life. *J Pediatr.* 1978;92:893.

Thomas DW, McGilligan K, Eisenberg LD, et al. Infant colic and type of milk feeding. *Am J Dis Child.* 1987; 141:451.

Vehaskari VM, Rapola M. Isolated proteinuria: analysis of a school-age population. *J Pediatr.* 1982;101:661– 668.

Pharmacology

Craig CR, Stitzel RE, eds. *Modern Pharmacology.* 4th ed. Boston: Little, Brown & Co Inc; 1994.

Hardman JG, Limbird LE, Molinoff PB, Ruddon RW, Gilman AG, eds. *Goodman & Gilman's The Pharmacological Basis of Therapeutics.* 9th ed. New York: McGraw-Hill; 1996.

Physiology

Ganong WF. *Review of Medical Physiology.* 17th ed. Norwalk, Conn: Appleton & Lange; 1995.

Guyton AC. *Textbook of Physiology.* 9th ed. Philadelphia, Pa: WB Saunders Co; 1996.

Preventive Medicine

Ahlbom A, Norell S. *Introduction to Modern Epidemiology.* Chestnut Hill, Mass: Epidemiology Resources, Inc; 1990.

Clark DW, MacMahon B. *Preventive and Community Medicine.* 2nd ed. Boston, Mass: Little, Brown & Co; 1981.

Kelley WN. *Textbook of Internal Medicine.* Philadelphia, Pa: JB Lippincott Co; 1989.

Kramer MS. *Clinical Epidemiology & Biostatistics: A Primer for Clinical Investigators and Decision-Makers.* Berlin, Germany: Springer-Verlag; 1988.

Last JM, Wallace R. *Maxcy-Rosenau-Last Public Health and Preventive Medicine.* 13th ed. Norwalk, CT: Appleton & Lange; 1992.

Levy BS, Wegman DH. *Occupational Health: Recognizing and Preventing Work Related Disease.* Boston, Mass: Little, Brown & Co; 1995.

Luft HS. Assessing the evidence of HMO performance. *Milbank Memorial Fund Quarterly; Health and Society.* 1980; (Oct-Dec):501–536.

Mausner JS, Bahn AK. *Epidemiology: An Introductory Text.* Philadelphia: WB Saunders Co; 1985.

Morton RF, Hebel JR. *A Study Guide to Epidemiology and Biostatistics.* Baltimore, Md: University Park Press; 1996.

Warren DG. *A Legal Guide for Rural Health Programs.* Cambridge, Mass: Ballinger Publishing Co; 1979.

Wyngaarden JB, Smith LM. *Cecil's Textbook of Medicine.* 18th ed. Philadelphia: WB Saunders Co; 1996.

Psychiatry

American Psychiatric Association (APA). *Diagnostic and Statistical Manual of Mental Disorders.* 4th ed. Washington DC: American Psychiatric Association; 1994.

Dunner DL, ed. *The Psychiatric Clinics of North America: Psychopharmacology II.* Philadelphia: WB Saunders Co., Dec 1993.

Halleck SL. *Law in the Practice of Psychiatry: A Handbook for Clinicians.* New York, NY: Plenum Medical Book Co, 1980.

Hales RE, Frances AJ, eds. *Psychiatry Update: American Psychiatric Association Annual Review.* Washington DC: American Psychiatric Press Inc; 1987;6.

Kaplan HI, Sadock BJ. *Comprehensive Textbook of Psychiatry VI.* 6th ed. Baltimore, Md: Williams & Wilkins; 1995; 2 vols.

Tupin JP, Shader RI, Harnett DS. *Handbook of Clinical Psychopharmacology.* 2nd ed. Northvale, NJ: Jason Aronson Inc; 1992.

Scheduled Appointments

Behrman RE. *Nelson Textbook of Pediatrics.* 15th ed. Philadelphia, Pa: WB Saunders Co; 1996.

Kursh ED. *Urology.* Oradell, NJ: Medical Economics Books; 1987.

Rakel RE. *Textbook of Family Practice.* 5th ed. Philadelphia, Pa: WB Saunders Co; 1995.

Wilson JD, Braunwald E, Isselbacher KJ, et al, eds. *Harrison's Principles of Internal Medicine.* 13th ed. New York, NY: McGraw-Hill Book Co Inc; 1994.

Woodley M. *The Washington Manual of Medical Therapeutics.* 28th ed. Boston, Mass: Little, Brown & Co Inc; 1995.

Jenson HP. *Pediatric Infectious Diseases, Principles and Practice.* Norwalk, Conn: Appleton & Lange; 1995.

Surgery

Braverman, LE, Utinger RD, eds., *Werner & Ingbar's The Thyroid: A Fundamental Clinical Text.* 6th ed. Philadelphia, Pa: Lippincott; 1991.

Cummings CW, et al, ed. *Otolarygology—Head and Neck Surgery.* 2nd ed. St. Louis, Missouri: Mosby Year Book; 1993.

David JA. *Wound Management.* Springhouse, Pa: Springhouse Corp. 1986.

Feliciano DV, Moore EE, Mattox KL, eds. *Trauma.* 3rd ed. Stamford, Ct: Appleton & Lange; 1996.

Greenfield LJ, et al. *Surgery: Scientific Principles and Practice.* Philadelphia, Pa: JB Lippincott Co; 1993.

Hardy JD, ed. *Hardy's Textbook of Surgery.* Philadelphia, Pa: JB Lippincott Co; 1988.

Juhl JH. *Paul and Juhl's Essentials of Roentgen Interpretation.* New York, NY: Harper & Row Publishers Inc; 1993.

Marini JJ. *Respiratory Medicine and Intensive Care for the House Officer.* Baltimore, Md: Williams & Wilkins; 1987.

Moore FA, Haenel JB, Moore EE. Alternatives to Swan-Ganz cardiac output monitoring. *Surg Clin N Am.* 1991;71:699–717.

Sabiston DC, ed. *Davis-Christopher Textbook of Surgery.* 14th ed. Philadelphia, Pa: WB Saunders Co; 1991.

Schwartz SI, Shires GT, Spencer FC, eds. *Principles of Surgery.* 6th ed. New York, NY: McGraw-Hill Book Co; 1994.

Schwartz SI, Ellis H, eds. *Maingot's abdominal operations,* 9th ed. Norwalk, Conn: Appleton & Lange; 1990.

Skinner DG, Lieskovsky G. *Genitourinary Cancer.* Philadelphia, Pa: WB Saunders Co; 1988.

Tanagho EA, McAninch JW. *Smith's General Urology.* 13th ed. Norwalk, Conn: Appleton & Lange; 1992.

Thompson NW, Cheung SY. Diagnosis and treatment of functioning and nonfunctioning adrenocortical neoplasms including incidentalomas. *Surg Clin North Am.* 1987;67(2):423–436.

Vander AJ. *Renal Physiology.* 5th ed. New York, NY: McGraw-Hill Book Co; 1995.

PRACTICE TEST SUBSPECIALTY LIST

ANATOMY

7. Central nervous system
14. Peripheral nervous system
21. Peripheral nervous system
28. Embryology
35. Embryology
42. Embryology
43. Skeletal system
49. Muscular system

BEHAVIORAL SCIENCES

13. Individual dynamics
20. Human sexuality
27. Human sexuality
34. Substance Abuse

41. Psychopathology
48. Alcoholism

BIOCHEMISTRY

3. Enzymes
9. Lipids
16. Lipids
23. Hormones
30. Vitamins
37. Energy metabolism
44. Carbohydrates
50. Small-molecule metabolism
51. Small-molecule metabolism
52. Small-molecule metabolism

INTERNAL MEDICINE

66. Cardiovascular system diseases
67. Gastroenterology
68. Gastroenterology
69. Cardiovascular system diseases
75. Gastroenterology
79. Nephrology
84. Cardiovascular system diseases
89. Nephrology
95. Endocrinology
101. Dermatology
107. Dermatology

MICROBIOLOGY

4. Virology
10. Physiology
17. Physiology
24. Pathogenic bacteriology
31. Pathogenic bacteriology
38. Immune deficiency syndrome
45. Virology

53. Virology
54. Pathogenic bacteriology
55. Virology

OBSTETRICS/GYNECOLOGY

93. Perinatal hazards
99. Clinical obstetrics, abnormal
105. Clinical gynecology
112. Prenatal gynecology
113. Prenatal gynecology

PATHOLOGY

5. Neoplasia
11. Alimentary system
18. Circulatory system
25. Musculoskeletal system
32. Nongenetic syndromes
39. Inflammation
46. Blood and lymphatic system
56. Miscellaneous
57. Miscellaneous

PEDIATRICS

61. Development
62. Development
63. Neonatology
64. Thoracic disease
65. Adolescent medicine
70. Eye, ear, nose, and throat
71. Infectious diseases
72. Genetics
74. Pharmacology
78. Neonatology
83. Oncology
88. Neurology
94. Neurology
100. Toxicology
106. Dermatology

PHARMACOLOGY

6. Central and peripheral nervous systems, sedatives and hypnotics
12. Chemotherapeutic agents
19. Rheumatology, anti-inflammatory drugs
26. Kidneys, bladder, fluids, and electrolytes, diuretics
33. Antibiotics
40. Endocrine system
47. Central and peripheral nervous systems, analgesics
58. Autonomic nervous system
59. Autonomic nervous system
60. Autonomic nervous system

PHYSIOLOGY

1. Temperature
2. Nervous system
8. Endocrinology
15. Gastrointestinal system
22. Endocrinology
29. Neurophysiology
36. Special senses

PREVENTIVE MEDICINE

77. Disease control
82. Disease control
87. Ethical and legal issues
92. Health services
98. Biostatistics
104. Epidemiology
110. Disease control
111. Disease control
118. Health services
119. Health services
120. Health services

PSYCHIATRY

73. Assessment
76. Psychopathology
81. Psychopathology
86. Intervention
91. Assessment
97. Psychopathology
103. Assessment
109. Legal issues
114. Intervention
115. Intervention

116. Intervention
117. Intervention

SURGERY

80. Gastroenterology
85. Genitourinary system
90. Cardiovascular system
96. Infection
102. Vascular system
108. Endocrine system

APPLETON & LANGE REVIEW SERIES

Health Related

Appleton & Lange's Review of Cardiovascular-Interventional Technology
Vitanza
1995, ISBN 0-8385-0248-2

Appleton & Lange's Review for the Chiropractic National Boards, Part I
Shanks
1992, ISBN 0-8385-0224-5

Appleton & Lange's Review for the Dental Assistant, 3/e
Andujo
1992, ISBN 0-8385-0135-4

Appleton & Lange's Review for the Dental Hygiene National Board Review, 4/e
Barnes and Waring
1995, ISBN 0-8385-0230-X

Appleton & Lange's Review for the Medical Assistant, 4/e
Palko and Palko
1994, ISBN 0-8385-0197-4

Medical Technology Examination Review, 2/e
Hossaini
1984, ISBN 0-8385-6283-3

Appleton & Lange's Review of Pharmacy, 5/e
Hall and Reiss
1993, ISBN 0-8385-0162-1
Appleton & Lange's Review for the

Appleton & Lange's Review for the Radiography Examination, 2/e
Saia
1993, ISBN 0-8385-0058-7

Radiography: Program Review & Exam Preparation (PREP)
Saia
1996, ISBN 0-8385-8244-3

Appleton & Lange's Review for the Surgical Technology Examination, 4/e
Allmers and Verderame
1996, ISBN 0-8385-0270-9

Appleton & Lange's Review for the Ultrasonography Examination, 2/e
Odwin
1993, ISBN 0-8385-9073-X

First Aid

1996 First Aid for the USMLE Step 1
A Student-to-Student Guide
Bhushan, Le, and Amin
1996, ISBN 0-8385-2597-0

First Aid for the USMLE Step 2
A Student-to-Student Guide
Go, Curet-Salim, and Fullerton
1996, ISBN 0-8385-2591-1

First Aid for the Wards
A Student-to-Student Guide
Le, Bhushan, and Amin
1996, ISBN 0-8385-2596-2

First Aid for the Match
A Student-to-Student Guide
Le, Bhushan, and Amin
1996, ISBN 0-8385-2596-2

Instant Exam

The Instant Exam Review for the USMLE Step 2, 2/e
Goldberg
1996, ISBN 0-8385-4328-6

The Instant Exam Review for the USMLE Step 3
Goldberg
1994, ISBN 0-8385-4334-0

Comprehensive A&L Reviews

Appleton & Lange's Review for the USMLE Step 1, 2/e
Barton
1996, ISBN 0-8385-0265-2

Appleton & Lange's Review for the USMLE Step 2, 2/e
Catlin
1996, ISBN 0-8385-0266-0

Appleton & Lange's Review for the USMLE Step 3, 2/e
Jacobs
1997, ISBN 0-8385-0305-5

Basic Science

Appleton & Lange's Review of Anatomy for the USMLE Step 1, 5/e
Montgomery
1995, ISBN 0-8385-0246-6

Appleton & Lange's Review of Epidemiology & Biostatistics for the USMLE
Hanrahan and Madupu
1994, ISBN 0-8385-0244-X

Appleton & Lange's Review of Microbiology and Immunology for the USMLE Step 1, 3/e
Yotis
1996, ISBN 0-8385-0273-3

Appleton & Lange's Review of General Pathology, 3/e
Lewis and Barton
1993, ISBN 0-8385-0161-3

Clinical Science

Appleton & Lange's Review of Internal Medicine
Goldlist
1996, ISBN 0-8385-0251-2

Appleton & Lange's Review of Obstetrics and Gynecology, 5/e
Julian, et al.
1995, ISBN 0-8385-0231-8

Appleton & Lange's Review of Pediatrics, 5/e
Lorin
1993, ISBN 0-8385-0057-9

Appleton & Lange's Review of Psychiatry, 5/e
Easson
1994, ISBN 0-8385-0247-4

Public Health and Preventive Medicine Review, 2/e
Penalver
1984, ISBN 0-8385-5936-2

Specialty Board Reviews

The MGH Board Review of Anesthesiology, 4/e
Dershwitz
1994, ISBN 0-8385-8611-4

(More on Reverse)

APPLETON & LANGE
QUICK REVIEW SERIES

Health Related
MEPC: Medical Assistant
Examination Review, 4/e
Dreizen and Audet
1989, ISBN 0-8385-5772-4

MEPC: Medical Record,
Examination Review, 6/e
Bailey
1994, ISBN 0-8385-6192-6

MEPC: Occupational Therapy
Examination Review, 5/e
Dundon
1988, ISBN 0-8385-7204-9

MEPC: Optometry
Examination Review, 4/e
Casser et al.
1994, ISBN 0-8385-7449-1

MEPC: Physician Assistant
Examination Review, 3/e
Rahr and Niebuhr
1996, ISBN 0-8385-8094-7

Comprehensive A & L Reviews
MEPC: USMLE Step 1 Review
Fayemi
1995, ISBN 0-8385-6269-8

MEPC: USMLE Step 2 Review
Jacobs
1996, ISBN 0-8385-6270-1, A6270-1

MEPC: USMLE Step 3 Review
Chan
1996, ISBN 0-8385-6339-2, A6339-4

Basic Science
MEPC: Anatomy, 10/e
A USMLE STEP 1 Review
Wilson
1995, ISBN 0-8385-6218-3

MEPC: Biochemistry, 11/e
A USMLE STEP 1 Review
Glick
1995, ISBN 0-8385-5779-1

MEPC: Microbiology, 11/e
A USMLE Step 1 Review
Kim
1995, ISBN 0-8385-6308-2

MEPC: Pathology, 10/e
A USMLE STEP 1 Review
Fayemi
1994, ISBN 0-8385-8441-1

MEPC: Pharmacology, 8/e
A USMLE STEP 1 Review
Krzanowski et al.
1995, ISBN 0-8385-6227-2

MEPC: Physiology, 9/e
A USMLE STEP 1 Review
Penney
1995, ISBN 0-8385-6222-1

Clinical Science
MEPC: Neurology, 10/e
A USMLE Step 2 Review
Slosberg
1993, ISBN 0-8385-5778-3

MEPC: Pediatrics, 9/e
A USMLE Step 2 Review
Hansbarger
1995, ISBN 0-8385-6223-X

MEPC: Preventive Medicine and Public Health, 10/e
A USMLE Step 2 Review
Hart
1996, ISBN 0-8385-6319-8

MEPC: Psychiatry, 10/e
A USMLE Step 2 Review
Chan and Prosen
1995, ISBN 0-8385-5780-5

MEPC: Surgery, 11/e
A USMLE Step 2 Review
Metzler
1995, ISBN 0-8385-6195-0

Specialty Board Reviews
MEPC: Anesthesiology, 9/e
Specialty Board Review
Dekornfeld and Sanford
1995, ISBN 0-8385-0256-3

MEPC: Otolaryngology
Specialty Board Review
Head & Neck Surgery
Willett and Lee
1995, ISBN 0-8385-7580-3

MEPC: Neurology, 4/e
Specialty Board Review
Giesser and Kanof
1995, ISBN 0-8385-8650-3

To order or for more information,
visit your local health science bookstore
or call Appleton & Lange toll free at
1-800-423-1359.

NAME _____
           Last   First   Middle

ADDRESS _____
          Street

_____
City   State   Zip

DIRECTIONS   Mark your social security number from top to bottom in the appropriate boxes on the right.
Use No. 2 lead pencil only.
Mark one and only one answer for each item.
Make each mark black enough to obliterate the letter within the parentheses.
Erase clearly any answer you wish to change.

1. (A) (B) (C) (D) (E)	25. (A) (B) (C) (D) (E)	49. (A) (B) (C) (D) (E)	73. (A) (B) (C) (D) (E)
2. (A) (B) (C) (D) (E)	26. (A) (B) (C) (D) (E)	50. (A) (B) (C) (D) (E)	74. (A) (B) (C) (D) (E)
3. (A) (B) (C) (D) (E)	27. (A) (B) (C) (D) (E)	51. (A) (B) (C) (D) (E)	75. (A) (B) (C) (D) (E)
4. (A) (B) (C) (D) (E)	28. (A) (B) (C) (D) (E)	52. (A) (B) (C) (D) (E)	76. (A) (B) (C) (D) (E)
5. (A) (B) (C) (D) (E)	29. (A) (B) (C) (D) (E)	53. (A) (B) (C) (D) (E)	77. (A) (B) (C) (D) (E)
6. (A) (B) (C) (D) (E)	30. (A) (B) (C) (D) (E)	54. (A) (B) (C) (D) (E)	78. (A) (B) (C) (D) (E)
7. (A) (B) (C) (D) (E)	31. (A) (B) (C) (D) (E)	55. (A) (B) (C) (D) (E)	79. (A) (B) (C) (D) (E)
8. (A) (B) (C) (D) (E)	32. (A) (B) (C) (D) (E)	56. (A) (B) (C) (D) (E)	80. (A) (B) (C) (D) (E)
9. (A) (B) (C) (D) (E)	33. (A) (B) (C) (D) (E)	57. (A) (B) (C) (D) (E)	81. (A) (B) (C) (D) (E)
10. (A) (B) (C) (D) (E)	34. (A) (B) (C) (D) (E)	58. (A) (B) (C) (D) (E)	82. (A) (B) (C) (D) (E)
11. (A) (B) (C) (D) (E)	35. (A) (B) (C) (D) (E)	59. (A) (B) (C) (D) (E)	83. (A) (B) (C) (D) (E)
12. (A) (B) (C) (D) (E)	36. (A) (B) (C) (D) (E)	60. (A) (B) (C) (D) (E)	84. (A) (B) (C) (D) (E)
13. (A) (B) (C) (D) (E)	37. (A) (B) (C) (D) (E)	61. (A) (B) (C) (D) (E)	85. (A) (B) (C) (D) (E)
14. (A) (B) (C) (D) (E)	38. (A) (B) (C) (D) (E)	62. (A) (B) (C) (D) (E)	86. (A) (B) (C) (D) (E)
15. (A) (B) (C) (D) (E)	39. (A) (B) (C) (D) (E)	63. (A) (B) (C) (D) (E)	87. (A) (B) (C) (D) (E)
16. (A) (B) (C) (D) (E)	40. (A) (B) (C) (D) (E)	64. (A) (B) (C) (D) (E)	88. (A) (B) (C) (D) (E)
17. (A) (B) (C) (D) (E)	41. (A) (B) (C) (D) (E)	65. (A) (B) (C) (D) (E)	89. (A) (B) (C) (D) (E)
18. (A) (B) (C) (D) (E)	42. (A) (B) (C) (D) (E)	66. (A) (B) (C) (D) (E)	90. (A) (B) (C) (D) (E)
19. (A) (B) (C) (D) (E)	43. (A) (B) (C) (D) (E)	67. (A) (B) (C) (D) (E)	91. (A) (B) (C) (D) (E)
20. (A) (B) (C) (D) (E)	44. (A) (B) (C) (D) (E)	68. (A) (B) (C) (D) (E)	92. (A) (B) (C) (D) (E)
21. (A) (B) (C) (D) (E)	45. (A) (B) (C) (D) (E)	69. (A) (B) (C) (D) (E)	93. (A) (B) (C) (D) (E)
22. (A) (B) (C) (D) (E)	46. (A) (B) (C) (D) (E)	70. (A) (B) (C) (D) (E)	94. (A) (B) (C) (D) (E)
23. (A) (B) (C) (D) (E)	47. (A) (B) (C) (D) (E)	71. (A) (B) (C) (D) (E)	95. (A) (B) (C) (D) (E)
24. (A) (B) (C) (D) (E)	48. (A) (B) (C) (D) (E)	72. (A) (B) (C) (D) (E)	96. (A) (B) (C) (D) (E)

97.	(A) (B) (C) (D) (E)	118.	(A) (B) (C) (D) (E)	139.	(A) (B) (C) (D) (E)	160.	(A) (B) (C) (D) (E)
98.	(A) (B) (C) (D) (E)	119.	(A) (B) (C) (D) (E)	140.	(A) (B) (C) (D) (E)	161.	(A) (B) (C) (D) (E)
99.	(A) (B) (C) (D) (E)	120.	(A) (B) (C) (D) (E)	141.	(A) (B) (C) (D) (E)	162.	(A) (B) (C) (D) (E)
100.	(A) (B) (C) (D) (E)	121.	(A) (B) (C) (D) (E)	142.	(A) (B) (C) (D)	163.	(A) (B) (C) (D) (E)
101.	(A) (B) (C) (D) (E)	122.	(A) (B) (C) (D) (E)	143.	(A) (B) (C) (D) (E)	164.	(A) (B) (C) (D) (E)
102.	(A) (B) (C) (D) (E)	123.	(A) (B) (C) (D) (E)	144.	(A) (B) (C) (D) (E)	165.	(A) (B) (C) (D) (E)
103.	(A) (B) (C) (D) (E)	124.	(A) (B) (C) (D) (E)	145.	(A) (B) (C) (D) (E)	166.	(A) (B) (C) (D) (E)
104.	(A) (B) (C) (D)	125.	(A) (B) (C) (D) (E)	146.	(A) (B) (C) (D) (E)	167.	(A) (B) (C) (D) (E)
105.	(A) (B) (C) (D) (E)	126.	(A) (B) (C) (D) (E)	147.	(A) (B) (C) (D) (E)	168.	(A) (B) (C) (D) (E)
106.	(A) (B) (C) (D) (E)	127.	(A) (B) (C) (D) (E)	148.	(A) (B) (C) (D) (E)	169.	(A) (B) (C) (D) (E)
107.	(A) (B) (C) (D) (E)	128.	(A) (B) (C) (D) (E)	149.	(A) (B) (C) (D) (E)	170.	(A) (B) (C) (D) (E)
108.	(A) (B) (C) (D) (E)	129.	(A) (B) (C) (D) (E)	150.	(A) (B) (C) (D) (E)	171.	(A) (B) (C) (D) (E)
109.	(A) (B) (C) (D) (E)	130.	(A) (B) (C) (D) (E)	151.	(A) (B) (C) (D) (E)	172.	(A) (B) (C) (D) (E)
110.	(A) (B) (C) (D) (E)	131.	(A) (B) (C) (D) (E)	152.	(A) (B) (C) (D) (E)	173.	(A) (B) (C) (D) (E)
111.	(A) (B) (C) (D) (E)	132.	(A) (B) (C) (D) (E)	153.	(A) (B) (C) (D) (E)	174.	(A) (B) (C) (D) (E)
112.	(A) (B) (C) (D) (E)	133.	(A) (B) (C) (D) (E)	154.	(A) (B) (C) (D) (E)	175.	(A) (B) (C) (D) (E)
113.	(A) (B) (C) (D) (E)	134.	(A) (B) (C) (D) (E)	155.	(A) (B) (C) (D) (E)	176.	(A) (B) (C) (D) (E)
114.	(A) (B) (C) (D) (E)	135.	(A) (B) (C) (D) (E)	156.	(A) (B) (C) (D) (E)	177.	(A) (B) (C) (D) (E)
115.	(A) (B) (C) (D) (E)	136.	(A) (B) (C) (D)	157.	(A) (B) (C) (D) (E)	178.	(A) (B) (C) (D) (E)
116.	(A) (B) (C) (D) (E)	137.	(A) (B) (C) (D) (E)	158.	(A) (B) (C) (D) (E)	179.	(A) (B) (C) (D) (E)
117.	(A) (B) (C) (D) (E)	138.	(A) (B) (C) (D) (E)	159.	(A) (B) (C) (D) (E)	180.	(A) (B) (C) (D) (E)